AF756455

CORONARY ARTERY DISEASE – CURRENT CONCEPTS IN EPIDEMIOLOGY, PATHOPHYSIOLOGY, DIAGNOSTICS AND TREATMENT

Edited by **David Gaze**

Coronary Artery Disease – Current Concepts in Epidemiology, Pathophysiology, Diagnostics and Treatment
Edited by David Gaze

Published by InTech

Janeza Trdine 9, 51000 Rijeka, Croatia

Copyright © 2012 InTech

All chapters are distributed under the Creative Commons Attribution 3.0 license, which allows users to download, copy and build upon published articles even for commercial purposes, as long as the author and publisher are properly credited, which ensures maximum dissemination and a wider impact of our publications. After this work has been published by InTech, authors have the right to republish it, in whole or part, in any publication of which they are the author, and to make other personal use of the work. Any republication, referencing or personal use of the work must explicitly identify the original source.

As for readers, this license allows users to download, copy and build upon published chapters even for commercial purposes, as long as the author and publisher are properly credited, which ensures maximum dissemination and a wider impact of our publications.

Notice

Statements and opinions expressed in the chapters are these of the individual contributors and not necessarily those of the editors or publisher. No responsibility is accepted for the accuracy of information contained in the published chapters. The publisher assumes no responsibility for any damage or injury to persons or property arising out of the use of any materials, instructions, methods or ideas contained in the book.

Publishing Process Manager Vedran Greblo

Technical Editor Teodora Smiljanic

Cover Designer InTech Design Team

Additional hard copies can be obtained from orders@intechopen.com

Coronary Artery Disease – Current Concepts in Epidemiology, Pathophysiology, Diagnostics and Treatment, Edited by David Gaze
p. cm.
ISBN 978-953-51-0262-5

We are IntechOpen, the world's leading publisher of Open Access books

Built by scientists, for scientists

4,100+
Open access books available

116,000+
International authors and editors

120M+
Downloads

151
Countries delivered to

Our authors are among the
Top 1%
most cited scientists

12.2%
Contributors from top 500 universities

WEB OF SCIENCE™

Selection of our books indexed in the Book Citation Index in Web of Science™ Core Collection (BKCI)

Interested in publishing with us?
Contact book.department@intechopen.com

Numbers displayed above are based on latest data collected.
For more information visit www.intechopen.com

For EU product safety concerns:
IN TECH d.o.o., Prolaz Marije Krucifikse Kozulić 3, 51000 Rijeka, Croatia,
info@intechopen.com or visit our website at intechopen.com.

Meet the editor

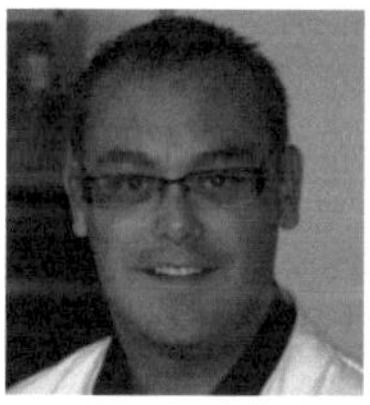

After undergraduate and postgraduate study in the North of England and London respectively, David Gaze works as a Research Biochemist in Clinical Blood Sciences at St George's Hospital and Medical School, London. His area of research interest is the development and clinical utility of cardiovascular biomarkers for assessment of patients with cardiovascular disease and cardiorenal disease. He has authored and co authored over 115 peer reviewed original papers, editorials and reviews, 145 conference proceedings and has authored two book chapters and a textbook on cardiac troponin. He has delivered over 25 invited international presentations. He received two NACB distinguished abstracts awards (2006/2008) and a diploma for oral presentation from the 17th IFCC–FESCC European Congress of Clinical Chemistry and Laboratory Medicine. He is a member of the American Association of Clinical Biochemistry, Association for Biochemistry, Institute of Biomedical Sciences, Fellow of the Royal Society of Medicine and a member of the Pathological Society of Great Britain.

Contents

Preface XI

Part 1 Epidemiology and Pathophysiology of Coronary Artery Disease 1

Chapter 1 **Epidemiology of Coronary Artery Disease 3**
John F. Beltrame, Rachel Dreyer and Rosanna Tavella

Chapter 2 **Gender Differences in Coronary Artery Disease 31**
Ryotaro Wake and Minoru Yoshiyama

Chapter 3 **Coronary Flow: From Pathophysiology to Clinical Noninvasive Evaluation 43**
Francesco Bartolomucci, Francesco Cipriani and Giovanni Deluca

Chapter 4 **Coronary Microvascular Dysfunction in CAD: Consequences and Potential Therapeutic Applications 65**
Alan N. Beneze, Jeffrey M. Gold and Betsy B. Dokken

Chapter 5 **Coronary Artery Disease and Pregnancy 81**
Titia P.E. Ruys, Mark R. Johnson and Jolien W. Roos-Hesselink

Part 2 Coronary Artery Disease Diagnostics 101

Chapter 6 **Cardiovascular Biomarkers for the Detection of Cardiovascular Disease 103**
David C. Gaze

Chapter 7 **Do We Need Another Look at Serum Uric Acid in Cardiovascular Disease? Serum Uric Acid as a Predictor of Outcomes in Acute Myocardial Infarction 123**
Siniša Car and Vladimir Trkulja

Chapter 8 **Stress Testing and Its Role in Coronary Artery Disease 147**
Rajkumar K. Sugumaran and Indu G. Poornima

Chapter 9 **Reassessing the Value of the Exercise Electrocardiogram in the Diagnosis of Stable Chest Pain 171**
Peter Bourdillon

Part 3 Treatment Regimens for Coronary Artery Disease 183

Chapter 10 **Effectiveness and Efficiency of Drug Eluting Stents 185**
José Moreu, José María Hernández, Juan M Ruiz-Nodar, Nicolás Vázquez, Ángel Cequier, Felipe Fernández-Vázquez and Carlos Crespo

Chapter 11 **Coronary Revascularization in Diabetics: The Background for an Optimal Choice 213**
Giuseppe Tarantini and Davide Lanzellotti

Chapter 12 **Diastolic Heart Failure After Cardiac Surgery 229**
Ahmed A. Alsaddique, Colin F. Royse, Mohammed A. Fouda and Alistair G. Royse

Chapter 13 **Spinal Cord Stimulation for Managing Angina from Coronary Artery Disease 257**
Billy Huh

Preface

Cardiovascular disease is ranked as the leading cause of death world wide. According to the World Heart Federation, cardiovascular disease is responsible for 17.1 million deaths globally each year. Surprisingly, 82% of these deaths occur in the developing world. Such numbers are often difficult to comprehend. The gravity of the situation is enhanced when portrayed as the following: Heart disease kills one person every 34 seconds in the USA alone. 35 people under the age of 65 die prematurely in the UK every day due to cardiovascular disease (12,500 deaths per annum). Although the leading killer, the incidence of cardiovascular disease has declined in recent years due to a better understanding of the pathology, implementation of lipid lowering therapy new drug regimens including low molecular weight heparin and antiplatelet drugs such as glycoprotein IIb/IIIa receptor inhibitors and acute surgical intervention.

The disease burden has a great financial impact on global healthcare systems and major economic consequences for world economies. Cardiovascular disease cost the UK healthcare system £14.4 billion (€16.7 billion; $22.8 billion) in 2006. Hospital care for patients with cardiovascular disease accounts for approximately 70% of the cost with 20% spent on pharmacological agents. The total cost should include non-healthcare costs such as production losses in the workforce and informal care of people with the disease. Production loss is estimated to cost the UK economy £8.2 billion in 2006 (55% due to death and 45% due to illness). Informal care cost the UK economy £8.0 billion in 2006. Overall cardiovascular disease is estimated to cost the UK economy £30.7 billion per annum.

This text aims to deliver the current understanding of coronary artery disease and is split into three main sections:

1. *Epidemiology and pathophysiology of coronary artery disease* where the spectrum of the disease will be described in relation to geographical location. Data from the industrialised countries on rates of myocardial infarction and angina are discussed in particular with reference to the wider healthcare and socioeconomic status. In the second chapter gender differences in rates and type of cardiovascular diseases are discussed. Often women view cardiovascular disease as a lower disease category than breast or cervical cancer. The differences in atherosclerotic pathology between men and women are discussed as well as the

different approaches to diagnostic regimens, treatment and mortality. Coronary blood flow is discussed with reference to the turbulence caused by atherosclerotic lesions and the clinical importance of Doppler Echocardiography in the evaluation of ischemic myocardium. In clinical practice, many patients present with angina and reduced coronary flow reserve despite normal coronary angiography of the large epicardial arteries. In this situation the vessels that limit flow to myocardium are the more distal epicardial prearterioles and intramyocardial arterioles typically too small to be visualized by conventional coronary angiography. Coronary microvascular dysfunction is poorly understood and difficult to manage. In addition, the presence of coronary microvascular dysfunction can be a confounding factor in the management of cardiac patients and is discussed in detail. The final chapter in this section deals with coronary artery disease during pregnancy. The incidence of pregnancy related acute coronary syndrome is 6 per 100,000 deliveries. One of the most important risk factors is maternal age. Pregnancy is a hypercoagulable state and has a major impact on hemodynamics. The presence of reduced left ventricular function increases the chance of an adverse maternal and fetal outcome. The underlying cause of an acute coronary syndrome may be different from outside pregnancy. The aetiology, pathophysiology and associated mortality as well as treatment options are discussed.

2. *Coronary artery disease diagnostics.* The first chapter of this section deals with the laboratory based biomarkers used to detect coronary artery disease. The challenge has been the identification of a cardiospecific biomarker. The cardiovascular biomarkers essentially fall into three categories. Those that identify patients at risk atherosclerosis; those associated with plaque destabilisation and those which indicate rupture of the plaque, necrosis and cardiac insufficiency. The use of serum uric acid as a predictive biomarker in myocardial infarction is discussed in the second chapter. A plethora of non-clinical, clinical and epidemiological studies have accumulated over the decades that aimed to elucidate molecular and cellular mechanisms of uric acid and its role as a diagnostic and prognostic aid or importantly, as a therapeutic target. This stems from its antioxidant potential. The role of serum uric acid on the cardiovascular system with respect to hypertension, stroke, renal failure, heart failure and coronary heart disease are discussed. Being able to identify patients with coronary artery disease early will help lower hospital costs and decrease mortality and morbidity. Stress testing has emerged as the sole non-invasive method for risk stratifying patients. Apart from highlighting the advantages and disadvantages of various stress testing modalities, the chapter reviews which patients should undergo stress testing based on appropriateness criteria; managed separately based on their risk factors and identifying those who may be at increased risk of acute myocardial infarction or death. The final chapter of this section discusses the role of exercise electrocardiography in patients with stable chest pain. A UK National Institute for Health and Clinical Excellence (NICE) guideline on the diagnosis of discomfort of suspected cardiac origin

published in 2010 proposes that Exercise ECG should not be used to diagnose or exclude angina for people without known coronary artery disease Historically exercise electrocardiography in the diagnosis of coronary artery disease has been questioned. However, the greater the ST segment changes on exercise electrocardiography, the greater the post-exercise probability of coronary artery disease. The chapter demonstrates the different impact the exercise electrocardiography has on subsequent management, depending on the method employed to analyse the data.

3. *Treatment regimens for coronary artery disease* The discovery of statins over 30 years ago comprised a revolution in the management of dyslipidaemia. Statins target hepatocytes and inhibit 3-hydroxy-3-methylglutaryl coenzyme A (HMG-CoA) reductase, the enzyme that converts HMG-CoA into mevalonic acid, a cholesterol precursor. They directly inhibit cholesterol synthesis. Statins exert several beneficial effects on patients with coronary artery disease, whether managed conservatively or undergoing surgical or percutaneous treatment. This chapter discusses the effects of optimal statin therapy in primary and secondary prevention, in particular clinical settings such as; acute coronary syndrome, and in patients undergoing percutaneous coronary intervention or coronary artery by-pass surgery. The second chapter in this section looks at the effectiveness and efficiency of drug eluting stents. With the use of data from stent registries in Europe and clinical trails in the field, this chapter discusses the benefit of drug eluting over bare metal stents with respect to restenosis rates, cardiac morbidity and mortality and provides an economic basis for their use. The third chapter tackles the impact of incomplete revascularisation on survival in systematic off-pump coronary artery bypass grafting surgery. It remains unclear whether the decreased number of grafts seen in off-pump versus on-pump bypass grafting is owing to patient selection. Incomplete revascularisation can derive from a surgical strategy of target vessel revascularisation in high-risk patients, where the impact of surgery is minimised to reduce perioperative mortality and morbidity, aiming to achieve the best feasible safe revascularisation. Revascularisation of diabetic patients is discussed in detail in the next chapter with the aid of case studies for illustration. Diabetes mellitus constitutes an independent predictor of early stent thrombosis, both in bare metal and drug eluting stents. Current guidelines favor coronary artery bypass graft surgery over percutaneous coronary intervention in most diabetic patients with multi-vessel disease; however, substantial variability exists in the current medical practice suggesting a lack of clinical consensus. The penultimate chapter of this section discusses diastolic heart failure following cardiac surgery; defining the clinical spectrum, the pathophysiology of diastole and contributing factors. The authors describe in detail methods to assess diastolic function. The final chapter discusses the role of spinal cord stimulation for the management of angina from coronary artery disease. Despite the recent advances in managing angina pectoris, many patients suffer from intractable pain. For those patients who have already failed optimal medical and surgical therapy, very few,

if any, therapeutic options are available. Spinal cord stimulation may play a unique role in managing such refractory anginal pain. This chapter details, the mechanisms of spinal cord stimulation, methodology employed as well as clinical outcomes.

Acknowledgements

I would like to acknowledge the tremendous efforts of the contributing authors to these chapters. The tireless work they have provided gives insight into the world of the basic and clinical sciences. It is their drive to continue to investigate and share their findings that drives forward science. In essence, through their work, we hope to provide help and treatment for the millions of people affected by coronary artery disease around the globe. I would also like to thank Mr Vedran Greblo of InTECH publishers for keeping the production of this book active and to for steering me to complete the editorial review by the appropriate deadlines. Lastly I have to say thank you to the true unsung heroes. The patients and their families who agree to participate in research programs; the benefits of which may not necessarily help themselves but could help their fellow humans in the future. It is these people who deserve the most credit.

David C. Gaze
Dept of Chemical Pathology Clinical Blood Sciences,
St George's Healthcare NHS Trust, London,
UK

Part 1

Epidemiology and Pathophysiology of Coronary Artery Disease

1

Epidemiology of Coronary Artery Disease

John F. Beltrame, Rachel Dreyer and Rosanna Tavella
Discipline of Medicine, University of Adelaide, The Queen Elizabeth Hospital, Australia

1. Introduction

Epidemiology involves the study of the frequency, distribution, and impact of diseases within a community in order to address potential prevention or treatment of these conditions. Accordingly, evaluating the epidemiology of coronary artery disease (CAD) constitutes a particularly wide spectrum that cannot be comprehensively covered in a solitary book chapter. Consequently this first section will provide an introductory broad overview of CAD including pathophysiological concepts, clinical manifestations, geographic variations and its impact on patient health. After defining the broader context of this large field, the specific scope of chapter will be outlined.

1.1 Defining coronary artery disease

The coronary circulation consists of coronary arteries, the microcirculation and the coronary veins. Its function is to supply oxygen and nutrients to the myocardium and remove carbon dioxide and waste products. The importance of this function is exemplified by the fact that a 50% or more reduction in this blood supply to the myocardium is incompatible with life. Thus, not surprisingly, dysfunction of the coronary circulation may result in significant morbidity and mortality.

Although beyond the scope of this chapter, it should be noted that disturbances of the coronary circulation may involve dysfunction within the microcirculation as well as the coronary arteries. Thus the all-encompassing term 'coronary heart disease' includes both CAD and microvascular dysfunction. The later may mimic the clinical manifestations of CAD and indeed may co-exist with CAD. However, defining the epidemiology of microvascular dysfunction is especially difficult since specialised investigations are required to confirm its presence, as it may occur in the absence of associated structural microvascular disease.

In contrast, CAD is more readily identifiable and the most common underlying pathophysiological process is coronary atherosclerotic disease. This may be identified by imaging techniques such as coronary angiography, or unequivocally at post-mortem autopsy. Accordingly, detailing the epidemiology of CAD is more readily achievable and the focus of this chapter.

1.2 Atherosclerotic coronary syndromes

Coronary atherosclerotic disease involves the epicardial coronary arteries and may manifest as an acute or chronic coronary syndrome. Acute coronary syndromes (ACS) typically arise from atherosclerotic plaque rupture with subsequent coronary thrombosis and/or spasm. The resulting coronary artery occlusion gives rise to intense myocardial ischaemia or even myocardial necrosis thereby manifesting as unstable angina or myocardial infarction. On occasions, the ischaemia/infarction may manifest as sudden cardiac death from malignant arrhythmias or acute pulmonary oedema in the compromised left ventricle. Hence ACS may have a spectrum of clinical manifestations ranging from unstable angina, acute myocardial infarction, acute pulmonary oedema or even sudden death, all arising from the same underlying pathophysiological process.

Chronic coronary syndromes (CCS) may also arise from coronary atherosclerotic disease. This typically manifests as exertional angina arising from a coronary atherosclerotic lesion that has progressed to the extent that it compromises coronary blood flow to the myocardium during the increased oxygen demand associated with exercise. As this obstructive lesion is non-occlusive, adequate oxygen supply is restored once the excess myocardial oxygen demand is removed with the cessation of exercise and thus the resolution of the ischaemic chest pain. Hence the principal manifestation of CCS is angina pectoris, which can be monitored in epidemiologic studies.

1.3 Geographic variations in coronary artery disease

The global prevalence of these CAD-related clinical manifestations is increasing although there are regional variations that are influenced by the extent of economic development and social organisation. With industrialisation, there is a shift from nutritional and infectious disorders to the chronic diseases such as CAD. This 'epidemiologic transition' has been described as involving 4 stages (Omran, 1971), as detailed in Table 1, (Yusuf et al, 2001). In developing countries, infectious disease and nutritional deficiency are responsible for most deaths (Stage 1) and cardiovascular disease plays only a minor role. The cardiovascular disorders (CVD) that are prevalent in these communities include infectious disease such as rheumatic heart disease or nutritional disorders such as beriberi. With improvements in public health and nutrition, these conditions become less prevalent and disorders related to uncontrolled hypertension become more common (Stage 2). With further industrialisation, lifestyle diseases become more evident. Thus smoking, high fat diets and obesity result in the rapid development of atherosclerosis so that CAD mortality is a major cause of death in middle-aged individuals (Stage 3). With further improvements in public health measures to address these lifestyle risk factors and advances in medical care, atherosclerotic disease associated mortality is delayed so that it is a condition of the elderly (Stage 4). Progression through each of these transition stages is associated with a greater life expectancy. Moreover as shown in Table 1, cardiovascular disease (and especially CAD) contributes proportionally more to the total population mortality.

As evident from Table 1, CAD is present across the globe although its frequency varies with geographic region. Consequently there is a wide spectrum in the prevalence of CAD in developing and industrialised countries; thus discussions relevant to one country may not be necessarily be pertinent to others. Hence it is important to report on the context of the findings when describing the epidemiology of CAD.

Transition Stage	%Deaths*	Cardiovascular Conditions	Countries
1. Infections & Nutritional Deficiency	5-10%	• Rheumatic Heart Disease • Nutritional Cardiomyopathy	• Sub-Saharan Africa • Rural South America • Rural Southern Asia
2. Hypertensive Diseases	10-35%	• Haemorrhagic Stroke • Hypertensive Heart Disease	• China • Urban Southern Asia
3. Atherosclerotic CVD in the Middle-aged	35-65%	• CAD • Atherothrombotic Stroke	• Urban India • Latin America • Former USSR
4. Atherosclerotic CVD in the Elderly	< 50%	• CAD • Atherothrombotic Stroke • Heart Failure	• Western Europe • North America • Australia, New Zealand

Adapted from Yusuf et al, Circulation 2001, 104:2746-53. (Yusuf et al, 2001)
*%Deaths from CVD, in relation to total deaths. CVD = Cardiovascular Disease.

Table 1. The Epidemiologic Transition of Cardiovascular Disease#.

1.4 Health status in coronary artery disease

Epidemiology not only involves monitoring diseases within the community but also their impact on health. Thus the focus should not only be on the disease manifestations of CAD (such as acute and chronic coronary syndromes) but also the patient's perception of the impact of these disorders on their health. The term '*health status*' (see Figure 1) is used to define the patient's perception (rather than the clinician's perception) of the disease process on their lifestyle. This incorporates the symptoms experienced (e.g. angina), the functional limitation from the symptom (eg reduced exercise tolerance) and quality of life (i.e. the

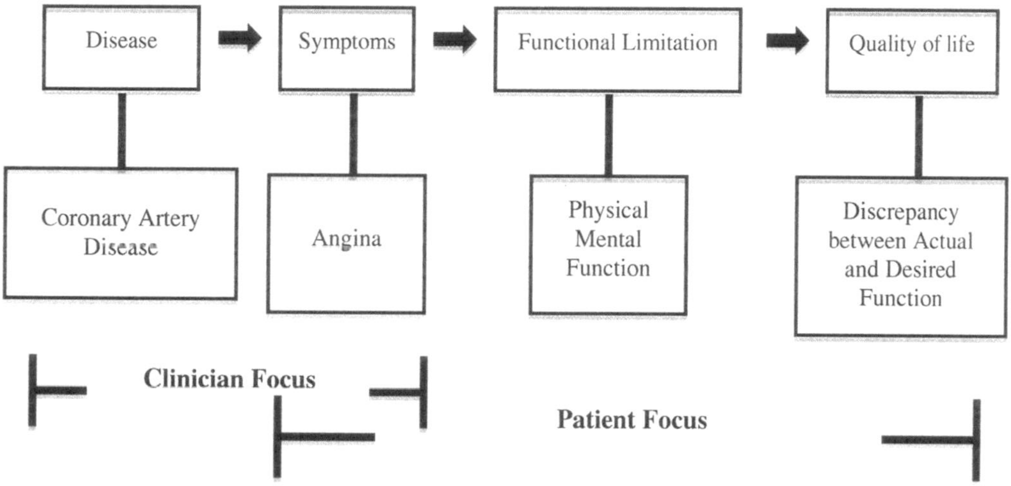

Rumsfeld, Circulation 2002, 106:5-7. (Rumsfeld, 2002). Copyright gained from Wolters Kluwer Health 04/08/2011

Fig. 1. Summary of Patient-centred Health Status.

discrepancy between actual and desired function) (Rumsfeld, 2002). Thus congruous with our evolving patient-centred health care, this chapter will not only focus on CAD in relation to the prevalence and incidence of disease processes but will also detail the impact of CAD on health status.

1.5 Scope of the chapter

Considering the wide spectrum encompassing CAD epidemiology, it is necessary to limit the topics covered in this chapter. Thus the chapter will evaluate overall CAD mortality, myocardial infarction as an example of an ACS and chronic stable angina as the example of a CCS. Within each of these areas, the discussion will focus on (1) the difficulty and limitations in defining the condition and thus its impact in interpreting the data, (2) the prevalence of the condition, (3) the incidence of the condition, where relevant, (4) and the impact of the condition on health status, when appropriate. This comprehensive approach will provide a detailed evaluation of the epidemiology of CAD.

Since the prevalence of CAD varies with geographic location, the discussion in this chapter will be largely focus on industrialised countries (i.e. Stage 4 countries, Table 1). Data from these countries are readily available, generally reliable and the prevalence of disease similar, although there are small differences even within these countries. Thus although the data presented in this chapter is comprehensive in relation to the industrialised countries, it is acknowledged that it is not globally inclusive.

2. Coronary artery disease mortality

2.1 Defining coronary artery disease mortality

Detailing mortality data may seem straightforward since the presence/absence of death is seldom a contentious issue, however whether the death can be attributed or indeed is associated with CAD is more problematic. Many epidemiologic studies derive mortality data from administrative death registries. In most of these registries, the cause of death is obtained from the death certificate completed by the treating doctor, who ascribes the cause of death based upon clinical impression. This contrasts to the more objective assignment of a cause of death from formally conducted autopsy studies. Since non-forensic national autopsy rates are about 5% in most industrialised countries, the cause of death derived from these registries may be unreliable and this should be considered when interpreting the mortality data detailed below.

2.2 Prevalence of coronary artery disease mortality

CVD encompasses not only CAD but also cerebrovascular disease, peripheral arterial disease as well as other cardiac disorders, and is currently the leading cause of death in the world, particularly amongst women. The World Health Organisation (WHO) estimates that such diseases caused almost 32% of all deaths in women and 27% in men in 2004 (World Health Organisation [WHO], 2008). CAD is the most common cause of CVD deaths (45% of all CVD deaths) accounting for 7.2 million deaths/year, or 12% of all deaths worldwide (Figure 2).

In many developed countries, CAD is the single leading cause of death. In the United Kingdom (UK) in 2008, CAD was responsible for about one in five male deaths and one in eight female deaths; a total of 88,000 CAD deaths (15% of total deaths) (British Heart

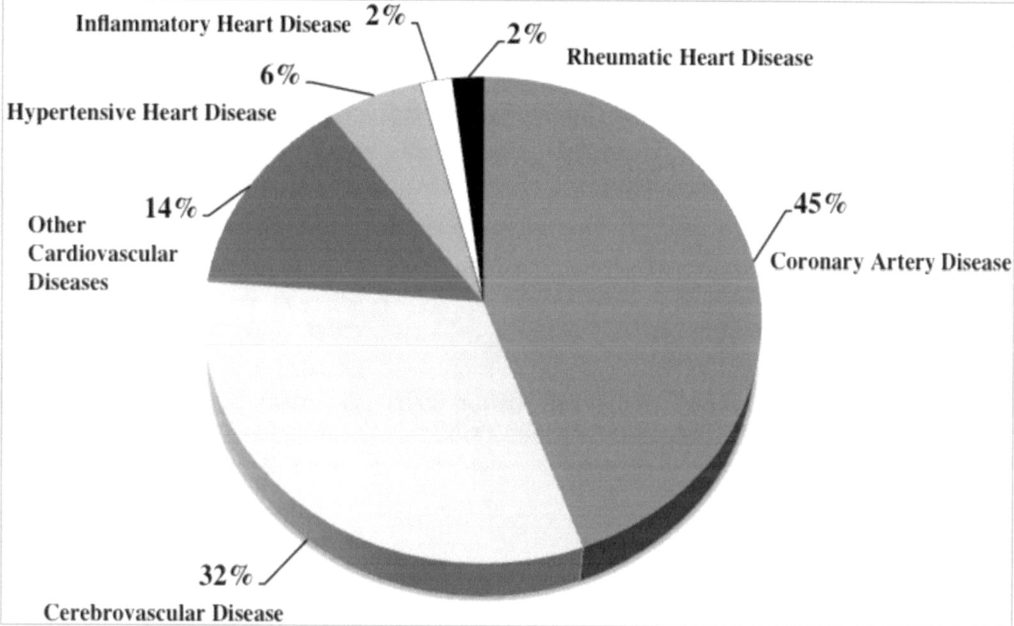

*Source World Health Organisation, Global Burden of Disease 2004 Update

Fig. 2. Distribution of Cardiovascular Diseases Accounting for Deaths Worldwide in 2004

Foundation [BHF], 2010). Similarly in the United States in 2005, CAD was responsible for one of every five deaths, accounting for 445,687 deaths (18% of total deaths) (Lloyd-Jones et al, 2009). In Australia in 2006, CAD accounted for 22,983 deaths (17% of all deaths) and once more was the most common condition responsible for Australian deaths (Australian Institute of Health and Welfare [AIHW], 2010).

2.3 Temporal changes in coronary artery disease mortality

The 'epidemiologic transition' described above (Table 1), not only accounts for geographic variations in CAD but also temporal changes. Over the past 30 years, two epidemiological trends have been observed in relation to CAD mortality. In many developed countries there has been an initial rise followed by a fall, while in developing countries there has mainly been a rise in CAD mortality.

In developed countries, there was a peak in CAD mortality in the 1950's with a progressive decline since the 1960's. The WHO Multinational MONItoring of trends and determinants in CArdiovascular disease (MONICA) project identified an annual 4% decline in CAD mortality rate trends over 10 years from the 1980's across 21 countries (Tunstall-Pedoe et al, 2000). For example, in 1996 Australia reported 29,637 deaths (23% of all deaths) due to CAD, and in 2006, the equivalent figure was 22, 983 (17% of all deaths). This decline in CAD deaths rates over the past 2 decades has been the most remarkable in Denmark, Australia, Sweden, the Netherlands and Canada, with the rate of CAD death falling by more than 60% (Figure 3). These trends are consistent with an 'epidemiologic transition' from Stage 3 to Stage 4 in these countries and reflect an increased life expectancy with the onset of CAD manifestations at an older age.

Figure 3 also highlights the heterogeneity between the countries in the improved CAD mortality. Thus while many Western European countries have shown substantial improvements in CAD mortality as described above, the Eastern European countries (such as Hungary) generally showed less improvement. These trends typically parallel socio-economic differences with the decline in CAD mortality being sharper in countries with a more favoured socio-economic status.

In contrast, some developing countries have an increasing rate of CAD mortality. Indeed, the WHO estimates that 60% of the global burden of CAD occurs in developing countries. Although mortality estimates are difficult to obtain in some of these countries, broad assessments of overall CVD epidemiology report rising CVD mortality in urban China, Malaysia, Korea and Taiwan. In China, CVD mortality increased as a proportion of total deaths from 12.8% in 1957 to 35.8% in 1990 (Khor, 2001). Like many developing countries, it has experienced rapid urbanisation, socioeconomic and health changes, together with an increase in life expectancy - features consistent with stage 2 of the epidemiologic transition.

2.4 Factors influencing coronary artery disease mortality

The landmark Framingham Heart Study was established in 1948 by the US Public Health Service to investigate the epidemiology of atherosclerotic CVD and hypertension. Its contribution to this field was huge as it precipitated a paradigm shift in the approach to CVD. This study transformed the popular belief at the time, which regarded atherosclerotic coronary artery disease as a normal aging process, to the ground-breaking concept of 'risk factors' thereby proposing that lifestyle modification could prevent CVD. This iconic longitudinal study demonstrated that advancing age, smoking, hypercholesterolaemia, hypertension and obesity increased the risk of CVD. Subsequently, these investigators developed the 'Framingham Risk Score', which predicts the 10 year risk of developing CAD based upon age, cholesterol profile, blood pressure level, diabetic and smoking status. They conclude that at the age of 40 years, the lifetime risk of CAD is 50% for men and 33% for women. Further insights into CAD continue to evolve from the study including the role of gender, depression, and socioeconomic status.

2.4.1 Age

Ageing is an unmodifiable risk factor for CAD, with males clinically manifesting this condition at 50-65 years of age and females about 10 years later, following menopause (Lerner & Kannel, 1986). The WHO reports that the principal cause of death of people over 65 years is CAD, and as age increases, a substantial proportion of deaths are among females. In many developed countries, the number and proportion of older people (i.e over 65 years) is increasing, which is largely explained by declines in fertility and mortality. The ageing population of many countries has accelerated the contribution of CAD to total disease burden. It is predicted that the global ageing population will maintain CAD as a predominant cause of death worldwide (Mensah, 2004).

Among countries with high but declining CAD mortality, it is suggested that these trends are changing with respect to younger age subgroups (O'Flaherty et al, 2009). A slowing or levelling of the decline in CAD mortality in young adults has now been reported in England and Wales, the US, France, Australia, and New Zealand. These findings are cause for concern, indicating that decades of progress in reducing deaths from CAD appear to be stalling. Changes in lifestyle factors in the young (increasing obesity and sedentary lifestyles) may account for this reduced improvement.

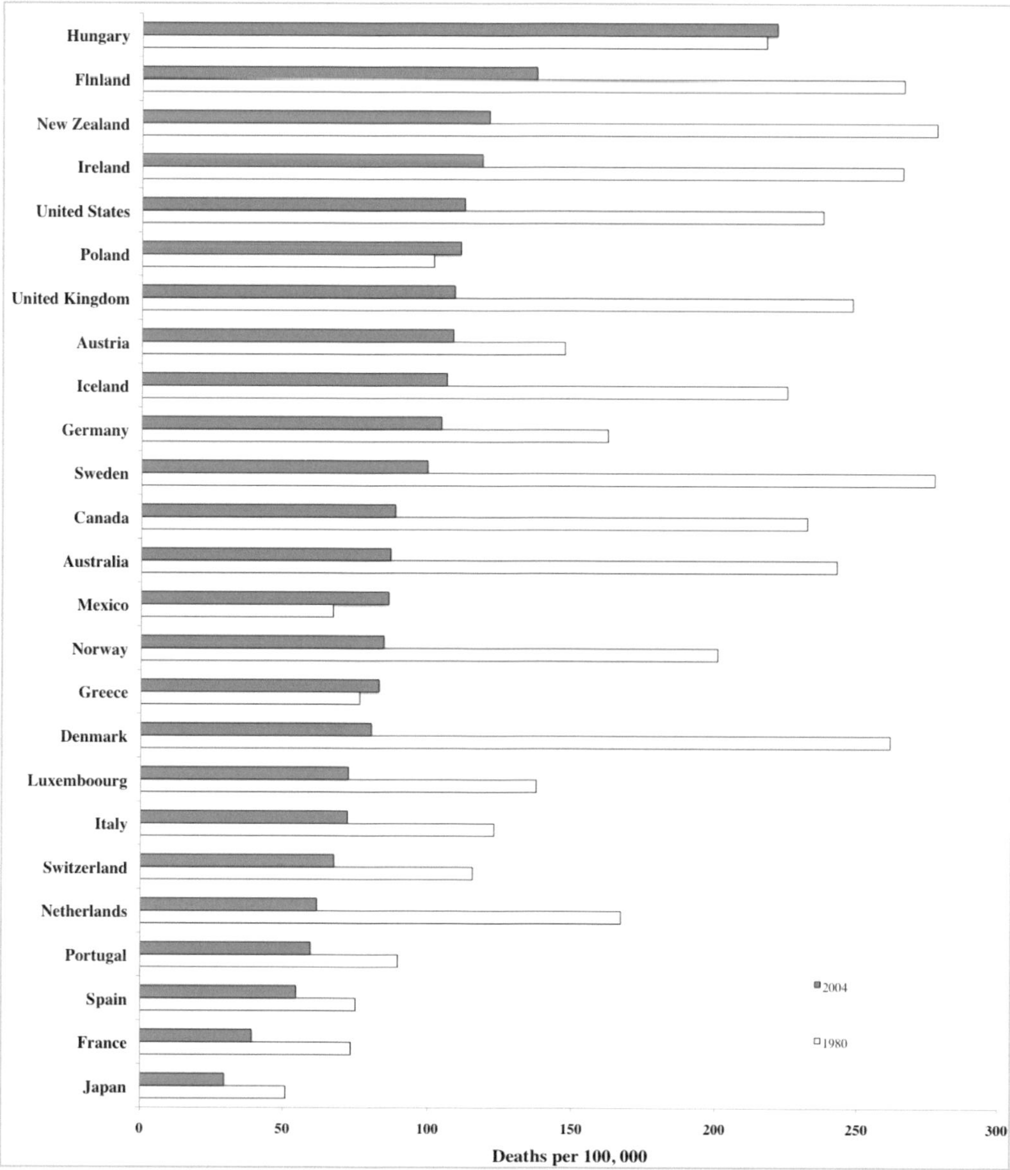

Source: Organisation for Economic Co-operation and Development (OECD), 2009.
Notes: Mexico (1981, 2004), Italy, Portugal (1980, 2003). Uses ICD-9 codes 410-414 and ICD-10 codes I20-I25

Source Organisation for Economic Co-operation and Development (OECD), 2009

Fig. 3. Age Standardised CAD Death Rates in Developed Countries in 1980 and 2004

2.4.2 Gender

CAD is the leading cause of mortality for both adult males and females alike worldwide. Although the initial manifestation of CAD is delayed in females by about ten years compared to males, there is not an abrupt increase in CAD mortality rates for females immediately following menopause but a progressive increase over subsequent years. Thus more elderly post-menopausal females succumb to CAD then men and have done so since 1984 (Castelli, 1988). Nonetheless, CAD is not solely a disease of elderly women.

In the US, among men aged 35 to 54, the average annual mortality rate from CAD fell by 6.2% in the 1980's, and levelled off between 2000 and 2002, with an annual decline of just 0.5%. Among women in the same age group, the annual rate of death from CAD dropped by 5.4% in the 1980's. Between 2000 and 2002, CAD mortality actually *increased* for females by an average of 1.5%. Furthermore, even in younger females (35 to 44 years), the CAD mortality increased by an average of 1.3% annually between 1997 and 2002. Overall within the transitional trends, the percentage decline in mortality rates has been far greater for men than women, particularly in the US, the UK, Australia and Sweden. The age-standardised mortality rate for males and females since 1978 for the UK is depicted in Figure 4. More alarming is the higher mortality rate observed for young females following myocardial infarction. Younger women, but not older women, have higher rates of death during hospitalisation for myocardial infarction than men of the same age (see Myocardial Infarction section below).

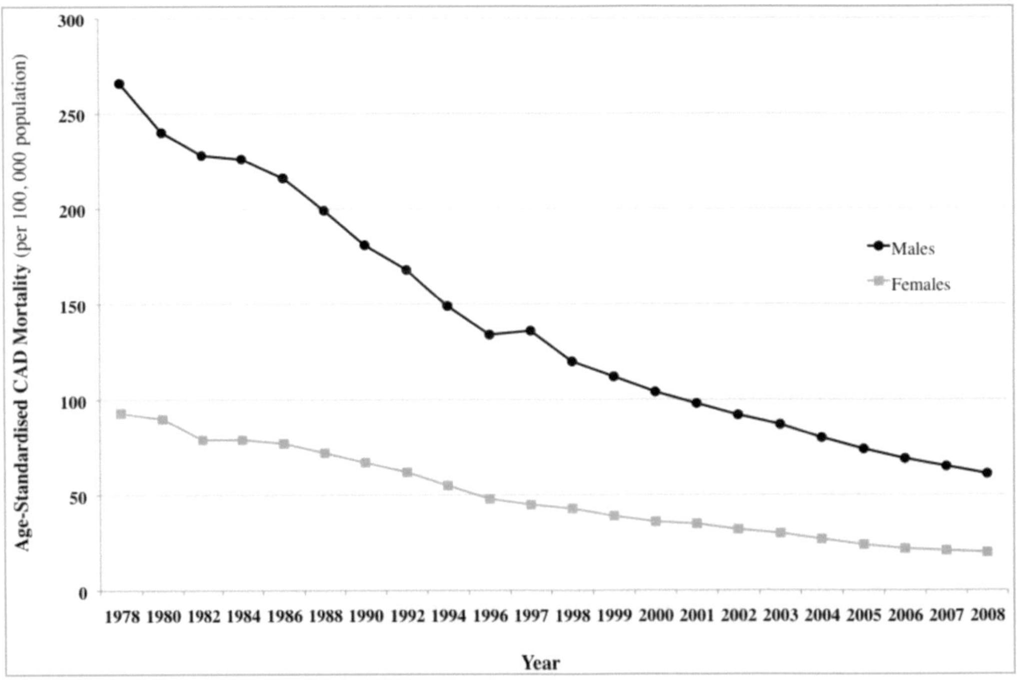

Source British Heart Foundation, Coronary Heart Disease Statistics, 2010.

Fig. 4. Age-standardised CAD Mortality in the United Kingdom for Males and Females from 1978 to 2008

2.4.3 Geographic differences

It is common to categorise CAD epidemiology by geographic region, however the natural history of CAD epidemics varies substantially between countries. For example, in Europe, the changes in CAD mortality in France and Southern European countries were smaller than that observed in the UK and Finland. The differences in industrialised nations are clearly evident in Figure 3. In Asia, CAD mortality is similar in Hong Kong and China, but it is different to trends in Thailand and South Korea, which report lower CAD mortality rates. These differences may be attributed to a low prevalence of CVD risk factors in the South-east Asian countries. Favourable trends observed in the US, Australia, Argentina, Chile and Cuba, who rates of CAD death are traditionally and substantially lower than in most other areas of the world, may in part be explained by improved control of hypertension, as well as better management of patients with CAD. In Eastern European countries, including Bulgaria, Croatia, Romania, and especially the Russian Federation, there is a persisting upward trend in mortality from CAD. Russian CAD mortality rates in the late 1990's were higher than those of Finland, the USA, or Australia three decades earlier.

Regional variation in Britain has been consistently reported for 25 years. In Scotland and Northern England, CAD death rates are the highest, Southern England the lowest and intermediate rates in Wales and Northern Ireland. The rate of sudden death for males in Scotland is 63% higher and for females it is 100% higher compared to the rates observed in South Western England. Furthermore, the highest mortality rates are concentrated in urban areas.

2.4.4 Socio-economic status

Socioeconomic status (SES) indicators, including education, income and occupation, are associated with CAD risk factors, morbidity, and mortality. Early studies beginning in the 1930's generally showed increased CAD prevalence with industrialisation and affluence in developed nations. However, contemporary data demonstrate that low SES, i.e. less education, lower income, and blue-collar occupations are associated with increased rates of CAD and increased risk of CAD mortality. Correspondingly, lower SES groups also have the least favourable lifestyle characteristics, including obesity, smoking, high cholesterol, hypertension, and lack of physical activity. It is suggested by some that these SES-related differences are increasing even as age-adjusted CAD mortality declines.

The British Heart Foundation reports a clear gradient in CAD mortality across low to high SES group. The inequality is more striking in females than males, with the CAD death rate being five times higher in female blue-collar workers compared to females in professional occupations.

2.4.5 Depression

Additional risk factors are continually being evaluated in order to identify their contribution to CAD mortality and thus potentially develop further targeted therapies. Research has consistently shown that depression is a risk factor contributing to both the development and complications of CAD. Depressive symptoms, regardless of a formal clinical diagnosis have an unfavourable impact on mortality in CAD patients. Both major depression and elevated depressive symptoms are associated with at least a doubling in risk of subsequent death in

CAD patients. The negative prognostic effect also remains in the long-term and after adjustment for other risk factors.

2.5 Summary comments

Epidemiologic data on CAD mortality is limited by the data source since most are derived from administrative registries where the cause of death is obtained from subjectively completed medical certificates rather than objectively performed autopsies. Considering this limitation, CAD is reported as the world's leading cause of mortality for men and women, being responsible for more than 7 million deaths each year. Although in developed nations CAD is the most common cause of death, globally over 60% of fatalities now occur in developing countries. It is clear that a wide spectrum in the prevalence of CAD mortality exits, and despite much effort to improve the disproportional mortality rates, a social gradient in CAD still remains. This is evident by the higher CAD death rates in lower SES areas within regions and even within countries, and also an apparent gender bias, particularly amongst younger women. With a slowing down of age-adjusted mortality, it is likely that social differences will increase. By 2030, it is projected that the number of CAD deaths will rise by up to 137% in developing nations, and by up to 48% in areas where CAD is in decline, as such CAD will remain the leading cause of death worldwide.

3. Myocardial infarction

3.1 Defining myocardial infarction

Acute myocardial infarction (AMI) remains a leading cause of worldwide mortality, being responsible for 12.6% of total deaths each year (Beaglehole, 2004). As described above, AMI and unstable angina constitute the CAD-related acute coronary syndromes. AMI differs to unstable angina as the former is associated with evidence of myocardial necrosis. A variety of methods are available to detect myocardial necrosis including changes on the electrocardiograph (ECG), plasma cardiac markers (creatine kinase, troponin), imaging techniques (cardiac magnetic resonance imaging, myocardial scintigraphy) and ultimately autopsy gross pathology and histology. The availability of these techniques allow for the definitive diagnosis of AMI to be made. In contrast, the diagnosis of unstable angina is more subjective relying on clinical impression and the absence of evidence of myocardial necrosis. Accordingly, investigating unstable angina epidemiologic data is less reliable and so this chapter will focus upon AMI data only.

The clinical diagnosis of AMI has evolved over the past 10-15 years with the need to make an early diagnosis so that prompt therapy can be instituted. Traditionally the diagnosis is made on the basis of chest pain symptoms, ECG changes and an abnormal plasma cardiac marker. These plasma cardiac markers are particularly pertinent as they are intracellular proteins that are released into the plasma when myocardial cell necrosis occurs. Previously the routine cardiac marker used was creatine kinase, which had limited sensitivity and specificity. The development of the more sensitive and specific troponin assay resulted in myocardial necrosis being detected in patients with a normal creatine kinase. When these troponin leaks were found to have prognostic implications, the clinical diagnosis of AMI was redefined to focus upon the troponin findings. Thus as shown on Table 2, a clinical diagnosis of AMI is primarily made on the basis of an abnormal troponin with at least one other feature; alternatively the diagnosis may be made on autopsy pathological examination (Thygesen et al, 2007).

This change in the diagnostic criteria for AMI, particularly with reference to the plasma cardiac marker, has resulted in more AMI's being detected. Hence any longitudinal study of AMI will be confounded by the change in the criteria and needs to be considered when interpreting the epidemiologic data. This problem will be further compounded in the future with the evolution of high-sensitivity troponin assays, which may potentially detect even more AMI's.

In addition to detecting myocardial infarction in the acute setting, a number of the above techniques may detect a previous myocardial infarct. Thus epidemiological studies may survey a population to detect the frequency of myocardial infarction by techniques mentioned in Table 2 relating to 'healed myocardial infarction'. Each of these methods has their advantages and disadvantages in relation to availability, cost and accuracy. These need to be considered when interpreting the epidemiologic data.

Clinically, AMI has been sub-classified on the basis of the presenting electrocardiograph (ECG) as either ST-elevation myocardial infarction (STEMI) or Non-ST elevation myocardial infarction (NSTEMI). Differentiating these two forms of AMI is important as the immediate clinical management differs. In STEMI, immediate coronary reperfusion strategies (either percutaneous coronary interventions or thrombolysis) on arrival to hospital are mandated in order to reduce the risk of death. In contrast, NSTEMI does not require immediate intervention although early invasive therapy (at least within days) is preferred. This nomenclature has replaced the previous classification of Q-wave and non-Q wave myocardial infarction since the later ECG findings do not occur until late in the course of AMI evolution and do not influence contemporary management strategies. However, as mentioned above, the Q wave can be used to diagnose the presence of a previous myocardial infarct.

Criteria for acute, evolving or recent Myocardial Infarction

Either one of the following satisfies the diagnosis for acute, evolving or recent MI:

1. Typical rise and/or fall in cardiac biomarkers (preferably troponin) with at least one of the following:
   - Ischaemia symptoms
   - Development of pathological Q waves in the ECG
   - Electrocardiographic changes indicative of ischaemia (ST-segment elevation or depression
   - Imaging evidence of new loss of viable myocardium or new regional wall motion abnormality.
2. Pathologic findings of an acute myocardial infarction

Criteria for healing or healed Myocardial Infarction

Any one of the following criteria satisfies the diagnosis for healing or healed myocardial infarction:

1. Development of new pathological Q waves with or without symptoms. Imaging evidence of a region of loss of viable myocardium that is thinned and fails to contract in the absence of a non-ischemic cause.
2. Pathological findings of a healed or healing myocardial infarction.

Adapted from Thygesen K et al. Universal definition of myocardial infarction. Eur Heart J 2007; 28: 2525.
Copyright permission gained from Oxford University Press 01/08/2011

Table 2. Revised Definition of Myocardial Infarction

In the following sections, the prevalence and incidence of myocardial infarction are described. The *prevalence* of a condition refers to its frequency within a given population at a particular point in time. The *incidence* of a condition refers to the number of new cases within a given population over a specified period of time. The estimates detailed in these sections are derived from several data sources including hospital discharge data, general practice registries and patient self-report from national survey data. Accordingly, the reliability of the data is dependent on the data source.

3.2 Prevalence of myocardial infarction

Based upon self-reported myocardial infarction in a UK national survey, the prevalence of myocardial infarction was reported as approximately 4.1% of men and 1.7% of women in 2006 (BHF, 2010). This represents some 1.5 million people within the UK. As shown in Figure 5, the prevalence is age-dependent, extending from 1% of men < 45 years of age to 17% of those ≥ 75 years old. Furthermore, there is local geographic variation for all ages in the United Kingdom the highest prevalence is seen in men from Wales (9%) and women from Scotland (2.4%).

Similarly, in the USA, the prevalence of myocardial infarction was 3.6% in 2006 based upon national survey data available from the American Heart Association (Lloyd-Jones et al, 2009). The prevalence was slightly higher in African American males (5.1%) compared with Caucasian males (4.9%) but lower in African American (2.2%) females compared with their Caucasian counterparts (3%). As with the UK data, the prevalence of myocardial infarction was greater in the elderly compared with those < 50 years of age.

In contrast to these developed countries, South Asian countries (such as India, Pakistan, Bangladesh, Sri Lanka, and Nepal) the highest prevalence of myocardial infarction is seen in those younger than 40 years of age, whereas it is less marked in those older than 60 years. These observations are consistent with Stage 3 of the epidemiologic shift (Table 1) and reflect the development of risk factors at younger ages (Joshi et al, 2007).

3.3 Incidence of myocardial infarction

While the prevalence of myocardial infarction reflects both previous and new (acute) myocardial infarcts, the incidence of myocardial infarction only reflects the later. The incidence of AMI has decreased in a number of developed countries during the past three decades, including the UK and remains the lowest in China and Japanese populations. Age adjusted data has indicated that for men and women between the ages of 35-64 years there are only 90/100,000 new cases for AMI in China and 20/100,000 new cases in Japan (Ueshima et al, 2008).

The most recent estimates of incidence of AMI in the UK are based on national level data from associated hospital and/or mortality statistics and suggest that in Scotland the incidence of AMI has decreased by about 25% between 2000 and 2009 in both men and women. Thus considering all ages in Scotland in 2006, approximately 252/100,000 males were newly diagnosed MI cases and 118/100,000 females.

In relation to the clinical type of AMI, it has been estimated that more than 3 million suffer from STEMI and 4 million people suffer from NSTEMI worldwide each year (White & Chew,

2008). The 6-month mortality rate following infarction has been reported as 4.8% for STEMI and 6.2% for NSTEMI in an international registry involving 14 countries (Goldberg et al, 2004). Other studies have also shown an adverse prognosis for NSTEMI compared with STEMI patients at 12 months post-infarction (Terkelsen et al, 2005; Montalescot et al, 2007).

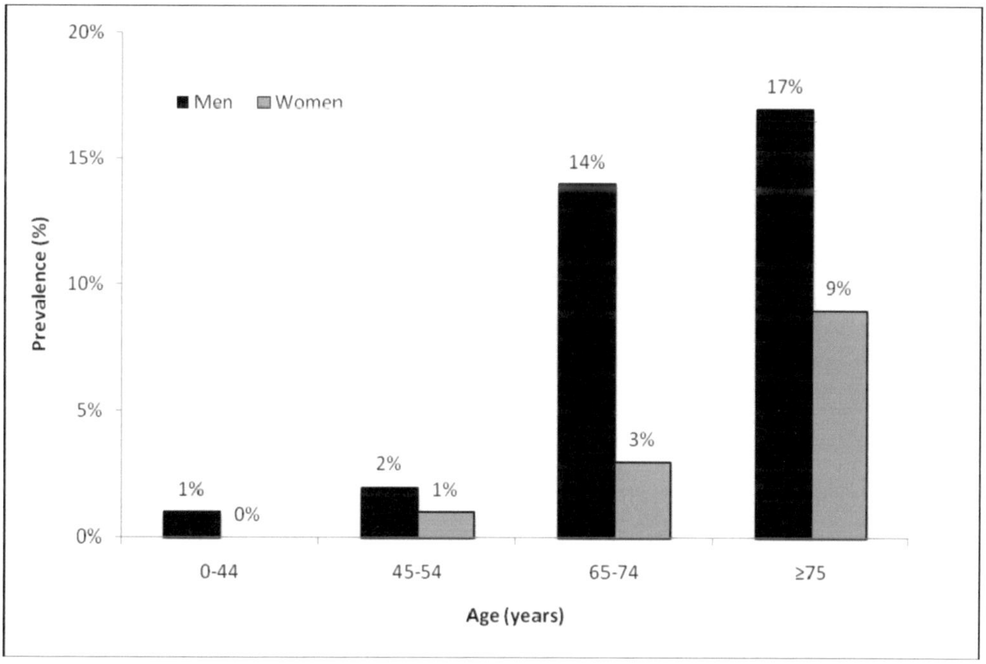

Adapted from the British Heart Foundation, 2010 report. Prevalence rates are weighted for non-response. Respondents were asked to recall whether they had ever been diagnosed with myocardial infarction by a doctor.

Fig. 5. Age specific prevalence of AMI in the United Kingdom, England, 2006

3.4 Factors influencing myocardial infarction

The prevalence and incidence of myocardial infarction can be influenced by demographic, biological and psychosocial factors, some of which are modifiable and thus potential therapeutic targets. These factors warrant further discussion.

3.4.1 Demographic factors

Acute myocardial infarction is rare in childhood and adolescent years but increases in prevalence in the middle decades, particularly in the developing countries. In developed countries it is increasingly becoming a disease of the elderly, which has important economic implications. For example, 70% of AMI admissions in Australia are for patient's ≥ 65 years old. These patients often have a complicated course as they have existing co-morbidities that complicate the therapy of their AMI.

Considerable interest has evolved in gender differences in CAD and is the focus of another chapter within this book. Epidemiologic data concerning AMI amongst women is now being revised as early data primarily focused on middle-aged males. It is well described that men experience myocardial infarction about 10 years younger than women (Figure 5) but in the post-menopausal years, women rapidly catch up to the men. Despite this, women have a larger in-hospital mortality from their AMI until about the age of 80 years when they are similar to men (Figure 6) (Vaccarino et al, 1999). Of particular concern is that the greatest disparity in this mortality is between young women and men (Figure 6). The cause for this gender difference is not apparent and the focus of ongoing investigations.

In addition to age and gender, geographic factors influence the incidence of AMI. These have been described above and are likely to be multifactorial in origin. Factors such as ethnicity, and following social economic class, industrialisation may all contribute to apparent geographic differences.

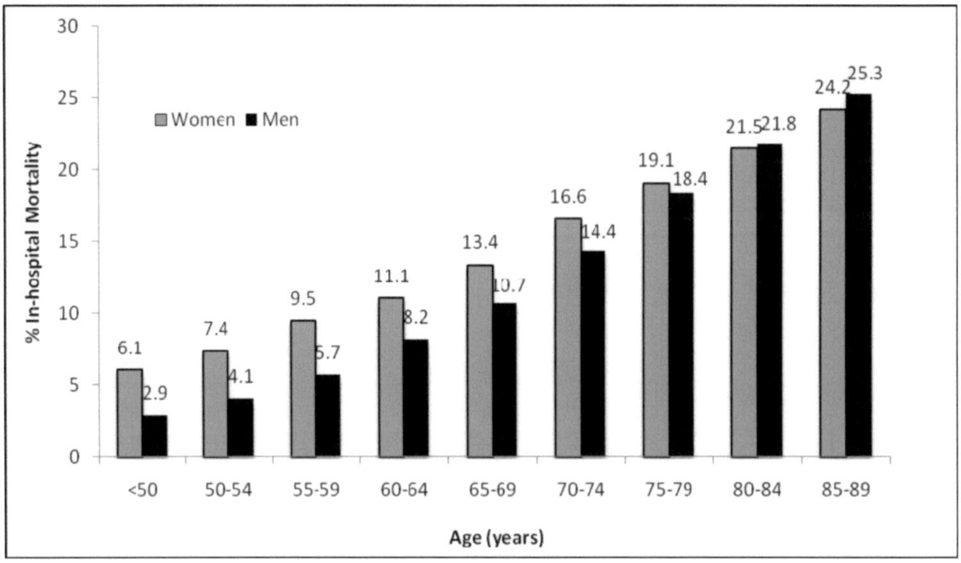

Adapted from Vaccarino et al. NRMI. N Engl J Med. 1999; 341: 217-225.

Fig. 6. Age & sex specific prevalence of AMI mortality

3.4.2 Biological/lifestyle risk factors

The Framingham Heart Study was instrumental in establishing modifiable biological risk factors that were associated with AMI. A plethora of subsequent therapeutic studies have since demonstrated that modifying these risk factors can prevent AMI thereby confirming the importance of these risk factors and establishing the practice of preventative cardiology. These risk factors have since been incorporated into many risk scores for predicting the risk of AMI.

A potential limitation of the Framingham study is the select population studied; an east coast USA community. More recently a large multinational study has been conducted to evaluate the association between the conventional modifiable risk factors and AMI (Yusuf et al, 2004). The INTERHEART study recruited patients from 52 countries in a case-control study. They reported that the traditional risk factors described in the Framingham study

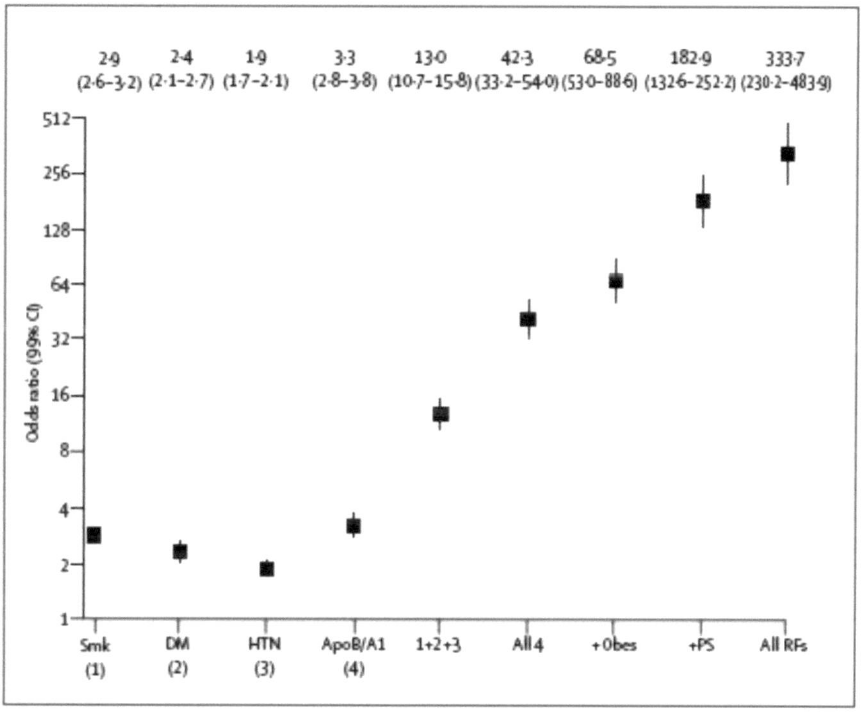

Smk = smoking, DM = diabetes mellitus, HTN = hypertension, Obes = obesity, PS = psychosocial, RFs = Risk Factors. Copyright Permission to use established from Elsevier 01/08/2011

Fig. 7. Acute Myocardial Infarction Risk Factors. (Adapted from Yusuf et al, 2004)

accounted for most of the risk of AMI, independent of the country (Yusuf et al, 2004). In particular, the risk of AMI increased with the following factors in descending order of their adjusted approximate odds ratio: dyslipidaemia (3.3-fold, as defined by apolipoprotein B/A1 ratio), smoking (2.9-fold), psychosocial factors (2.7-fold), diabetes (2.4-fold), hypertension (1.9-fold) and abdominal obesity (1.6-fold). Reduced exercise and daily fruit/vegetable intake also increased the risk. Figure 7 highlights the importance of these factors and in particular the exponential risks when these factors are combined.

The prevalence of these biological factors within the community varies with age and gender, as shown in Figure 8. In relation to smoking rates, the UK prevalence is around 20% with the prevalence having peaked for men and even begun to decline; however for women they continue to climb. In contrast, hypercholesterolaemia, hypertension and diabetes all remain prevalent (Figure 8). Whereas the prevalence of hypertension and diabetes increases with age, the prevalence of hypercholesterolaemia plateau's/declines in the elderly.

3.4.3 Psychosocial factors

Both social and psychological factors are associated with AMI risk. Socioeconomic factors such as shorter education and lower income (particularly in women), and unmarried cohabitation have been shown to contribute towards the risk of AMI (Nyboe et al, 1989). In particular, socioeconomic status, work and home roles may play an important prognostic role, particularly in young women (Lacey & Walters, 2003). Women often work outside the home, in addition to their roles within the household as wives, mothers and caregivers to elderly parents. There is also mounting evidence that age, gender, and social class affect health related quality of life (HRQoL) in the general population, with women reporting a poorer HRQoL than men, particularly following a cardiac event.

Depression is the leading cause of disability worldwide affecting more than 120 million people every year. It is known to be an independent risk factor for the onset and subsequent poor prognosis of CAD (Schrader et al, 2004; Schrader et al, 2006) and can be a precursor to AMI and even cardiac death. Following AMI, 65% of patients report experiencing symptoms of depression and major depression is present in 15-22% of these patients (Guck, 2001). Depressed patients, particularly women, are also at an increased risk of mortality, experience a greater likelihood of cardiac hospitalisation and suffer from poor HRQOL in the first year post AMI (Frasure-Smith et al, 1999).

Depression has a significant, negative impact on psychological and social functioning, as well as on work and leisure-related activities. Patients who are depressed are more likely to experience social problems over the first year of post-MI recovery, are slower in returning to work, experience more frequent episodes of angina, report more physical impairment and are less likely to attend cardiac rehabilitation than are non-depressed patients (Carney and Freedland, 2003).

3.5 Health status in myocardial infarction

Mortality associated with myocardial infarction is well described and reflected in the CAD mortality figures described in section 2. However the impact on this disorder also must be considered in relation to health status. In a recent study, Maddox et al (Maddox et al, 2008) reported that almost 1 in 5 patients with AMI experienced ongoing angina 12 months following an infarct. The clinical determinants of this ongoing chest pain included cardiac variables such as a prior history of angina, post-infarct angina during the index hospital admission and previous coronary bypass surgery. Additionally, non-cardiac variables such as younger age, female gender, continued smoking post-infarction, and depression were also important. Indeed depression is not only associated with ongoing symptoms following AMI but is also an important determinant of subsequent HRQoL (Rumsfeld et al, 2001).

3.6 Summary comments

The diagnostic methods and criteria for AMI have evolved in recent years so that more infarcts can be detected with the current technologies. This needs to be considered when interpreting data (especially longitudinal data) concerning myocardial infarction. Despite this, it is clear that AMI is a leading cause of morbidity and mortality worldwide and is responsible for over 12% of deaths each year, with a larger majority of the population suffering from NSTEMI than STEMI. The incidence of AMI has decreased in the industrialised world due to lifestyle changes and therapeutics; however, rates are rising in developing countries such as Asia, Eastern Europe and parts of Latin America. Although the prevalence of AMI is higher in men of all age groups, it is concerning and unexplained why the in-hospital myocardial infarct mortality is higher in women, particularly in the premenopausal era. The factors influencing the occurrence of myocardial infarction have been well addressed over the past 4-5 decades however the management of factors that influence health status in patients with a recent myocardial infarct require further development.

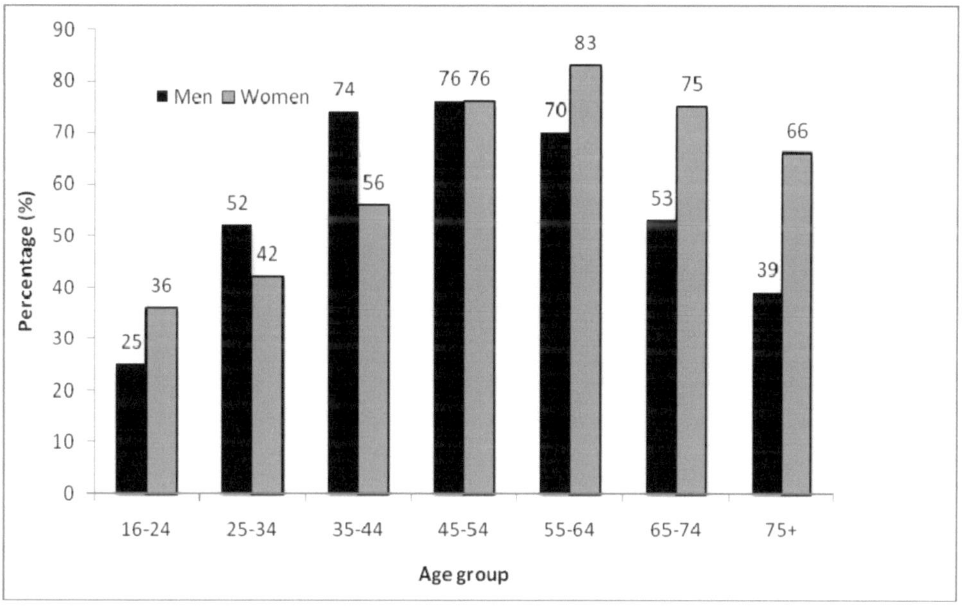

Percentage of adults with blood cholesterol levels ≥ 5.0mmol/l.

Fig. 8A. Prevalence of major biological risk factors by age and sex, in England in 2008.

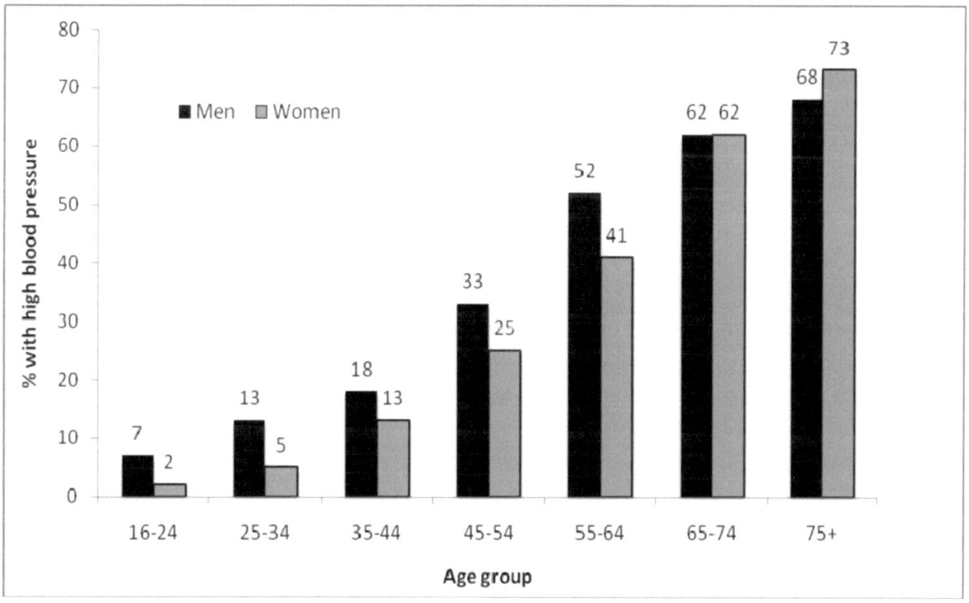

Hypertension - blood pressure > 140/80.

Fig. 8B. Prevalence of major biological risk factors by age and sex, in England in 2008.

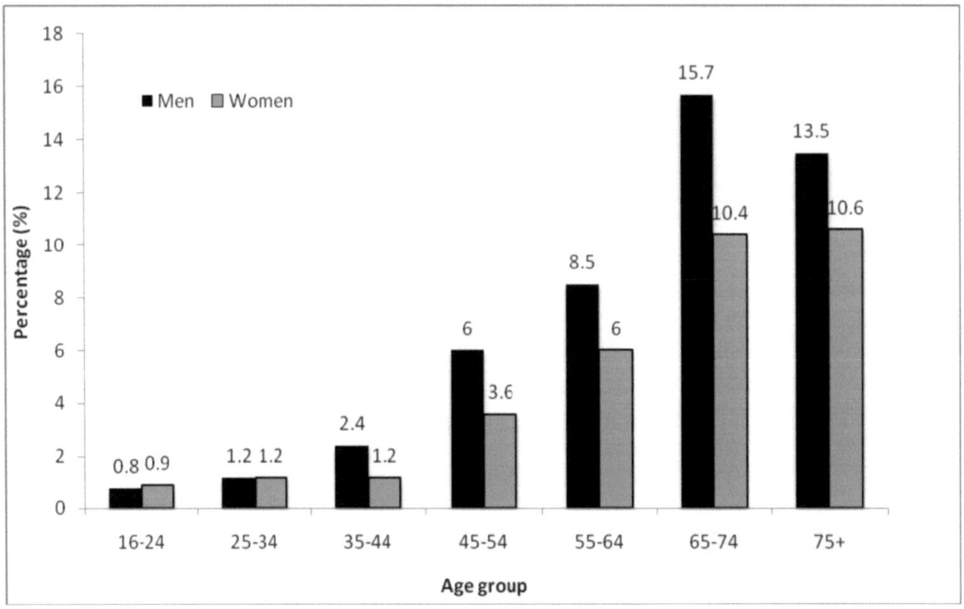

Diabetes mellitus - both Type I and II. Source a, b & c - British Heart Foundation 2010 report.

Fig. 8C. Prevalence of major biological risk factors by age and sex, in England in 2008.

4. Chronic stable angina

4.1 Defining chronic stable angina

The evaluation of epidemiologic data concerning chronic stable angina is more challenging than assessing CAD mortality or myocardial infarction data. Unlike these other conditions, the diagnosis of chronic stable angina is largely based upon clinical criteria and can only be objectively assessed with specialised investigations such as invasive coronary angiography. As these techniques may not be performed in all individuals with chest pain or angina, the background frequency of the disease is difficult to quantitate. Accordingly, interpretation of data concerning chronic stable angina must be made in the context of the data collected, which may be merely on clinical impression in many studies. This limitation should be considered when reviewing this data.

There exists a certain ambiguity in defining the term 'angina pectoris' which has arisen from its use to describe a group of clinical disorders rather than a symptom. First clinical characterised by William Heberden in his 1772 publication entitled 'Some account of a disorder of the breast'(Heberden, 1772), it refers to a strangling sensation, which usually occurs on exertion, however patients may experience angina without physical activity whereupon it is referred to as rest angina (Maseri, 1995) .

In contemporary medicine, 'angina' may be used in a more generic context, referring to any coronary heart disease syndrome that results in myocardial ischaemia. These angina syndromes may have different coronary pathophysiological mechanisms responsible for initiating the myocardial ischaemia, including coronary artery spasm and microvascular dysfunction. They may manifest as exertional or rest angina, depending upon the underlying mechanism. The clinical angina syndromes are summarised in Table 3 below.

Angina Syndrome	Clinical Features
Unstable Angina	• Characterised by crescendo or rest angina • An acute coronary syndrome manifestation (may progress on to myocardial infarction) • Typically due to an unstable atherosclerotic plaque
Stable Angina	• Characterised by exertional angina • Typically due to a stable but tight obstructive coronary artery stenosis
Prinzmetal Variant Angina	• Characterised by rest or nocturnal angina • Typically due to coronary artery spasm
Decubitus Angina	• Characterised by angina when lying down • Typically due to left ventricular dysfunction resulting in redistribution of pulmonary fluids and thus increased cardiac workload.
Silent Ischaemia	• Absence of angina in the presence of documented ischaemia • May occur with coronary artery or microvascular dysfunction
"Syndrome X"	• Includes classical syndrome X, microvascular angina, coronary slow flow phenomenon • Characterised by prolonged episodes of exertional or rest angina • Typically due to coronary microvascular dysfunction

Table 3. **Types of Angina.** Source British Heart Foundation, Coronary Heart Disease Statistics, 2010

Despite these diverse implications for the term 'angina', it is most commonly used to refer to patients with chronic stable angina. Although the initial description of exertional angina by Heberden still holds true today, a more operational version has been detailed by the American College of Physicians (Diamond, 1983) . As summarised in Table 4, this definition describes angina as either 'typical' or 'atypical' on the basis of how many of the clinical features are consistent with exertional angina. In those patients with features of typical angina, the sensitivity and specificity for detecting significant coronary artery disease on angiography is respectively 91% and 87% in males, and correspondingly 89% and 63% in females (Detry et al, 1977).

Chest Pain Features	
1. Substernal chest discomfort - characteristic quality (tightness) & duration (minutes) **2. Provoking Factors** - exertion or emotional stress **3. Relieving Factors** - rest or sublingual nitrates	
ACP Classification:	**Typical Angina** - all 3 of above criteria met. **Atypical Angina** - only 2 of above criteria **Non-cardiac Chest Pain** - only 1 of above criteria

Table 4. American College of Physicians (ACP) Angina Pectoris Definition

In this section, the data presented concerning 'angina' will predominantly focus on patients with chronic stable angina. It will concentrate on the prevalence, incidence, clinical profile, associated morbidity and mortality with this condition. Although the clinical features of the other forms of angina have been alluded to, their epidemiological aspects are less clearly described and unfortunately there are no studies that directly compare the prevalence or incidence of the various forms of angina.

4.2 Prevalence of chronic stable angina

Despite the declining incidence of myocardial infarction, the prevalence of angina remains high with direct costs in the United States in 2000 estimated at over $75 billion (Javitz et al, 2004). Although the exact prevalence of stable angina is unclear, in the UK in 2009, it is estimated that 2.1 million people suffered from angina thus representing a prevalence of approximately 5% of men and 4% of women (BHF, 2010). Coronary heart disease accounts for 1 in 4 deaths in the UK and the lifetime risk for those over 40 years is 49% in men and 32% in women.

Similarly, in the United States, approximately 10.2 million Americans were reported to have angina in 2006 with 4.7% of Caucasian men and 4.5% of Caucasian women over the age of 20 years affected (Lloyd-Jones et al, 2010). These data are primarily based upon patient self-report of a history of angina and thus subject to limited validity.

Although the prevalence of angina in the UK and USA are similar, it is affected by age, gender, ethnicity, and geographic region. As shown in (Figure 9), within the UK, the prevalence is almost 17% amongst males and 12% in females over the age of 75 years but is less than 1% of all those under 45 years of age. Furthermore for all ages, the prevalence of angina in men from Northern Ireland is approximately 6% whereas amongst Welshman it is 4% (BHF, 2010). Ethnic differences in angina occurrence are well illustrated in the United States where the prevalence in men over the age of 20 years is 3.8% in Caucasians, 3.3% in African Americans, and 3.6% in the Hispanic population. The equivalent prevalence amongst females is 3.7%, 5.6% and 3.7%.

4.3 Incidence of chronic stable angina

Based upon surveying general practitioner patient case records, the incidence of newly diagnosed angina in the UK was estimated at 28,000 new cases in 2009 (BHF, 2010). Thus overall, approximately 49/100,000 males were newly diagnosed angina cases and 28/100,000 females. Figure 10 illustrates the age-specific incidence of angina.

4.4 Factors influencing chronic angina

Several large prospective epidemiological studies have provided important insights into the characteristics of patients with chronic stable angina. One of these was the Coronary Artery Disease in gENeral practiCE (CADENCE) study (Beltrame et al, 2009), which recruited 2,031 chronic stable angina patients from general practices across Australia. The sample was representative of this population based upon geographic location. It particularly focussed upon continuing angina symptoms in these patients and surprisingly found that almost 1 in 3 continued to experience angina at least once a week, despite contemporary therapies. This

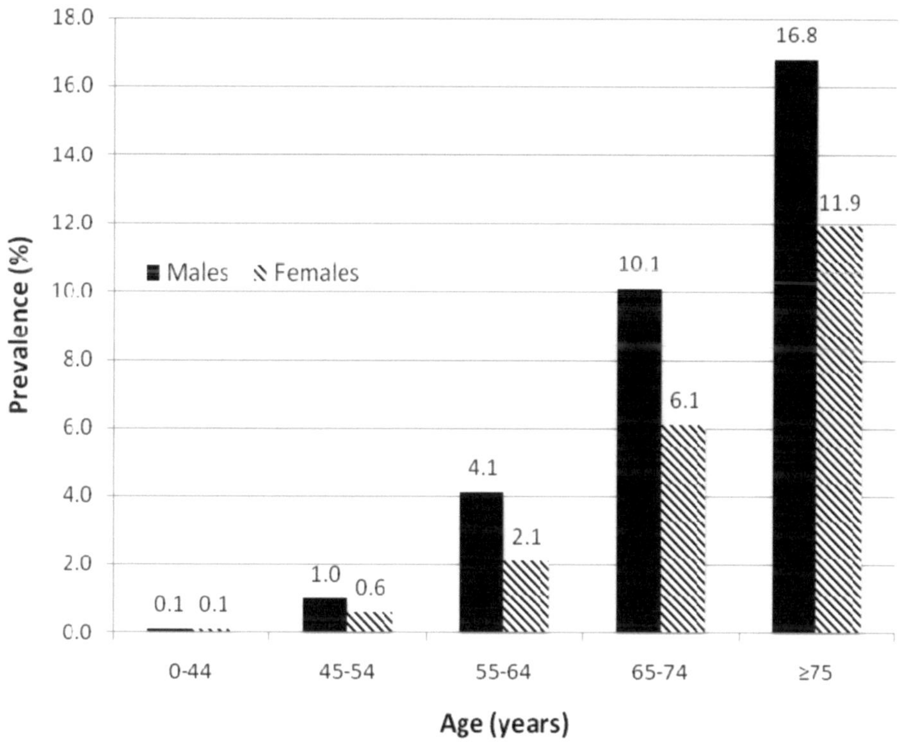

Source British Heart Foundation, Coronary Heart Disease Statistics, 2010

Fig. 9. Age-specific Prevalence of Angina in the United Kingdom in 2009.

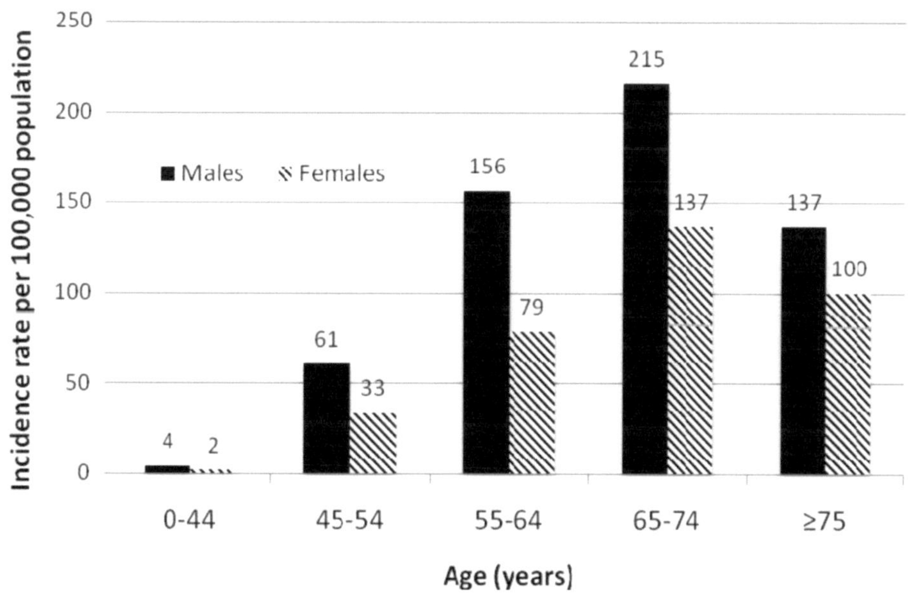

Source British Heart Foundation, Coronary Heart Disease Statistics, 2010

Fig. 10. Age-specific Incidence of Angina in the United Kingdom in 2009.

was similar to that reported in United States (Wiest et al, 2004) and in an international multicentre study (Kirwan et al, 2008).

The clinical characteristics of the chronic stable angina population in the CADENCE study, is summarised in Table 5. As would expected, these are predominantly elderly males with many having conventional cardiovascular risk factors. Their angina symptoms were consistent with ACP defined angina in 72% of the patients. Most had experienced an episode of ACS at some stage of their chronic illness with almost half having experienced an acute myocardial infarction.

Importantly, this study reported that gender or the presence of heart failure or peripheral arterial disease, were independent clinical determinants of ongoing weekly angina in patients with chronic stable angina (Beltrame et al, 2009).

Clinical Characteristic	Prevalence
Coronary Artery Disease Risk Factors	
Age	71 ± 11 years
Male gender	64%
Diabetes mellitus	30%
Hypertension	72%
Hypercholesterolaemia	78%
Previous or current smoker	59%
Obesity (BMI and/or waist circumference)	85%
Associated Cardiovascular Disease	
Previous acute coronary syndrome	70%
Cardiac Failure	22%
Peripheral Artery Disease	17%
Atrial Fibrillation	10%
Angina Characteristics	
Substernal chest discomfort	93%
Pain provoked by exertion	73%
Pain provoked by emotional stress	26%
Pain relieved by rest	54%
Pain relieved by sublingual nitrates	51%

Table 5. Clinical Characteristics in Stable Angina Patients. Data from (Beltrame, Weekes et al. 2009).

4.4.1 Gender

In a gender sub-analysis of the CADENCE study, significant gender disparities in coronary risk factors, clinical features, diagnostic investigations and management were observed as well as differences in angina-related health outcomes (Dreyer et al, 2011). Although women had more frequent angina which was associated with greater physical impairment and a poorer quality of life, they were less extensively investigated, prescribed fewer cardio-protective agents, less likely to achieve guideline lipid or weight targets and were less likely to receive any specialist cardiology review (Figure 11). The predilection for women having more frequent angina is likely to be multi-factorial and may include biological, clinical presentation and assessment differences between genders (Bairey Merz et al, 2006). For example, women may have smaller coronary arteries that are less amenable to revascularisation therapies. Furthermore, coronary microvascular dysfunction is more prevalent in women and angina resulting from this is less responsive to conventional anti-anginals.

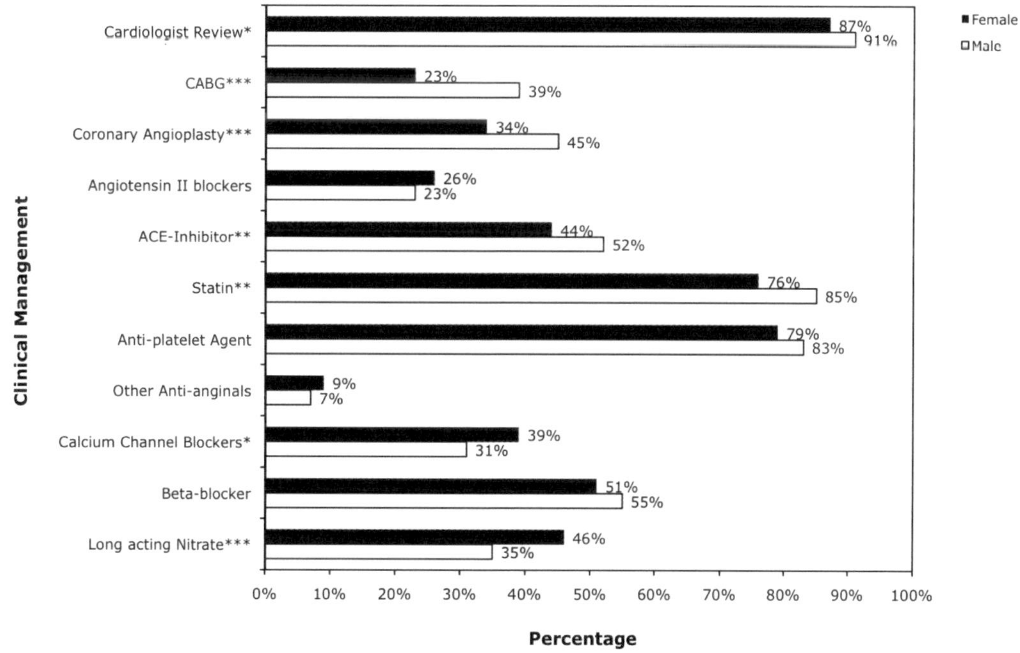

Fig. 11. Gender comparisons in the clinical management of stable angina patients. Age adjusted frequency data for (a) cardiology review, (b) pharmacological therapy and (c) revascularisation therapy, in 2005 stable angina patients categorised by gender. (male vs. female: *p < 0.05, **p < 0.01, ***p < 0.001). Data from Dreyer et al (2011). Copyright permission gained Elsevier 30/09/2011

4.4.2 Co-morbidities

As shown in Table 5, many chronic stable angina patients have a history of a previous MI and their cardiac prognosis will be influenced by this event. In chronic stable angina patients who have not previously experienced a myocardial infarct, the risk of myocardial infarct or all-cause death has been described as 1.7%/year and 1.9%/year, respectively (Lampe et al, 2000).

Co-existing heart failure and/or peripheral arterial disease have been shown to be important determinants of on-going angina symptoms in patients with chronic stable angina (Beltrame et al, 2009). This potentially reflects the more extensive disease in these patients. Certainly, patients with chronic stable angina and co-existing peripheral arterial disease were more physically limited and a poorer quality of life than those without co-existing peripheral arterial disease (Wilson et al, 2011).

4.5 Impact of chronic stable angina on health status

The CADENCE study not only demonstrated that many patients with chronic stable angina have frequent ongoing symptoms but also that frequent angina is associated with reduced physical limitations and a poorer quality of life (Beltrame et al, 2009). Although the CADENCE study utilised a threshold of angina of at least once week, the relationship is a continuum as shown in Figure 12. Thus the more frequent the angina, the greater the impairment in physical limitation and quality of life. Hence enquiring about angina frequency may provide useful clinical insights into the impact of the disorder on the patient's quality of life.

While enquiring about the frequency of angina provides some insights into the disability associated with the disorder, it does not replace a detailed history and evaluation identifying the full impact of the condition on the patient. Unfortunately clinicians may not be completely aware of the angina burden experienced by their patients as alluded to in the CADENCE study. In this study, the clinicians reported that 80% of their patients had optimally controlled angina and that 61% had minimal impairment in their physical activity by the angina. In contrast, patient questionnaires demonstrated that only 52% of patients reported being angina-free and only 47% described their angina as not limiting their enjoyment in life. Hence further efforts are required to bridge this gap between the patient's experience and the clinician's perception of the disability associated with angina.

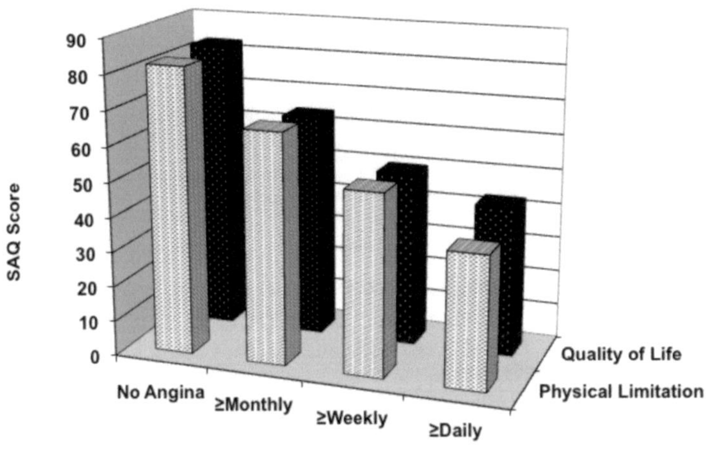

SAQ = Seattle Angina Questionnaire. Adapted from (Beltrame et al, 2009). Copyright gained 30/09/2011.

Fig. 12. Relationship between Angina Frequency and Patient-assessed Quality of Life Indices.

4.6 Summary comments

Although data concerning the epidemiology of chronic stable angina must be interpreted with caution considering the objectivity of the data source, substantial information is available primarily based upon patient self-report and general practitioner clinic surveys. In developed countries, the estimated prevalence of stable angina is 4-5% and the incidence of new cases approximately 46/100,000 population. The chronic nature of this condition results in significant impairment in patient health status with a recent study reporting that almost a third of patients have angina once a week. Since there is an inverse relationship between symptom frequency and its related physical limitation and quality of life, these patients have substantial health status impairment that warrants more attention.

5. Key facts in the epidemiology of coronary artery disease

Coronary artery disease (CAD) is the global leading cause of death and may manifest clinically as an acute coronary syndrome such as AMI, or a chronic coronary syndrome such as chronic stable angina.

Concerning CAD Mortality:

- It is estimated that 7.2 million people died world-wide in 2004 from CAD (i.e. approximately 12%of all deaths).
- In developing countries the CAD mortality is rising but in developed countries it has been falling since the 1960's.
- CAD mortality varies with age, gender, geographic region, socioeconomic status and depression.

Concerning Myocardial Infarction:

- The prevalence of myocardial infarction within developed countries is approximately 3-4%.
- The incidence of new myocardial infarction within developed countries is approximately 200/100,000 population.
- Factors influencing the frequency of myocardial infarction within the community include (a) demographic - age, gender, (b) lifestyle/biological - lipid profile, smoking status, blood pressure, diabetic status, obesity, fruit/vegetable intake, alcohol consumption, and (c) psychosocial factors.
- Approximately 1 in 5 patients continue to experience angina 12 months following an AMI. The frequency of these ongoing symptoms is not only influenced by cardiac factors (such as a pre-infarction history of angina) but also non-cardiac factors such as age, gender and depression.

Concerning Chronic Stable Angina:

- The prevalence of chronic stable angina within developed countries is approximately 4-5%
- The incidence of newly diagnosed angina within developed countries is approximately 46/100,000 population.
- Factors that influence the frequency of angina symptoms in patients with chronic stable angina include female gender and co-existing heart failure or peripheral arterial disease.
- Despite contemporary therapies in developed countries, almost 1 in 3 patients with chronic stable angina continue to experience angina at least once a week. Since angina frequency is inversely related to physical limitation and quality of life, these patients have a considerably impaired health status.

6. Appendix: definitions

ANGINA PECTORIS - a strangling sensation in the chest resulting from myocardial ischaemia.

CORONARY HEART DISEASE - a group of clinical disorders involving coronary circulatory dysfunction resulting in impaired coronary blood flow and thus myocardial ischaemia. This includes coronary atherosclerosis, coronary artery spasm and/or microvascular dysfunction.

CRESCENDO ANGINA - angina pectoris that is occurring more frequently or with greater intensity, or with less provocation. It is a form of unstable angina.

EXERTIONAL ANGINA - angina pectoris precipitated by exertion.

INCIDENCE - the number of new episodes of a disorder over a period of time (eg new myocardial infarcts in 2007)

MIXED PATTERN ANGINA - angina pectoris occurring during exertion but also on occasions at rest.

MYOCARDIAL INFARCT - a pathological condition where inadequate coronary blood flow results in myocardial necrosis.

MYOCARDIAL ISCHAEMIA - a pathological condition where an insufficient coronary blood flow results in inadequate oxygen supply and the accumulation of wastes products in the myocardium

PREVALENCE - the number of patients with the disorder at any particular time (eg patients with a myocardial infarct in Britain).

REST ANGINA - angina pectoris occurring at rest.

7. References

Australian Institute of Health and Welfare [AIHW]. (2010). Cardiovascular Disease Mortality: Trends at Different Ages. Date of access: 18/07/11, Available from: www.aihw.gov.au/WorkArea/DownloadAsset.aspx?id=6442455116

Bairey Merz, CN., Shaw, LJ et al. (2006). Insights from the NHLBI-Sponsored Women's Ischemia Syndrome Evaluation (WISE) Study: Part II: gender differences in presentation, diagnosis, and outcome with regard to gender-based pathophysiology of atherosclerosis and macrovascular and microvascular coronary disease. *J Am Coll Cardiol* 47(3 Suppl): S21-29.

Beaglehole, R. (2004). The World Health Report 2004- changing history. World Health Organistation (WHO). 120-124.

Beltrame, JF, Weekes, AJ et al. (2009). The prevalence of weekly angina among patients with chronic stable angina in primary care practices: The Coronary Artery Disease in General Practice (CADENCE) Study. *Arch Intern Med* 169(16): 1491-1499.

British Heart Foundation [BHF]. (2010). Coronary heart disease statistics 2010. Oxford, British Heart Foundation Health Promotion Research Group. Date of access: 15/07/11, Available from: www.bhf.org.uk/publications/view-publication.aspx?ps=1001546

Carney, RM and Freedland, KE. (2003). Depression, mortality, and medical morbidity in patients with coronary heart disease. *Biol Psychiatry* 54(3): 241-247

Castelli, WP. (1988). Cardiovascular disease in women. *Am J Obstet Gynecol* 158(6 Pt 2): 1553-1560, 1566-1557.

Detry, JM. Kapita, BM et al. (1977). Diagnostic value of history and maximal exercise electrocardiography in men and women suspected of coronary heart disease. *Circulation* 56(5): 756-761.

Diamond, GA. (1983). A clinically relevant classification of chest discomfort. *J Am Coll Cardiol* 1(2 Pt 1): 574-575.

Dreyer, R. Arstall, M et al. (2011). Gender Differences in Patients with Stable Angina attending Primary Care Practices. *Heart Lung Circ* 20(7): 452-459.

Frasure-Smith, N. Lesperance, F et al. (1999). Gender, depression, and one-year prognosis after myocardial infarction. *Psychosom Med* 61(1): 26-37.

Goldberg, RJ. Currie, K et al. (2004). Six-month outcomes in a multinational registry of patients hospitalized with an acute coronary syndrome (the Global Registry of Acute Coronary Events [GRACE]). *American Journal of Cardiology* 93(3): 288-293.

Guck, TP. Kavan, MC. Elsasser, GN. & Barone, EJ. (2001). Assessment and treatment of depression following myocardial infarction. *Am Fam Physician* 15(64): 641-648.

Heberden, W. (1772). Some account of a disorder of the breast. *Medical Transactions* 2: 59-67.Javitz, HS. Ward, MM et al. (2004). Cost of illness of chronic angina. *Am J Manag Care* 10(11 Suppl): S358-369.

Joshi, P. Islam, S et al. (2007). Risk factors for early myocardial infarction in South Asians compared with individuals in other countries. *JAMA* 297(3): 286-294.

Khor, GL. (2001). Cardiovascular epidemiology in the Asia-Pacific region. *Asia Pac J Clin Nutr* 10(2): 76-80.

Kirwan, BA., Lubsen, J et al. (2008). Quality management of a large randomized double-blind multi-centre trial: the ACTION experience. *Contemp Clin Trials* 29(2): 259-269.

Lacey, EA. and Walters, SJ (2003). Continuing inequality: gender and social class influences on self perceived health after a heart attack. *J Epidemiol Community Health* 57(8): 622-627.

Lampe, F.C. Whincup, PH et al. (2000). The natural history of prevalent ischaemic heart disease in middle-aged men. *Eur Heart J* 21(13): 1052-1062.

Lerner, DJ. and Kannel, WB (1986). Patterns of coronary heart disease morbidity and mortality in the sexes: a 26-year follow-up of the Framingham population. *Am Heart J* 111(2): 383-390.

Lloyd-Jones, D. Adams, RJ et al. (2009). Heart disease and stroke statistics--2009 update: a report from the American Heart Association Statistics Committee and Stroke Statistics Subcommittee. *Circulation* 119(3): e21-181.

Lloyd-Jones, D. Adams, RJ et al. (2010). Heart disease and stoke statistics-2010 update: a report from the American Heart Association Statistics Committee and Stroke Statistics Subcommittee. *Circulation* 121(7):46-e215.

Maddox, TM. Reid, KJ et al. (2008). Angina at 1 year after myocardial infarction: prevalence and associated findings. *Arch Intern Med* 168(12): 1310-1316.

Maseri, A. (1995). Transient myocardial ischemia and angina pectoris: classification and diagnostic assessment. *In: Ischemic Heart Disease: A rational Basis for Clinical Practice and Clinical Research.* N. Y. C. Livingstone: 451-476.

Mensah, MJ. (2004). Atlas of Heart Disease and Stroke: World Health Organisation (WHO).

Montalescot, G. Dallongeville, J et al. (2007). STEMI and NSTEMI: are they so different? 1 year outcomes in acute myocardial infarction as defined by the ESC/ACC definition (the OPERA registry). *Eur Heart J* 28(12): 1409-1417.

Nyboe, J. Jensen, G et al. (1989). Risk factors for acute myocardial infarction in Copenhagen. I: Hereditary, educational and socioeconomic factors. Copenhagen City Heart Study. *Eur Heart J* 10(10): 910-916.

O'Flaherty, M. Bishop, J et al. (2009). Coronary heart disease mortality among young adults in Scotland in relation to social inequalities: time trend study. *BMJ* 339: b2613.

Omran, AR. (1971). The epidemiologic transition. A theory of the epidemiology of population change. *Milbank Mem Fund* Q 49(4): 509-538.

Rumsfeld, JS. (2002). Health status and clinical practice: when will they meet? *Circulation* 106(1): 5-7.

Rumsfeld, JS. Magid, DJ et al. (2001). Predictors of quality of life following acute coronary syndromes. *Am J Cardiol* 88(7): 781-784.

Schrader, G. Cheok, F et al. (2004). Predictors of depression three months after cardiac hospitalization. *Psychosom Med* 66(4): 514-520.

Schrader, G. Cheok, F et al. (2006). Predictors of depression 12 months after cardiac hospitalization: the Identifying Depression as a Comorbid Condition study. *Aust N Z J Psychiatry* 40(11-12): 1025-1030.

Terkelsen, CJ. Lassen, JF et al. (2005). Mortality rates in patients with ST-elevation vs. non-ST-elevation acute myocardial infarction: observations from an unselected cohort. *Eur Heart J* 26(1): 18-26.

Thygesen, K. Alpert, JS et al. (2007). Universal definition of myocardial infarction. *Eur Heart J* 28(20): 2525-2538.

Tunstall-Pedoe, H. Vanuzzo, D et al. (2000). Estimation of contribution of changes in coronary care to improving survival, event rates, and coronary heart disease mortality across the WHO MONICA Project populations. *Lancet* 355(9205): 688-700.

Ueshima, H. Sekikawa, A et al. (2008). Cardiovascular disease and risk factors in Asia: a selected review. *Circulation* 118(25): 2702-2709.

Vaccarino, V. Parsons, L et al. (1999). Sex-based differences in early mortality after myocardial infarction. National Registry of Myocardial Infarction 2 Participants. *N Engl J Med* 341(4): 217-225.

White, HD. and Chew, DP (2008). Acute myocardial infarction. *Lancet* 372(9638): 570-584.

World Health Organisation [WHO] (2008). The global burden of disease: 2004 update. Geneva, World Health Organisation. Date of Access: 15/07/11, Available from: http://www.who.int/healthinfo/global_burden_disease/2004_report_update/en/

Wiest, FC. Bryson, CL et al. (2004). Suboptimal pharmacotherapeutic management of chronic stable angina in the primary care setting. *Am J Med* 117(4): 234-241.

Wilson, WR. Fitridge, RA et al. (2011). Quality of Life of Patients With Peripheral Arterial Disease and Chronic Stable Angina. Angiology (In press).

Yusuf, S. Hawken, S et al. (2004). Effect of potentially modifiable risk factors associated with myocardial infarction in 52 countries (the INTERHEART study): case-control study. *Lancet* 364(9438): 937-952.

Yusuf, S. Reddy, S et al. (2001). Global burden of cardiovascular diseases: part I: general considerations, the epidemiologic transition, risk factors, and impact of urbanization. *Circulation* 104(22): 2746-2753.

2

Gender Differences in Coronary Artery Disease

Ryotaro Wake and Minoru Yoshiyama
*Osaka City University Graduate School of Medicine,
Japan*

1. Introduction

Coronary artery disease (CAD) is a leading cause of mortality and morbidity in most developed countries [1]. Many studies have found gender-related differences in the presentations, prevalence, and clinical outcomes of CAD [2-4]. CAD first presents itself in women approximately 10 years later than in men, most commonly after menopause [5]. The worldwide INTERHEART study, a large study of more than 52000 individuals with MI, first demonstrated that this approximate 8 to 10 year difference in age at onset holds widely around the world, across various socioeconomic, climatic, and cultural environments. Although coronary artery disease in general is manifestated earlier in less developed countries, the age gap in time of onset between men and women is universal (Table 1) [6].

Region	Median age, women	Median age, men
Western Europe	68 (59-76)	61 (53-70)
Central and eastern Europe	68 (59-74)	59 (50-68)
North America	64 (52-75)	58 (49-68)
South America and Mexico	65 (56-73)	59 (50-68)
Australia and New Zealand	66 (59-74)	58 (50-67)
Middle East	57 (50-65)	50 (44-57)
Africa	56 (49-65)	52 (46-61)
South Asia	60 (50-66)	52 (45-60)
China and Hong Kong	67 (62-72)	60 (50-68)
Southeast Asia and Japan	63 (56-68)	55 (47-64)

Table 1. Comparison of age at first myocardial infarction among women and men across geographic regions: Effect of potentially modifiable risk factors associated with myocardial infarction in 52 countries (the INTERHEART study): Case-control study [6].

Compared to women, men present with ST-segment elevation myocardial infarction (MI) more often and have a higher prevalence of CAD adjusted for age [7,8]. However, younger women experience more adverse outcomes after MI and coronary artery bypass grafting surgery than men [9]. A greater proportion of women than men with MI die of sudden cardiac arrest before reaching hospital [3,10]. Previous reports have shown a 20% reduction in total mortality among patients randomized to exercise-based cardiac rehabilitation compared with controls receiving usual care [11]. The outcome was however similar between men and women, although only 20% of all participants were women in many reports. Women are less likely than men to participate in cardiac rehabilitation after acute MI [11].

The prevalence of microvascular angina is higher in women than men. Takotsubo cardiomyopathy is more prevalent in women than in men [12]. These findings indicate that gender difference may have an important influence on cardiovascular physiology and pathology [13,14].

In many developing countries, a large budget is expended for the treatment of CAD, and it is necessary to minimize the influence of risk factors. The burden of CAD on women and the global economy will continue to increase [5]. In addition to population-based and macroeconomic interventions, interventions in individual patients are key to reducing the incidence of CAD globally [15]. Prevention of CAD is paramount to the health of every woman and every nation.

There have been numerous clinical trials that have a bearing on CAD prevention in women [16]. Women and men differ in their genetic complement by a single chromosome out of the 46 that are present in the human species. However, this single chromosomal difference affects both the expression of disease and the psychosocial and behavioral characteristics and work environments of individuals, which may reduce or increase the susceptibility to cardiovascular diseases.

In future, novel drugs for tailor-made therapy of CAD based on gender differences may be developed. This review discusses gender differences in the features of ischemic heart disease and the possibilities of future developments in treatments.

2. Clinical risk factors of coronary artery disease in women

It is important to classify women as being at high, intermediate, or low risk for CAD. Classification may be based on clinical criteria and the Framingham global risk score [17]. A woman found to have coronary calcification or increased carotid intimal thickness may be at low risk for CAD on the basis of the Framingham risk score, but she may be actually at intermediate or high risk for a future CAD event.

We should take several factors into consideration, including medical and lifestyle histories, Framingham risk score, family history of CAD, and other genetic conditions (e.g., familial hypercholesterolemia), since these affect the decisions about the aggressiveness of preventive therapy. Novel CAD risk factors (e.g., high-sensitivity C-reactive protein [18]) and novel screening technologies (e.g., coronary calcium scoring) should help guide preventive interventions. Further research is needed on the benefits, risks, and costs associated with such strategies. There are many unique opportunities for early detection of CAD in women; for example, in pregnancy, preeclampsia may be an early indicator of CAD risk [19,20]. In addition, maternal placental syndromes in combination with traditional cardiovascular risk factors, such as pre-pregnancy hypertension or diabetes mellitus, obesity, dyslipidemia, and metabolic syndrome, may be additive in defining CAD risk in women [19]. Future research should evaluate the potential for events or medical contact during unique phases in a woman's life, such as adolescence, pregnancy, and menopause, to identify women at high risk, and determine the effectiveness of preventive interventions during critical periods.

The diagnosis of CAD in women presents challenges not observed in case of men. Differences in the epidemiology of CAD between men and women show that women are generally at a lower risk than their male counterparts until the seventh decade of life. For both asymptomatic and symptomatic women, the choice of initial test is guided by classification into low, intermediate, or high pretest risk categories. Asymptomatic intermediate-risk women have lower event rates. In symptomatic women, noninvasive diagnostic studies (exercise electrocardiography (ECG) and cardiac imaging studies) are recommended for those who are at an intermediate to high pretest likelihood of CAD [21]. Therapeutic decision-making is guided by the extent and severity of inducible ischemia. Thus, referral of low-likelihood women (for example, premenopausal women with less than one risk factor and non-anginal/atypical symptoms) will be associated with a high rate of false positives.

Smoking is an important risk factor for vascular diseases. Vascular disease risk was most quickly reduced by cessation of smoking compared with other associated factors. The beneficial effect of quitting on the risk for death from CHD was realized within 5 years, whereas the risks for death from chronic obstructive pulmonary disease and lung cancer did not approach those of women who had never smoked until the age of 20 and 30 years, respectively [22]. It may never be too late for women to quit smoking in order to reduce the risk for vascular diseases.

A blood pressure-lowering treatment provided similar protection against major cardiovascular events in men and women [23].

3. Features of coronary artery pathology in women

Men have a greater burden of atheroma and eccentric atheroma in coronary arteries compared to women. A study reported that plaque rupture in patients with sudden coronary death was more frequent in men than in women [24].

Men have more severe structural and functional abnormalities in the epicardial coronary arteries than women. These factors may influence the higher incidence rates of CAD and ST-segment MI (STEMI) in men compared to women. With regard to the lower cardiac event rate in female patients, several mechanisms have been proposed to explain the cardioprotective effect of sex hormones in women [13]. We show the effect of sex hormones in ischemic heart disease in table 2.

Women had lower rates of obstructive CAD at angiography when evaluated for symptoms suggestive of myocardial ischemia [25]. Among angiographic CAD patients, atheroma volume in women is less than that in men, despite the presence of more cardiovascular risk factors in women. Women had slightly lower coronary vasodilator reserve even with normal coronary angiographic results [26]. Endothelial-independent microvascular dysfunction was an independent predictor of adverse outcomes in patients with mild CAD [27]. It has been suggested that the mechanism of myocardial ischemia in women may be localized to the microvascular coronary arteries and that abnormal microvascular function may have prognostic implications [28].

	Favorable	Unfavorable
Lipids	↓ LDL - cholesterol ↑ HDL -cholesterol	↑ Trigriceride
Coagulation Fibrinolysis	↓ PAI-1 ↓ Fibrinogen	↑ Factor VII ↓ AT III
Inflammation Adhesion	↓ Adhesion molecules	↑ CRP
Endothelial function Blood pressure	↓ ACE activity ↑ Nitric oxide ↓ Endothelin-1 ↑ Plasminogen I2 ↓ VSMC migration, proliferation	↑ Angiotensinogen

PAI-1: plasminogen activator inhibitor-1, AT III: antithrombin III, ACE: angiotensinogen converting enzyme, VSMC: vascular smooth muscle cell.

Table 2. Effect of estrogen on atherosclerosis.

4. Takotsubo cardiomyopathy

Takotsubo cardiomyopathy (or transient LV apical ballooning syndrome) is more prevalent in women than in men. Because the onset of this syndrome is often preceded by emotional or physical stress, catecholamine-mediated multivessel epicardial spasm, microvascular coronary spasm, or possible direct catecholamine-mediated myocyte injury have been advocated as possible pathophysiological mechanisms [12]. Electrocardiographic findings are like myocardial infarction. The left ventricular wall motion is akinetic from the middle to apex of the left ventricle on the left ventriculography and echocardiography [29]. The epicardial coronary artery stenosis is absent in the coronary angiography. Cardiac magnetic resonance can be useful for differentiating apical ballooning syndrome from an acute coronary event [12]. Late gadolinium enhancement in this setting represents a disproportionate expansion of extracellular matrix with increased collagen I deposition on immunohistochemical tissue staining [30].

5. Diagnosis and prognosis

5.1 Electrocardiography

Changes in ECG during exercise have been reported to be of diminished accuracy in women as a result of more frequent changes in resting ST-T wave, lower ECG voltage, and hormonal factors such as endogenous estrogen in premenopausal women and hormone replacement therapy in postmenopausal women [31-33]. In a meta-analysis of exercise ECG studies in women, sensitivity was 61% and specificity was 70%, compared to 72% and 77%, respectively, in men [21]. From a cohort of symptomatic women who were referred for exercise treadmill testing followed by coronary angiography, significant coronary stenosis (more than 75%) was observed in 19%, 35%, and 89% of low-, moderate-, and high-risk women, respectively, based on Duke treadmill score risk categories [34].

Maximal exercise capacity and heart rate recovery measurements can aid in estimation of near- and long-term outcome in large cohorts of women [35]. Recent reports have noted that a simple measure such as heart rate recovery (at 1 or 2 min after exercise) have substantial prognostic value.

Women engage less often in physical exercise programs, have lower functional capacity, and show a greater functional decline during their menopausal years. Because of their lower work capacity on exercise tests (on average 5–7 min) as a result of premature peripheral fatigue, it is difficult to provoke myocardial ischemia [36]. Women who exercise less than 5 metabolic equivalents (METs) are at an increased risk for death [37]. Women expected to perform less than 5 METs may be better evaluated by pharmacological stress imaging. However, women who have inducible ischemia at low workloads (less than 5 METs) have a higher likelihood of obstructive CAD and may be referred for coronary angiography.

The exercise ECG test has a high negative predictive value in women with a low pretest probability of CAD and a low-risk Duke treadmill score [21]. The diagnostic and prognostic accuracy of the exercise ECG stress test in symptomatic women with suspected CAD is increased by the inclusion of additional parameters in the interpretation of the ST-segment response to exercise.

5.2 Echocardiography

Stress echocardiography can provide information about the presence of left ventricular systolic or diastolic dysfunction, valvular heart disease, and the extent of infarction and stress-induced ischemia. Exercise echocardiography may be performed with a treadmill or by supine or upright bicycle exercise. Exercise stress echocardiography is a physiological investigation and the most widely available method for evaluation of CAD. However, exercise capacity is often impaired in aged or diabetic patients and the workload required to produce stress-induced myocardial ischemia might not be achieved by such patients.

Stress echocardiography provides significantly higher specificity and accuracy than the standard exercise ECG testing in women [38].

Stress echocardiography has demonstrated good diagnostic accuracy for detecting or excluding significant CAD, with a mean sensitivity of 81%, specificity of 86%, and an overall accuracy of 84% [38-41]. There appears to be no significant effect of gender on the diagnostic accuracy of exercise echocardiography.

A study of dobutamine stress echocardiography (DSE) revealed an overall sensitivity of 80% and specificity of 84% [39]. To exercise stress echocardiography, DSE appears to have similar diagnostic accuracy in detecting CAD in both women and men.

Cardiac events occur less frequently in women than in men. This difference is compatible with the lower prevalence and lesser sensitivity of detection of CAD in women compared to men. No gender differences have been reported in the prognostic value of exercise stress echocardiography in a large population.

The low specificity of exercise ECG testing in women, especially in young and middle-aged women, may lead to a higher rate of unnecessary angiography and higher expense, particularly if stress imaging is not used before coronary angiography in a sequential testing strategy.

Stress echocardiography with exercise or dobutamine is an effective and highly accurate noninvasive means of detecting ischemic heart disease and risk-stratifying symptomatic women with an intermediate to high pretest likelihood of CAD. Stress echocardiography provides incremental value over exercise ECG and clinical variables in women with suspected or known coronary heart disease. Stress echocardiography is recommended for symptomatic women with an intermediate or high pretest probability of CAD (women with suspected CAD must also have an abnormal resting ECG). Previous reports demonstrated that pharmacological stress echocardiography provides independent prognostic information in both men and women [42,43].

5.3 Myocardial perfusion

Gated myocardial perfusion single-photon emission computed tomography (SPECT) is a nuclear-based technique that provides a combination of test elements that are used to diagnose and risk-stratify women. Myocardial perfusion imaging, however, has been reported to have technical limitations in women, including false-positive results due to breast attenuation and small left ventricular chamber size [44].

The accuracy of 201Tl SPECT imaging, for example, is reduced in patients with small hearts, and these patients are more likely to be women than men. When 201Tl is used as the radioisotope in women, false-positive test results may occur due to soft tissue attenuation (e.g., breast attenuation) in the anterior and anterolateral segments [44].

For women, the lower-energy isotope 201Tl has been largely supplanted by technetium-based imaging agents that improve accuracy. In comparing the diagnostic accuracy of 201Tl with gated 99mTc-sestamibi SPECT in women, the sensitivity for detecting CAD was 80%, and test specificity improved dramatically from 67% for 201Tl to 92% for gated 99mTc-sestamibi SPECT [45].

Pharmacological stress SPECT also merits consideration, given the higher incidence of decreased exercise capacity and advanced age for women, as discussed previously [44,46]. Vasodilator pharmacological stress perfusion imaging has been shown to be more accurate than exercise perfusion imaging in identification of CAD in both men and women with left bundle-branch block [46]. Adenosine 99mTc-sestamibi imaging was reported to have 91% sensitivity and 86% specificity for detecting significant coronary artery stenoses of more than 50% [47].

Myocardial perfusion imaging has powerful predictive value with regard to the development of subsequent cardiac death or MI or the need for coronary revascularization [48-50], regardless of sex [36]. Prognosis worsens commensurate with the number of vascular territories involved, with 3-year survival rates ranging from 99% for women without ischemia to 85% in women who had three-vessel ischemia [36].

In addition, pharmacological stress was recently shown to be effective in the risk stratification of diabetic women with suspected and known CAD. The CAD mortality for non-diabetic women with a moderately abnormal scan was 2.8% compared with 4.1% in diabetic women [48].

6. Treatment

Studies have shown that percutaneous coronary intervention (PCI) is a more effective reperfusion strategy for acute coronary syndrome than intravenous thrombolysis [51]. The advantage of primary PCI over thrombolytic therapy was greater for women than men [52]. Primary PCI reduced the risk of intracranial bleeding and improved survival in women [53].

Mortality from acute MI (AMI) was higher in women than in men, consistent with the results of most previous studies [52,54,55]. This poorer outcome in women was likely related to the facts that compared to men, women with AMI were older, underwent PCI less frequently, and had higher incidences of coronary risk factors, such as hyperlipidemia, diabetes mellitus, and hypertension.

The use of a drug-eluting stent makes the outcome after PCI better than that after the use of a bare metal stent. There is no difference between men and women in the outcome [56].

On the other hand, the most important benefit of PCI in chronic stable CAD may be the relief of symptoms [57]. Statin therapy is effective for chronic stable CAD [58].

Women experience more bleeding than men with antiplatelet therapy and/or anticoagulant therapy as they often have a smaller body size, resulting in excessive dosing. These agents should be used with regard to the patient's body size [59]. In a primary prevention trial in women, aspirin lowered the risk of stroke without affecting the risk of MI. On the other hand, in men, aspirin lowered the risk of MI without affecting the risk of stroke [60,61].

Angiotensin-converting enzyme inhibitors, angiotensin receptor blockers and warfarin for blood pressure control are contraindicated in women contemplating pregnancy and in those who are pregnant.

The perception of the risks and benefits of hormone replacement therapy (HRT) and the time when the therapy should be initiated has changed dramatically since the publication of the Women's Health Initiative trial in 2002. This study of women in whom HRT was initiated on average 13 years after menopause did not reveal long-term benefits for cardiovascular outcomes [62]. However, combined HRT started many years after menopause can improve health-related quality of life [63].

Reports show 20% reduction in total mortality among patients randomized to exercise-based cardiac rehabilitation compared with controls receiving usual care. The outcome is similar between men and women, although only 20% of all participants were women in many reports. Women are less likely than men to participate in cardiac rehabilitation after acute MI [11]. This may be one reason for the poor outcome in women with AMI. Cardiac rehabilitation should be recommended to more women after AMI.

7. Conclusions

Appropriate diagnosis, prevention, and treatment will improve the care of all CAD patients. Since there are gender differences in ischemic heart disease, it is necessary to consider these differences when examining men and women with ischemic heart disease. We have found many gender differences in CAD. The development of novel drugs and therapeutic methods for tailor-made therapy of CAD based on gender differences is required.

8. References

[1] Rosamond, W. et al. (2007) Heart disease and stroke statistics--2007 update: a report from the American Heart Association Statistics Committee and Stroke Statistics Subcommittee. Circulation 115 (5), e69-171

[2] Bairey Merz, C.N. et al. (2006) Insights from the NHLBI-Sponsored Women's Ischemia Syndrome Evaluation (WISE) Study: Part II: gender differences in presentation, diagnosis, and outcome with regard to gender-based pathophysiology of atherosclerosis and macrovascular and microvascular coronary disease. J Am Coll Cardiol 47 (3 Suppl), S21-29

[3] Shaw, L.J. et al. (2006) Insights from the NHLBI-Sponsored Women's Ischemia Syndrome Evaluation (WISE) Study: Part I: gender differences in traditional and novel risk factors, symptom evaluation, and gender-optimized diagnostic strategies. J Am Coll Cardiol 47 (3 Suppl), S4-S20

[4] Wake, R. et al. (2007) Effects of gender on prognosis of patients with known or suspected coronary artery disease undergoing contrast-enhanced dobutamine stress echocardiography. Circ J 71 (7), 1060-1066

[5] Yusuf, S. et al. (2001) Global burden of cardiovascular diseases: part I: general considerations, the epidemiologic transition, risk factors, and impact of urbanization. Circulation 104 (22), 2746-2753

[6] Yusuf, S. et al. (2004) Effect of potentially modifiable risk factors associated with myocardial infarction in 52 countries (the INTERHEART study): case-control study. Lancet 364 (9438), 937-952

[7] Heer, T. et al. (2002) Gender differences in acute myocardial infarction in the era of reperfusion (the MITRA registry). Am J Cardiol 89 (5), 511-517

[8] Kosuge, M. et al. (2006) Differences between men and women in terms of clinical features of ST-segment elevation acute myocardial infarction. Circ J 70 (3), 222-226

[9] Vaccarino, V. et al. (2002) Sex differences in hospital mortality after coronary artery bypass surgery: evidence for a higher mortality in younger women. Circulation 105 (10), 1176-1181

[10] Thom, T. et al. (2006) Heart disease and stroke statistics--2006 update: a report from the American Heart Association Statistics Committee and Stroke Statistics Subcommittee. Circulation 113 (6), e85-151

[11] Taylor, R.S. et al. (2004) Exercise-based rehabilitation for patients with coronary heart disease: systematic review and meta-analysis of randomized controlled trials. Am J Med 116 (10), 682-692

[12] Wittstein, I.S. et al. (2005) Neurohumoral features of myocardial stunning due to sudden emotional stress. N Engl J Med 352 (6), 539-548

[13] Mendelsohn, M.E. and Karas, R.H. (2005) Molecular and cellular basis of cardiovascular gender differences. Science 308 (5728), 1583-1587

[14] Pepine, C.J. (2004) Ischemic heart disease in women: facts and wishful thinking. J Am Coll Cardiol 43 (10), 1727-1730

[15] Strong, K. et al. (2005) Preventing chronic diseases: how many lives can we save? Lancet 366 (9496), 1578-1582
[16] Kotseva, K. et al. (2009) Cardiovascular prevention guidelines in daily practice: a comparison of EUROASPIRE I, II, and III surveys in eight European countries. Lancet 373 (9667), 929-940
[17] (2002) Third Report of the National Cholesterol Education Program (NCEP) Expert Panel on Detection, Evaluation, and Treatment of High Blood Cholesterol in Adults (Adult Treatment Panel III) final report. Circulation 106 (25), 3143-3421
[18] Ridker, P.M. et al. (2009) Reduction in C reactive protein and LDL cholesterol and cardiovascular event rates after initiation of rosuvastatin: a prospective study of the JUPITER trial. Lancet 373 (9670), 1175-1182
[19] Ray, J.G. et al. (2005) Cardiovascular health after maternal placental syndromes (CHAMPS): population-based retrospective cohort study. Lancet 366 (9499), 1797-1803
[20] Wilson, B.J. et al. (2003) Hypertensive diseases of pregnancy and risk of hypertension and stroke in later life: results from cohort study. Bmj 326 (7394), 845
[21] Gibbons, R.J. et al. (2002) ACC/AHA 2002 guideline update for exercise testing: summary article: a report of the American College of Cardiology/American Heart Association Task Force on Practice Guidelines (Committee to Update the 1997 Exercise Testing Guidelines). Circulation 106 (14), 1883-1892
[22] Kenfield, S.A. et al. (2008) Smoking and smoking cessation in relation to mortality in women. Jama 299 (17), 2037-2047
[23] Turnbull, F. et al. (2008) Do men and women respond differently to blood pressure-lowering treatment? Results of prospectively designed overviews of randomized trials. Eur Heart J 29 (21), 2669-2680
[24] Virmani, R. et al. (2000) Lessons from sudden coronary death: a comprehensive morphological classification scheme for atherosclerotic lesions. Arterioscler Thromb Vasc Biol 20 (5), 1262-1275
[25] Sharaf, B.L. et al. (2001) Detailed angiographic analysis of women with suspected ischemic chest pain (pilot phase data from the NHLBI-sponsored Women's Ischemia Syndrome Evaluation [WISE] Study Angiographic Core Laboratory). Am J Cardiol 87 (8), 937-941; A933
[26] Kern, M.J. et al. (1996) Variations in normal coronary vasodilatory reserve stratified by artery, gender, heart transplantation and coronary artery disease. J Am Coll Cardiol 28 (5), 1154-1160
[27] Britten, M.B. et al. (2004) Microvascular dysfunction in angiographically normal or mildly diseased coronary arteries predicts adverse cardiovascular long-term outcome. Coron Artery Dis 15 (5), 259-264
[28] Johnson, B.D. et al. (2004) Prognosis in women with myocardial ischemia in the absence of obstructive coronary disease: results from the National Institutes of Health-National Heart, Lung, and Blood Institute-Sponsored Women's Ischemia Syndrome Evaluation (WISE). Circulation 109 (24), 2993-2999
[29] Hurst, R.T. et al. (2006) Transient midventricular ballooning syndrome: a new variant. J Am Coll Cardiol 48 (3), 579-583
[30] Rolf, A. et al. (2009) Immunohistological basis of the late gadolinium enhancement phenomenon in tako-tsubo cardiomyopathy. Eur Heart J 30 (13), 1635-1642

[31] Rosano, G.M. et al. (2000) Natural progesterone, but not medroxyprogesterone acetate, enhances the beneficial effect of estrogen on exercise-induced myocardial ischemia in postmenopausal women. J Am Coll Cardiol 36 (7), 2154-2159

[32] Schulman, S.P. et al. (2002) Effects of acute hormone therapy on recurrent ischemia in postmenopausal women with unstable angina. J Am Coll Cardiol 39 (2), 231-237

[33] Waters, D.D. et al. (2004) Women's Ischemic Syndrome Evaluation: current status and future research directions: report of the National Heart, Lung and Blood Institute workshop: October 2-4, 2002: Section 4: lessons from hormone replacement trials. Circulation 109 (6), e53-55

[34] Alexander, K.P. et al. (1998) Value of exercise treadmill testing in women. J Am Coll Cardiol 32 (6), 1657-1664

[35] Mora, S. et al. (2003) Ability of exercise testing to predict cardiovascular and all-cause death in asymptomatic women: a 20-year follow-up of the lipid research clinics prevalence study. Jama 290 (12), 1600-1607

[36] Marwick, T.H. et al. (1999) The noninvasive prediction of cardiac mortality in men and women with known or suspected coronary artery disease. Economics of Noninvasive Diagnosis (END) Study Group. Am J Med 106 (2), 172-178

[37] Hlatky, M.A. et al. (1989) A brief self-administered questionnaire to determine functional capacity (the Duke Activity Status Index). Am J Cardiol 64 (10), 651-654

[38] Cheitlin, M.D. et al. (2003) ACC/AHA/ASE 2003 guideline update for the clinical application of echocardiography: summary article: a report of the American College of Cardiology/American Heart Association Task Force on Practice Guidelines (ACC/AHA/ASE Committee to Update the 1997 Guidelines for the Clinical Application of Echocardiography). Circulation 108 (9), 1146-1162

[39] Kim, C. et al. (2001) Pharmacologic stress testing for coronary disease diagnosis: A meta-analysis. Am Heart J 142 (6), 934-944

[40] Kwok, Y. et al. (1999) Meta-analysis of exercise testing to detect coronary artery disease in women. Am J Cardiol 83 (5), 660-666

[41] Lewis, J.F. et al. (1999) Dobutamine stress echocardiography in women with chest pain. Pilot phase data from the National Heart, Lung and Blood Institute Women's Ischemia Syndrome Evaluation (WISE). J Am Coll Cardiol 33 (6), 1462-1468

[42] Biagini, E. et al. (2005) Seven-year follow-up after dobutamine stress echocardiography: impact of gender on prognosis. J Am Coll Cardiol 45 (1), 93-97

[43] Cortigiani, L. et al. (1998) Prognostic value of pharmacological stress echocardiography in women with chest pain and unknown coronary artery disease. J Am Coll Cardiol 32 (7), 1975-1981

[44] Mieres, J.H. et al. (2003) American Society of Nuclear Cardiology consensus statement: Task Force on Women and Coronary Artery Disease--the role of myocardial perfusion imaging in the clinical evaluation of coronary artery disease in women [correction]. J Nucl Cardiol 10 (1), 95-101

[45] Taillefer, R. et al. (1997) Comparative diagnostic accuracy of Tl-201 and Tc-99m sestamibi SPECT imaging (perfusion and ECG-gated SPECT) in detecting coronary artery disease in women. J Am Coll Cardiol 29 (1), 69-77

[46] Klocke, F.J. et al. (2003) ACC/AHA/ASNC guidelines for the clinical use of cardiac radionuclide imaging--executive summary: a report of the American College of Cardiology/American Heart Association Task Force on Practice Guidelines

(ACC/AHA/ASNC Committee to Revise the 1995 Guidelines for the Clinical Use of Cardiac Radionuclide Imaging). Circulation 108 (11), 1404-1418

[47] Amanullah, A.M. et al. (1997) Identification of severe or extensive coronary artery disease in women by adenosine technetium-99m sestamibi SPECT. Am J Cardiol 80 (2), 132-137

[48] Berman, D.S. et al. (2003) Adenosine myocardial perfusion single-photon emission computed tomography in women compared with men. Impact of diabetes mellitus on incremental prognostic value and effect on patient management. J Am Coll Cardiol 41 (7), 1125-1133

[49] Galassi, A.R. et al. (2001) Incremental prognostic value of technetium-99m-tetrofosmin exercise myocardial perfusion imaging for predicting outcomes in patients with suspected or known coronary artery disease. Am J Cardiol 88 (2), 101-106

[50] Sharir, T. et al. (1999) Incremental prognostic value of post-stress left ventricular ejection fraction and volume by gated myocardial perfusion single photon emission computed tomography. Circulation 100 (10), 1035-1042

[51] Weaver, W.D. et al. (1997) Comparison of primary coronary angioplasty and intravenous thrombolytic therapy for acute myocardial infarction: a quantitative review. Jama 278 (23), 2093-2098

[52] Tamis-Holland, J.E. et al. (2004) Benefits of direct angioplasty for women and men with acute myocardial infarction: results of the Global Use of Strategies to Open Occluded Arteries in Acute Coronary Syndromes Angioplasty (GUSTO II-B) Angioplasty Substudy. Am Heart J 147 (1), 133-139

[53] Stone, G.W. et al. (1995) Comparison of in-hospital outcome in men versus women treated by either thrombolytic therapy or primary coronary angioplasty for acute myocardial infarction. Am J Cardiol 75 (15), 987-992

[54] Lansky, A.J. et al. (2005) Gender differences in outcomes after primary angioplasty versus primary stenting with and without abciximab for acute myocardial infarction: results of the Controlled Abciximab and Device Investigation to Lower Late Angioplasty Complications (CADILLAC) trial. Circulation 111 (13), 1611-1618

[55] Vakili, B.A. et al. (2001) Sex-based differences in early mortality of patients undergoing primary angioplasty for first acute myocardial infarction. Circulation 104 (25), 3034-3038

[56] Moses, J.W. et al. (2003) Sirolimus-eluting stents versus standard stents in patients with stenosis in a native coronary artery. N Engl J Med 349 (14), 1315-1323

[57] Trikalinos, T.A. et al. (2009) Percutaneous coronary interventions for non-acute coronary artery disease: a quantitative 20-year synopsis and a network meta-analysis. Lancet 373 (9667), 911-918

[58] Baigent, C. et al. (2005) Efficacy and safety of cholesterol-lowering treatment: prospective meta-analysis of data from 90,056 participants in 14 randomised trials of statins. Lancet 366 (9493), 1267-1278

[59] Alexander, K.P. et al. (2006) Sex differences in major bleeding with glycoprotein IIb/IIIa inhibitors: results from the CRUSADE (Can Rapid risk stratification of Unstable angina patients Suppress ADverse outcomes with Early implementation of the ACC/AHA guidelines) initiative. Circulation 114 (13), 1380-1387

[60] (2009) Aspirin for the prevention of cardiovascular disease: U.S. Preventive Services Task Force recommendation statement. Ann Intern Med 150 (6), 396-404

[61] Ridker, P.M. et al. (2005) A randomized trial of low-dose aspirin in the primary prevention of cardiovascular disease in women. N Engl J Med 352 (13), 1293-1304
[62] Rossouw, J.E. et al. (2002) Risks and benefits of estrogen plus progestin in healthy postmenopausal women: principal results From the Women's Health Initiative randomized controlled trial. Jama 288 (3), 321-333
[63] Welton, A.J. et al. (2008) Health related quality of life after combined hormone replacement therapy: randomised controlled trial. Bmj 337, a1190

3

Coronary Flow: From Pathophysiology to Clinical Noninvasive Evaluation

Francesco Bartolomucci[1], Francesco Cipriani[1] and Giovanni Deluca[2]
[1]*U.O.C. - Cardiologia - UTIC, Ospedale "L. Bonomo", Andria (BT)*
[2]*U.O.C. di Cardiologia, Ospedale Civile Bisceglie (BT)*
Italy

1. Introduction

Coronary artery disease is the leading cause of mortality in western countries. Myocardial contraction is indeed closely connected to coronary flow and oxygen delivery; the balance between oxygen supply and demand is a crucial determinant of the normal function of the heart. Acute impairment of this relationship due to coronary blood flow reduction results in a vicious cycle, where ischemia-induced contractile dysfunction causes hypotension and further myocardial ischemia.

The presence of an atheromatous plaque modifies the normal pressure profile of the epicardial coronary vessels, obstructing its lumen and stimulating the circulation counter-measures to face it properly. An accurate knowledge of the coronary flow is essential to fully understand the nature and pathophysiological bases of many disorders. Systolic and diastolic variations in coronary blood flow are markers of myocardial oxygen demand due to the various flow control systems, such as mechanic, anatomic, hemodynamic. Microcirculation disorders affect the coronary flow controls too. The availability of high effective therapies able to prevent major cardiac events raised great interest in early diagnosis and widened the indications of Doppler Echocardiography in the evaluation of the ischemic cardiomyopathy.

2. CFR: the invasive assessment

The Coronary Flow Reserve (CFR) assessment via Trans-Thoracic Echo-color Doppler is nowadays a reality in clinical practice: it is a reliable, cheap, non-invasive and easy to perform test to assess the coronary flow at rest and after the administration of drugs. Other techniques, such as thermodiluition, Magnetic Resonance (MR), Positron Emission Tomography (PET) and intracoronary Doppler Flow Wire have limited indications, because they are time and money consuming and, of course, because they are invasive techniques[1].

PET is considered the *gold standard* among all invasive methods to estimate the CFR[2]. Newer techniques recently introduced in clinical practice are Thermodiluition, Fractional Flow Reserve and Doppler Flow Wire.

Thermodilution is an indicator-dilution method of measuring blood flow. This method is based on the premise that when an indicator substance is added to circulating blood, the rate of blood flow is inversely proportional to the change in concentration of the indicator over time. CFR assessment with the thermodiluition method requires a pressure wire introduced into a coronary vessel for at least 5-7 in. using a guiding catheter during a coronary catheterization. 70 I.U. of heparin intravenously and 100-200 mg of intracoronaric nitroglycerin have to be given before starting the procedure, to reduce vasoconstriction. The pressure sensor is located 1 in. far from the wire soft tip, being the distal sensor, while the proximal one is the wire shaft. A software program calculates all the gathered data to provide information about the *mean transit time* of a determined quantity of saline solution injected at ambient temperature. The baseline value is the mean of 3 consecutive injections of 3 ml of saline solution; the operator must repeat this procedure immediately after the administration of a pharmacological stressor, obtaining the *hyperemic mean transit time*. Hyperemic peak value is inducible with the intracoronaric administration of papaverine (12 mg for the right coronary artery; 20 mg for the left coronary artery) or using a continuous administration of adenosine (140 mg/Kg/min). Being the vessel volume invariable, the mean transit time is inversely proportional to the flow: the mean hyperemic on the mean baseline time ratio provides the CFR estimation. This is a fast and cheap assessment, which can be performed with the simultaneous Fractional Flow Reserve (FFR) estimation using the Doppler technique without any additional hardware[3]. Its limits are in being invasive, in the mismatch with the CFR Doppler Flow Wire values (the variability range is 20%) and the usual over estimated values in distal coronary vessels.

The FFR **(FIG 1)** is a technique used in coronary catheterization, allowing the pressure and the flow measurement in a defined coronary artery. Measuring the pressure differences across a stenosis means understanding if that stenosis impedes the oxygen delivery to the heart muscle. The FFR itself is the ratio between maximum post-stenotic flow and maximum pre-stenotic flow. The assessment is performed after coronary catheterization and during maximal blood flow, using a pressure flow wire pulled back as the pressures are detected by the sensors on it. The CFR values obtained are well related with PET data[4]. The obtained values are considered normal if above 0.80 **(FIG 2)**. The combined use of FFR and thermodiluition give answers on the state of myocardial microcirculation in patients with diffuse vessel injuries[5].

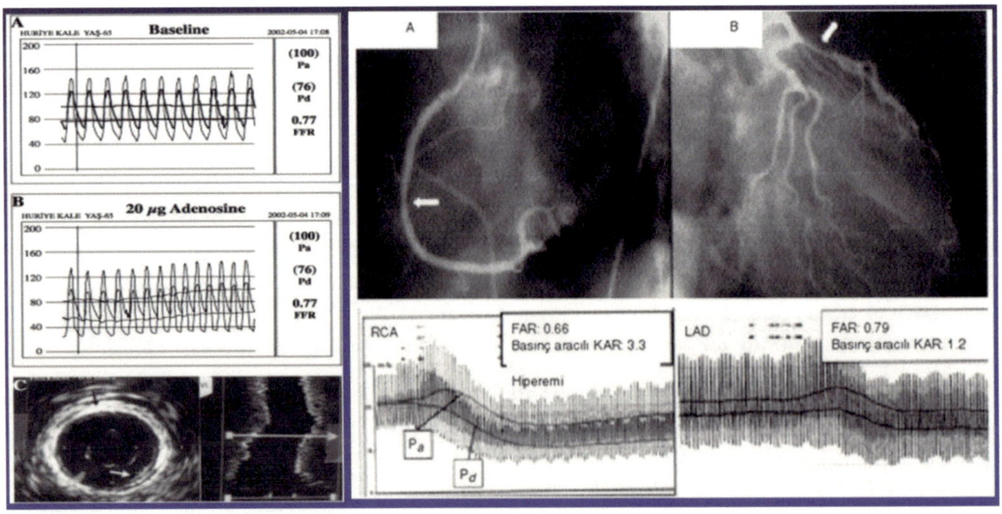

Fig. 1.

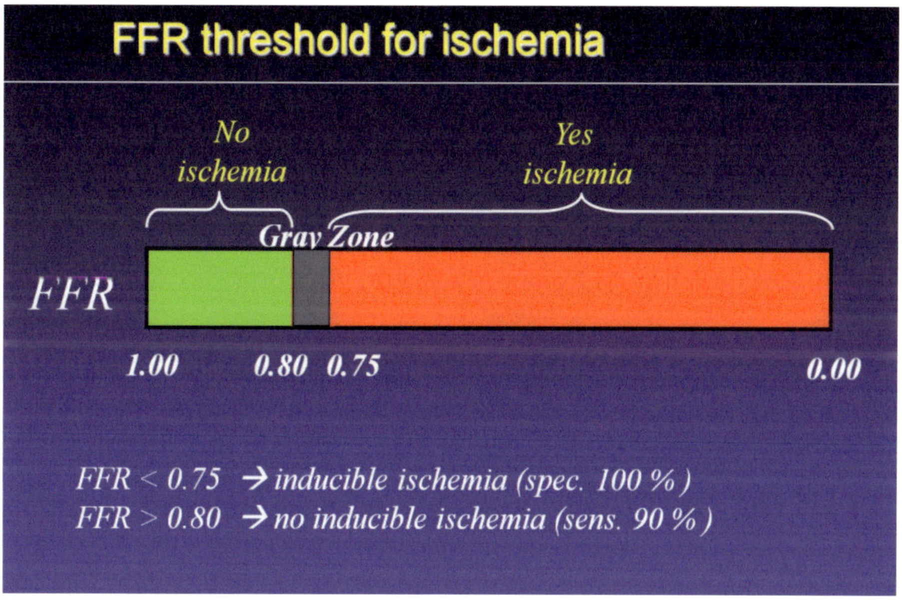

Fig. 2.

The Doppler Flow Wire **(FIG 3)** allows an invasive measurement of CFR and coronary flow speed at rest and during maximal blood flow. The Flow Wire is a floppy and flexible tipped wire, whose top carries a Doppler transducer to assess peak and mean flow speed within the vessels. Flow and flow speed are directly proportional, so it is possible to obtain a CFR estimation using the flow ratio. Doppler Flow Wire (DFW) and CFR are well related with other, already diffused techniques[6].

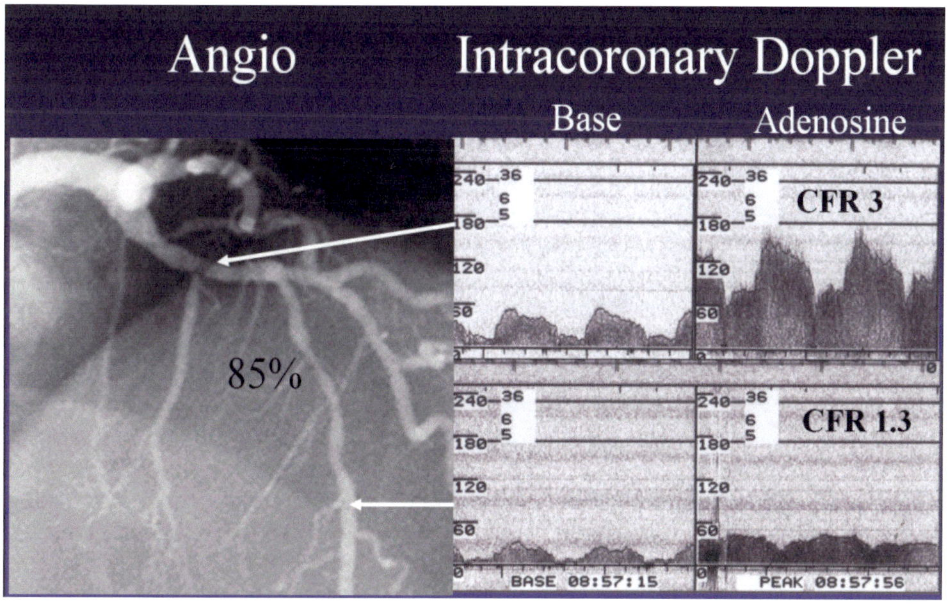

Fig. 3.

3. Echocardiography and CFR: from trans-esophageal to trans-thoracic approach

Non invasive techniques are attractive methods to quantify pathophysiology.

The assessment of coronary flow reserve with trans-thoracic doppler echocardiography **(FIG 4)**, measured as the ratio between hyperaemic and baseline coronary flow velocities, is a new tool for coronary artery disease and coronary microcirculation evaluation.

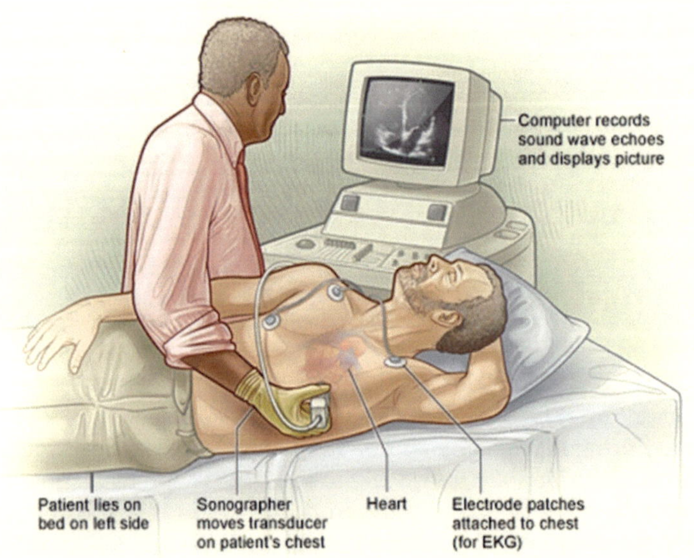

Fig. 4.

For the proximity of the heart to the thoracic wall and the wide spaces between the ribs, echocardiography always provided lots of useful information about cardiac morphology and functionality. The Trans-Esophageal Echocardiography (TEE) uses an even closer point of view on the heart **(FIG 5)** and then it expanded the diagnostic capabilities of echocardiography. This happened thanks to multi-planar, high frequency (7 MHz) transducers, capable of color Doppler and Pulsed Wave Doppler visualization of the coronary flow. The superior resolution and the lack of anatomical obstacles are the best advantages of this technique[7]: TEE allows the visualization of the ascending aorta and the first segments of the coronary arteries. There are Authors who documented the stenosis of the proximal part of the common trunk using TEE[8]. Anterior descending artery is almost parallel to the ultrasound beam, thus being ideal for a Doppler assessment: resting flow speeds are normal before to a stenosis, faster within the stenosis and significantly slower after it[7]. The most important information are provided by the TEE-CFR assessment with the intravenous administration of adenosine or dipyridamole[9]. This kind of evaluation is very easy to perform and its prognostic value, concerning the proximal segment of the anterior descending artery, is very high[10], allowing the common trunk cross-sectional area and the coronary flow measurement[11] **(FIG 6)**. The clinical usefulness of TEE-CFR is limited by an important factor: the difficulty, for the patient, to undergo such an invasive assessment. The evaluation of CFR in cases of distal coronary stenoses still remains impossible and this is another important limitation.

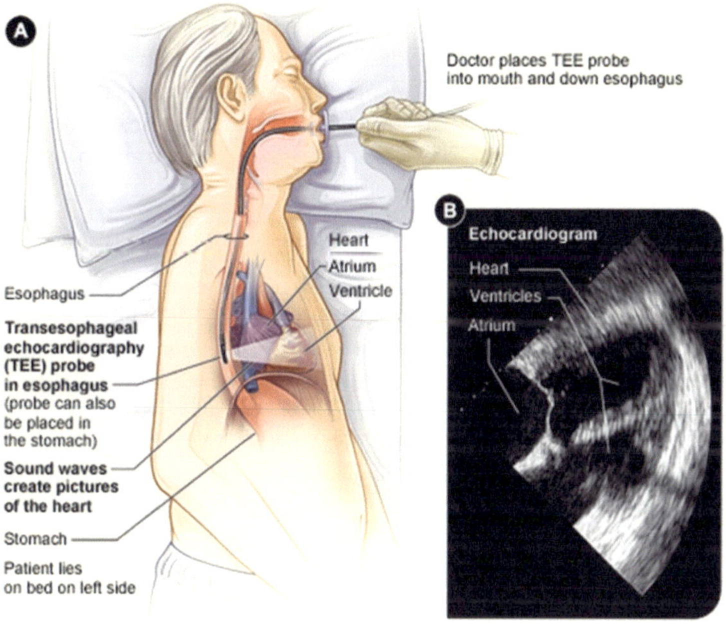
A
Doctor places TEE probe into mouth and down esophagus
Heart
Atrium
Ventricle
Esophagus
Transesophageal echocardiography (TEE) probe in esophagus
(probe can also be placed in the stomach)
Sound waves create pictures of the heart
Stomach
Patient lies on bed on left side
B
Echocardiogram
Heart
Ventricles
Atrium

Fig. 5.

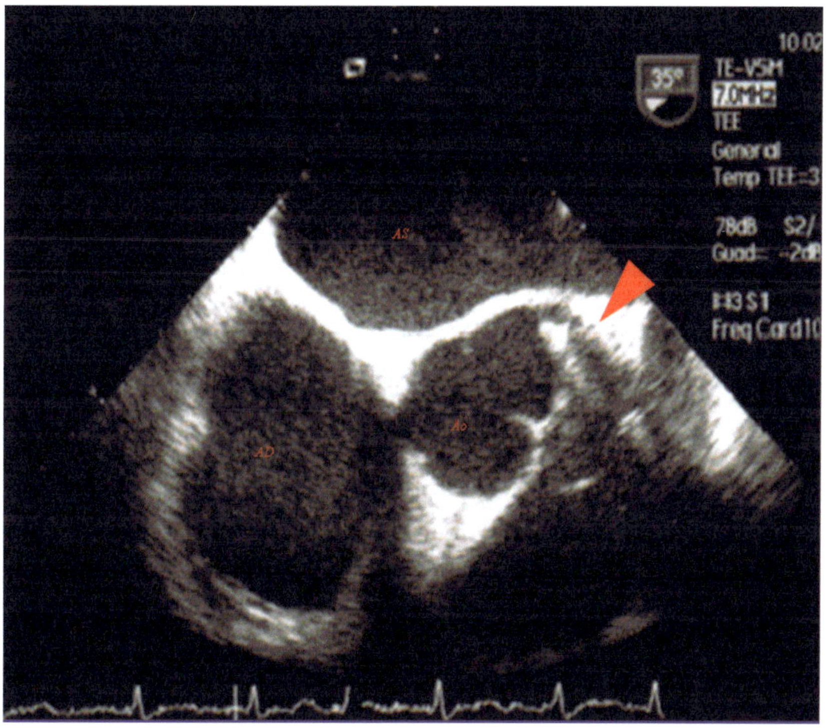
35°
TEE
General

Fig. 6.

Trans Thoracic Echocardiography (TTE), especially after the introduction of Tissue Harmonic Imaging (THI), made possible the evaluation of the coronary flow via pulsed-wave Doppler, color Doppler guided[12]. Anterior descending artery, in its intermediate and terminal parts is ideal for this kind of assessment: it is very close to the thoracic wall, while the circumflex branch of left coronary and posterior descending artery are less reachable by the ultrasonic beam **(FIG 7)**. The frames are acquired through an apical 2-chambers modified echocardiographic view, using the color-Doppler guidance to optimize the targeting of the vessel with the probe. The Doppler signal itself can be enhanced, if necessary, giving a contrast agent (e.g.: SonoVue, Levovist). In this specific projection a craniad tilting of the probe is requested: at first the operator must target the anterior interventricular groove, looking for the anterior descending artery, with the color-Doppler function active. Then, rotating the transducer counterclockwise and tilting it craniad, the requested point of view should be reached. All this procedure is ECG-gated **(FIG 8)**, being the images much sharper during the diastole; moreover, it is noticeable that the coronary blood flow is continuous and its diastolic part is wider than the systolic. The diastolic coronary flow speeds usually span the range 15 to 30 cm/sec. It's crucial to identify the internal mammary artery, which, for its close proximity to the anterior descending one, can be a confounding factor for the assessment: this is easily possible because for that artery there are no heartbeat movements and the systolic part of the flow is wider than the diastolic **(FIG 9)**. TTE-CFR assessment is made possible by a main factor: the easy sampling of anterior descending artery, both in resting and hyperemic conditions **(FIG 10)**. Each cardiac ultrasound unit is equipped with the right hardware to perform this kind of analysis, however, the operators must take care of some parameters: using low color Doppler rates (PRF 11-25 cm/sec); keeping a constant Doppler angle between the probe and

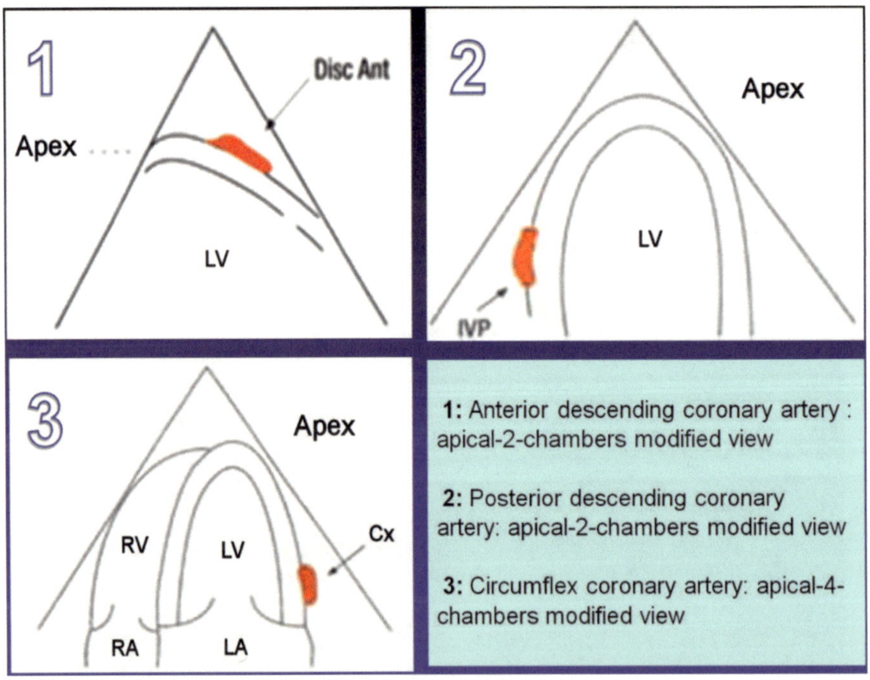

Fig. 7.

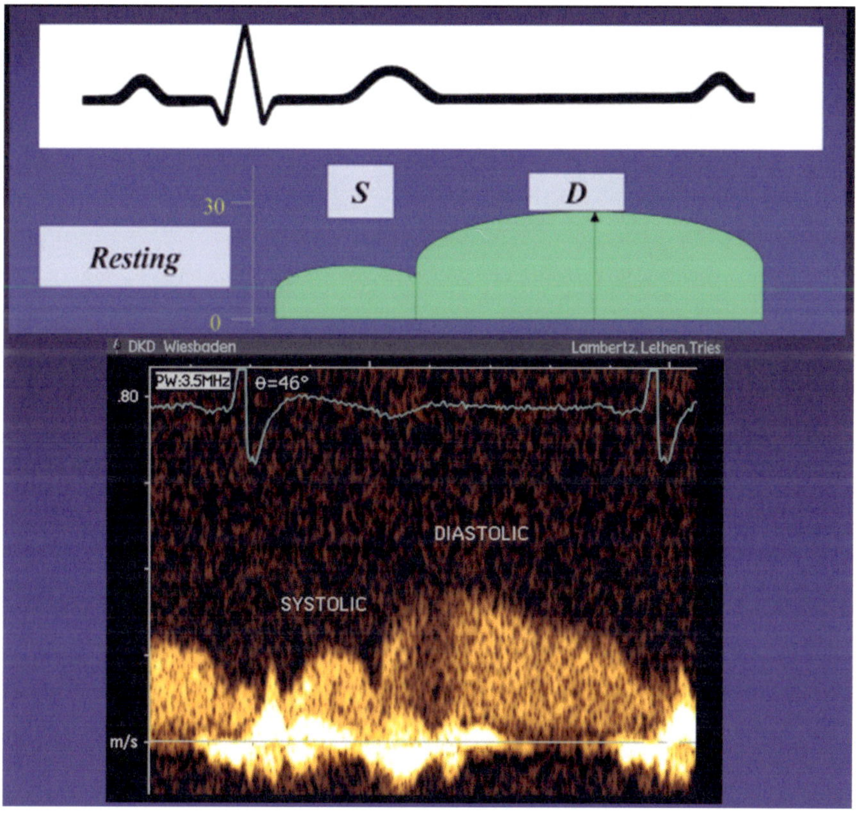
S
D
30
Resting
0
DKD Wiesbaden
Lambertz, Lethen, Tries
PW:3.5MHz
θ=46°
.80
DIASTOLIC
SYSTOLIC
m/s

Fig. 8.

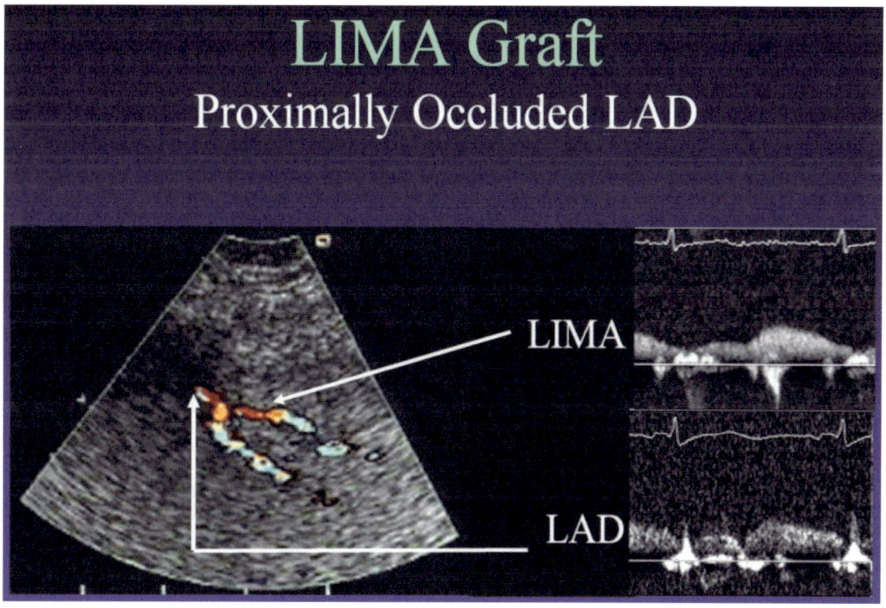
LIMA Graft
Proximally Occluded LAD
LIMA
LAD

Fig. 9.

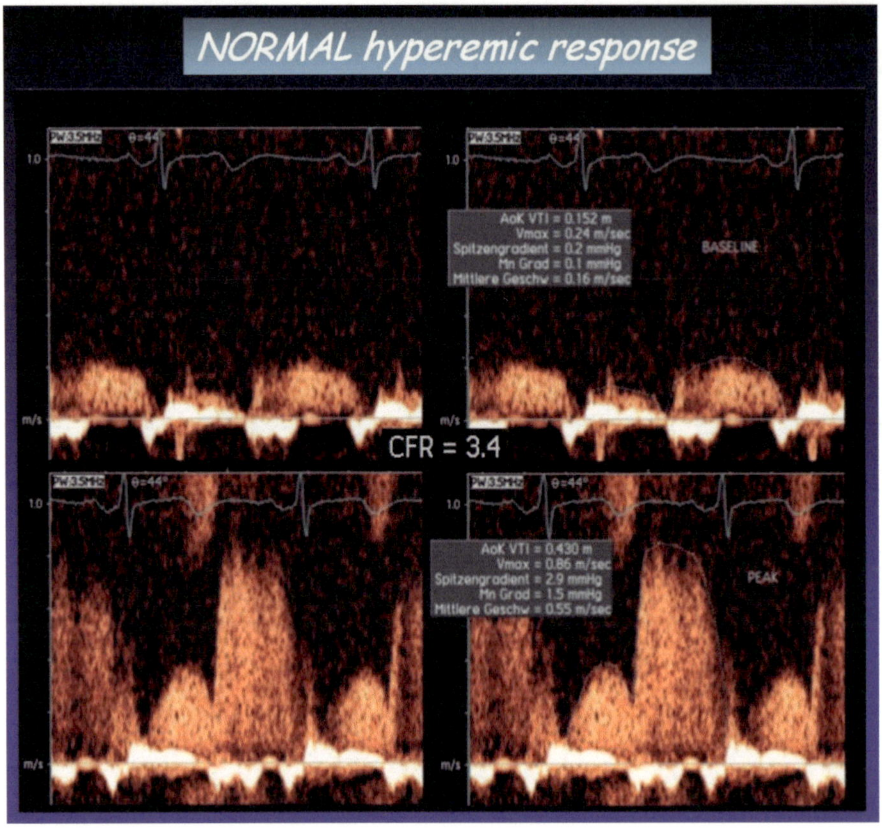

Fig. 10.

the observed flow for the duration of the exam in order to compare the baseline and the hyperemic Doppler patterns; using a pulsed-wave Doppler volume dimension wider than 2 mm, in order to overcome the sampling problems due to hyperventilation. TTE-CFR assessment feasibility is up to 98% and it is highly repeatable: for these reasons Doppler signal enhancement and contrast agents as well are not necessary. All collected data are strictly congruent with DFW. Using an apical, 2-chambers echocardiographic view is also possible to check the posterior interventricular artery: the feasibility of this examination is clearly worse, in this case, due to the over breathing induced by adenosine and for the use of common transducers (while for the anterior descending artery is already mandatory the use of dedicated probes). The overall feasibility of the TTE-CFR assessment is quite good in all the main epicardial coronary arteries: 98% for the anterior descending artery; 81% for the posterior interventricular one; 73% for the circumflex[13].

TTE-CFR assessment limitations: TTE-CFR has limited spatial resolution, making it impossible to evaluate the vessel cross-sectional area. According to some Authors'[14] opinion, a CFR estimation is not fully reliable, if only based on flow speed data collection, but the reality is that adenosine-induced diameter variation of epicardial coronary arteries is always less than 5%, which means there is no statistical significance in such values[15]. Like in each Doppler analysis, CFR assessment is angle-dependant and it's important that this angle should be >30°, to avoid an underestimation of the factors, and it must be kept constant before and after the hyperemic stimulation. The production of sampling artifacts is possible too: when a big marginal artery is mistaken for the anterior descending one; when the anterior descending artery is affected by a very distal stenosis, causing a CFR assessment which is exclusively based on a pre-stenotic data acquisition.

4. Stressors used in CFR assessment

There are various stressors used to induce myocardial ischemia and they all act these ways: the steal effect and the increased myocardial oxygen demand. The most commonly used stressors are drugs and non-pharmacologic stressors.

Non pharmacological stressors are: exercise, which is the most commonly used, and pacing. Exercise test echocardiography is the closest to every day conditions: coronary flow increases as the double product of heart rate and systolic blood pressure (HR x SBP), which is used as an estimate of myocardial work and is proportional to myocardial oxygen consumption.

The steal effect is caused by dipyridamole, while the increased myocardial oxygen demand is caused by the administration of dobutamine, by the pacing[16] and by transient coronary obstruction[17].

Drugs used to induce coronary vasodilation are: dipyridamole, adenosine and papaverine, being this last one, the least commonly used. Dipyridamole reduces myocardial oxygen demand acting on the A2 adrenergic receptors placed on the smooth muscle cells and on the endothelial cells: it causes a bad blood flow distribution, thus a "steal effect". The fact is that it also indirectly raises the adenosine concentration, limiting its re-uptake and consumption[18]. Dipyridamole must be given in an intravenous administration of 0.84 mg/Kg: in the *traditional protocol*[19] this happens in 10 minutes, divided in 2 infusions (0.56 mg/Kg over 4 minutes; 4 minutes of no dose and, if still negative, an additional 0.28 mg/Kg over 2 minutes) and eventually followed by the delivery of up to 1 mg of atropine in order to maximize the accuracy of the test. The sensitivity of the test increases using the *fast protocol*, that consists in the administration of a one-shot dose of 0.84 mg/Kg of dipyridamole in 6 minutes[20] **(FIG 11)**. This is useful to limit the duration of the test too. Wall Motion Score Index (WMSI) and anterior descending artery coronary flow are further parameters evaluable during CFR assessment with the fast protocol. Dipyridamole effects are quite long-lasting: up to 30 minutes and the peak effect can last up to 6-16. For this reason the main side effects of its use are hypotension, headache, nausea, flushing, then a fast administration of the right antidote, aminophylline[21], should be considered. Contraindications to dipyridamole use are: third degree atrio-ventricular block, sick sinus syndrome, asthma. No more adenosine must be administered in the 24 hours following a CFR assessment, for its long lasting blood concentration; during the 24 hours before the examination the patient must avoid the use of coffee or tea-based drinks in order to test the largest number of free adenosine receptors.

Adenosine acts through specific A2 inhibitor receptors located on the surface of smooth muscle cells and on the endothelium of epicardial coronary vessels. Its ischemia-inducing action is similar to dipyridamole, but for the direct and short-lasting effects (only a few seconds)[22]. Even side effects are the same, but really brief, in these cases and no aminophylline

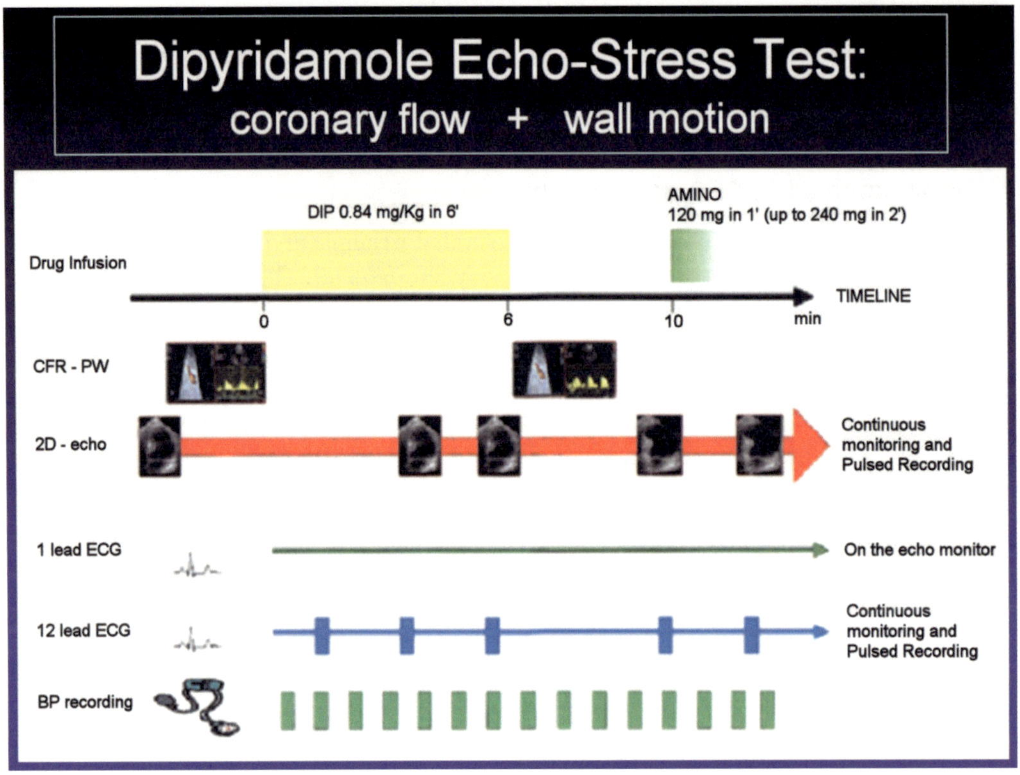

Fig. 11.

is usually required. In normal patients adenosine administration raises up to 4-5 times the coronary flow, just like high-dose dipyridamole[23], however always much more than after dobutamine or after stress exercise. Dipyridamole can be manually injected using a syringe, but for adenosine an infusion pump is necessary and the starting dose is 100 µg/Kg/min, slowing raising up to 200 µg/Kg/min. The final administration of atropine at the end of the test to reach the maximal heart rate, raises its sensitivity in these cases too. To evaluate the CFR via TTE a dose of 140 µg/Kg/min in an endovenous infusion of 5 minutes is ideal[24]: imaging is performed prior and after the starting of the injection. Even better, because significantly cheaper, is the IV injection of only 6 mg of drug in 10-15 seconds **(FIG 12)**. Adenosine test is always safe and reliable for the assessment of anterior descending artery stenoses[25].

Dobutamine is a sympathomimetic drug, directly acting on the β_1 adrenergic myocardial receptors increasing heart rate and contractility and also acting on the β_2 receptors on the epicardial coronary vessels, as a vasodilator[26]. Chronotropic and inotropic response to the dobutamine stimulation raises myocardial oxygen consumption, inducing ischemia: coronary flow increases 3 times the baseline value to face this condition. The drug is administered intravenously in incremental doses spanning the range 5 to 40 µg/Kg/min in repeated stages, each one lasting 3 minutes. If the maximal heart rate is not reached is possible a final administration of atropine. The feasibility of these tests is about 90%[27], being also possible a WMSI and a anterior descending artery flow assessment.

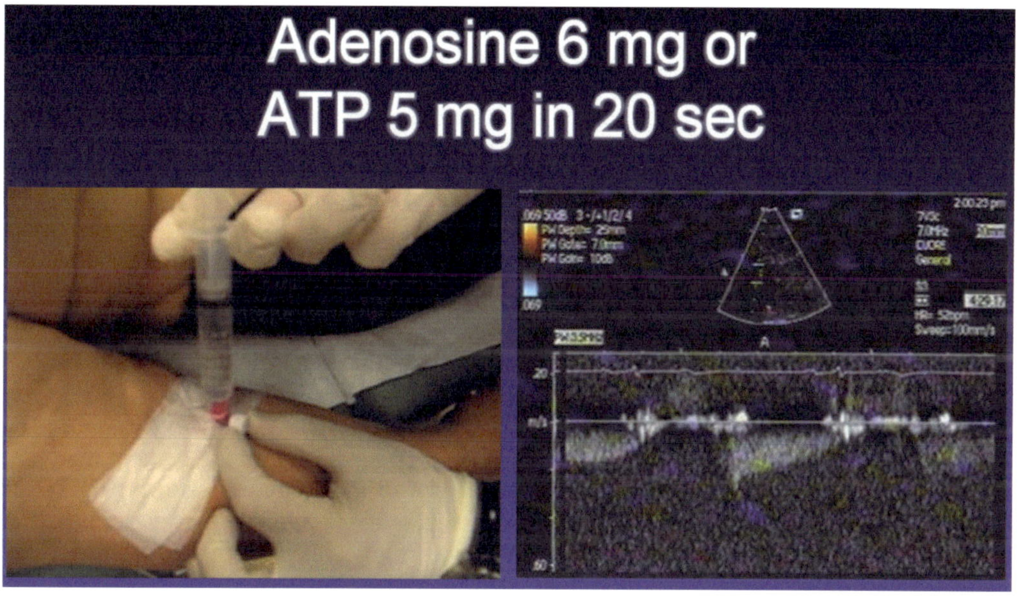

Fig. 12.

The most commonly used non-pharmacologic stressors are physical exercise, cardiac pacing and the Cold Pressure Test (CPT).

Exercise echocardiography can be performed using either a treadmill or a bicycle protocol: when using a treadmill, scanning during exercise is not feasible, so it's mandatory an immediate post-exercise imaging as soon as possible (<1 minute from cessation of exercise). Bicycle exercise is performed during either an upright or a recumbent posture: in every moment during the various levels of exercise the collection of data is possible. Physical exercise acts raising the heart rate, the blood pressure values and the inotropic state, then raising the myocardial oxygen consumption as well: as a consequence, the CFR values raise too, because the coronary flow is controlled by the oxygen demand. The stress CFR is easier to assess using nuclear medicine techniques, such as Single-Photon Emission Computed Tomography (SPECT) or PET, than using ultrasound due to hyperventilation and chest wall movements.

Cardiac pacing allows the induction of a controlled myocardial stress raising the heart rate, which is the main determinant of the oxygen demand. This result can be achieved via right atrium direct pacing during a catheterization procedure, via transesophageal atrial pacing or via atrial or ventricular noninvasive pacing exploiting the presence of a permanent pacemaker. External cardiac pacing requires the use of the standard echo-stress protocol: starting from 110 beats per minute, the heart rate should be increased by 10 beats every 3 minutes until the target heart rate is reached (85% of age-predicted maximal heart rate). The same goals can be achieved in an accelerated fashion, increasing the heart rate every 30 seconds[16]. A limiting factor is that several pacemakers cannot be programmed to reach the target heart rate. Echocardiographic image acquisition is performed at baseline conditions and throughout the test; the final data collection is made after 3 minutes of pacing at the highest heart rate or at the target heart rate. The diagnostic accuracy of this stress test is remarkable.

The CPT is based on an endothelial dependant response to a thermal stimulation. The exam is performed putting a patient's hand in the cold water for 2-3 minutes, inducing a reactive hyperemia. This vasodilator response is caused by endothelial NO release, due to an *a frigore* sympathetic nervous system activation. With the subsequent reduced NO bioavailability, α-adrenergic effects are no longer balanced and the ischemia prevails. The CPT assessed endothelial dysfunction is a good predictor of major cardiac events and is useful in prognostic stratification[28]. Nowadays normal reference ranges for CFR assessed via CPT still don't exist, so this test cannot be used to diagnose inducible ischemia yet[29].

5. Coronary Flow Reserve and epicardial coronary stenoses

Estimating the patients' coronary reserve allows to estimate the rate at which this reserve may disappear: as a direct consequence it become possible to pronounce a correct prognosis and to give a proper therapy, directed to increase this reserve, preventing or eliminating the stresses that might compromise it. Downstream to an epicardial coronary stenosis there is a pressure drop directly proportional to the obstruction itself. If the stenosis is little or moderate, the blood flow is maintained by the vasodilation activated as a reaction. For an hemodynamically significant stenosis, angina symptoms start to appear. Over 70% of stenosis the coronary flow reserve cannot increase over the factor of 2x, defined as the normality cutoff. 85-90% stenoses can reduce the coronary blood flow even at rest, because the adaptive capabilities of coronary flow are completely lost: this is why CFR assessment is important in order to identify the least important obstructions, being an estimation of the functionality of compensatory mechanisms **(FIG 13)**. The CFR dissolves for >90% obstructions. These data are true for isolated stenoses of a single vessel, without the involvement of microcirculation, nor side branches **(FIG 14)**. Many more confounding factors may arise: the main one is certainly the microcirculatory dysfunction. TTE-CFR can be used in clinical practice to collect data comparable with that from invasive tests[30]. CFR normality cutoff is >2. This technique samples the blood flow typically from the anterior

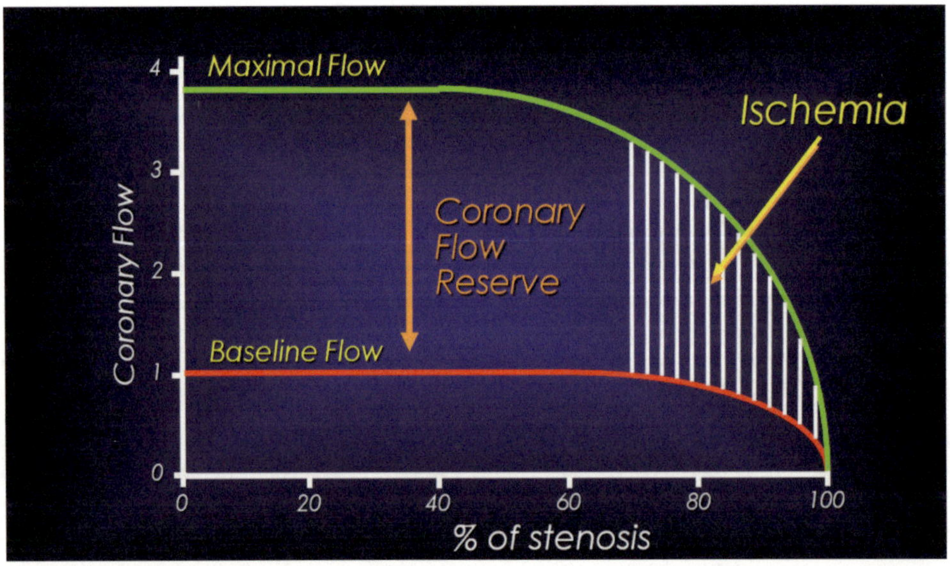

Fig. 13.

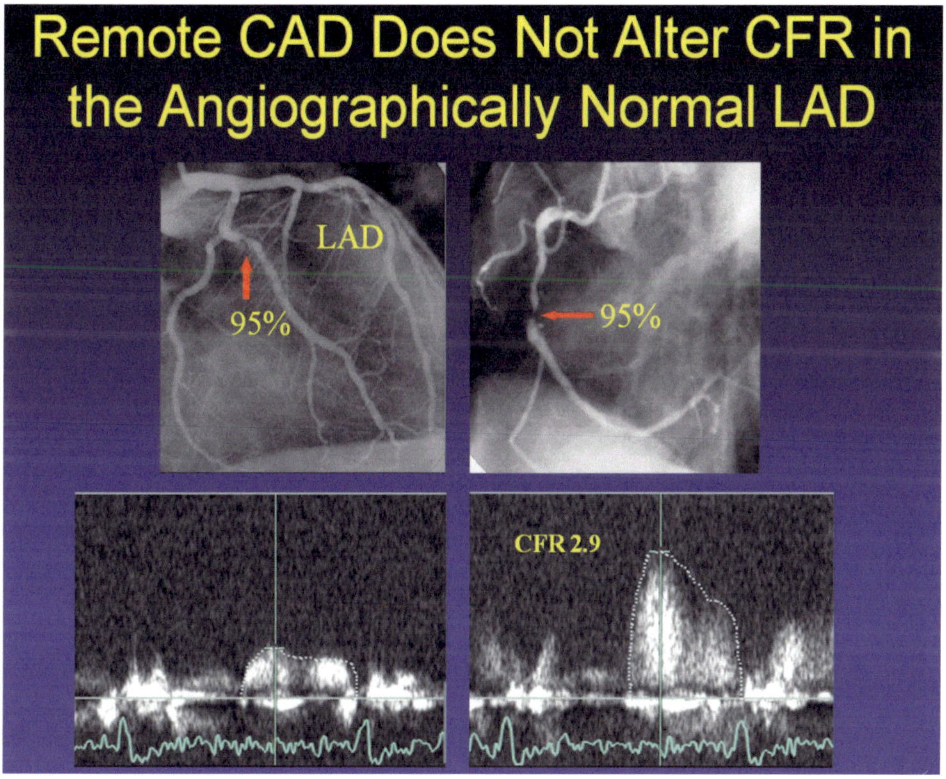

Fig. 14.

descending artery, neglecting microcirculatory conditions: for this reason it should be integrated in a classic pharmacologic echocardiographic stress test to evaluate the regional wall motion. Both tests can be conducted using the same pharmacological stressor: dipyridamole. The combined Wall motion and CFR assessment, then, adds more sensitivity without a significant loss of specificity to the echocardiographic stress examination **(FIG 15)**. Dipyridamole is a stressor drug particularly suitable for this use. A skilled operator can exploit another chance, assessing not only the anterior descending, but also the posterior descending and the circumflex arteries[31]. Performing the TTE-CFR assessment requires a skilled operator because of hyperventilation too: from 5 to 10 seconds after the administration of the pharmacological stressor the maximal hyperemia is observable and a significant hyperventilation occurs, making difficult to focus the ultrasonic beam on the assessed coronary artery. After all, without hyperventilation the test is not acceptable and the risk of an underestimation of CFR becomes very high (maybe because of the inadequate dose of drug or for a peculiar pool of cardiac receptors in the evaluated patient). Angiography may be unable to determine intermediate (40-70%) stenoses, revealing the need for a revascularization: a functional evaluation of the stenoses appears then crucial. Only the functionally significant stenoses, which are related to scintigraphically observable regional myocardial perfusion defects should be addressed to revascularization[32]. Moreover, CFR, if between 1.8 and 2.0, have a positive predictive value of 88-100% and a negative predictive value of 77-95% when there is a scintigraphically evident myocardial perfusion defect **(FIG 16)**. CFR, then, recovers very early, even in the next few hours after the

Diagnostic value of 2D Echo-Stress test and CFR

	Sensitivity	Specificity	Accuracy
Echo 2D	74%	91%	86%
CFR (cut-off=2)	89%	77%	81%
CFR (cut-off=1.9)	81%	84%	83%
CFR (cut-off=1.8)	69%	90%	83%
CFR (cut-off=1.7)	63%	97%	86%
CFR (cut-off=1.6)	50%	100%	85%
CFR (cut-off=1.5)	30%	100%	79%
2D Echo+CFR cutoff = 1.9	90%	94%	93%

Fig. 15.

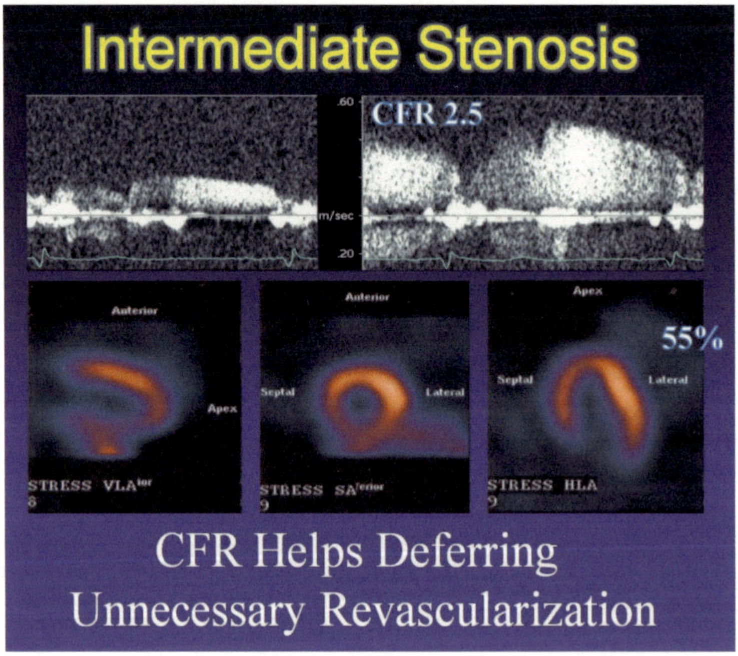

Fig. 16.

procedure if all epicardial coronary stenoses are treated. TTE-CFR is also useful to evaluate the outcomes of revascularization procedures after acute events: it's very important during the follow-up of a stenting procedure to assess the eventual in-stent restenosis with a sensitivity of 78% and a specificity of 93% for each restenosis[33] **(FIG 17)**. It should be remembered that post surgical procedures a flow competition from the native coronary artery can reduce the blood stream even without a bypass stenosis. In these cases the best choice is to perform the TTE-CFR directly on the native anterior descending artery[34] **(FIG 18)(FIG 19)**.

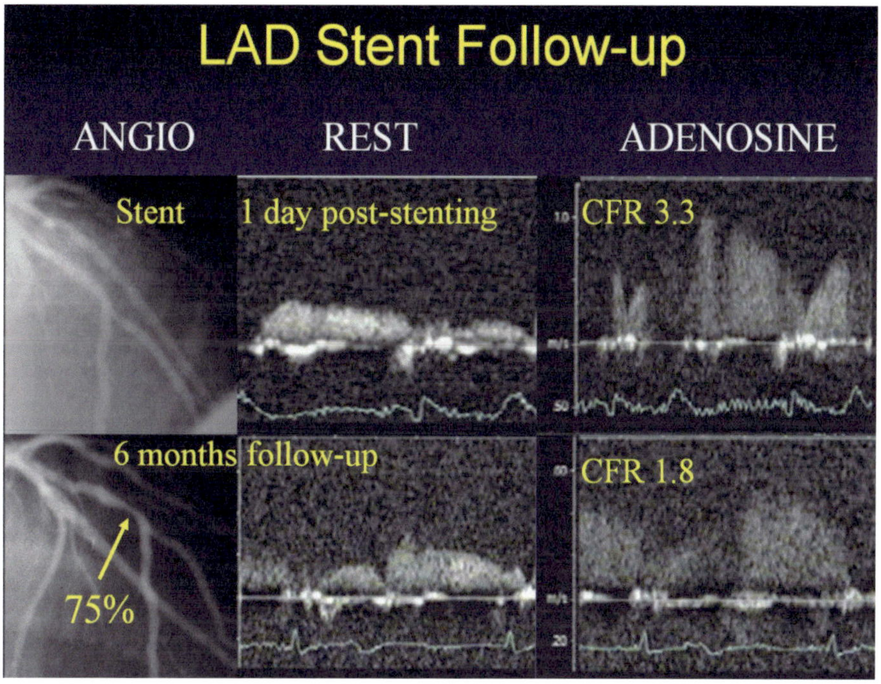
LAD Stent Follow-up
ANGIO
REST
ADENOSINE
Stent
1 day post-stenting
CFR 3.3
6 months follow-up
CFR 1.8
75%

Fig. 17.

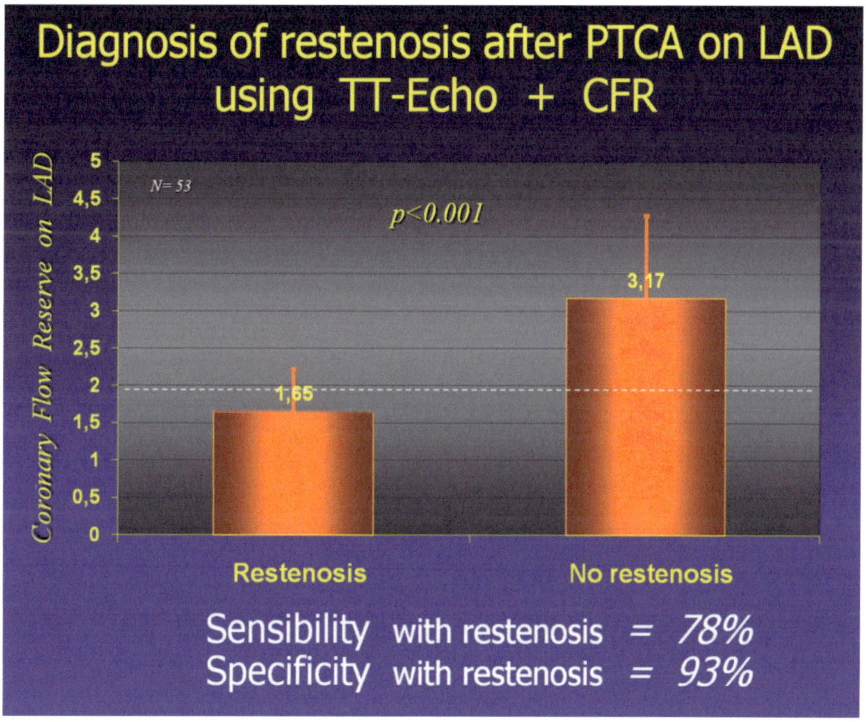
Diagnosis of restenosis after PTCA on LAD using TT-Echo + CFR
Coronary Flow Reserve on LAD
N= 53
p<0.001
1,65
3,17
Restenosis
No restenosis
Sensibility with restenosis = 78%
Specificity with restenosis = 93%

Fig. 18.

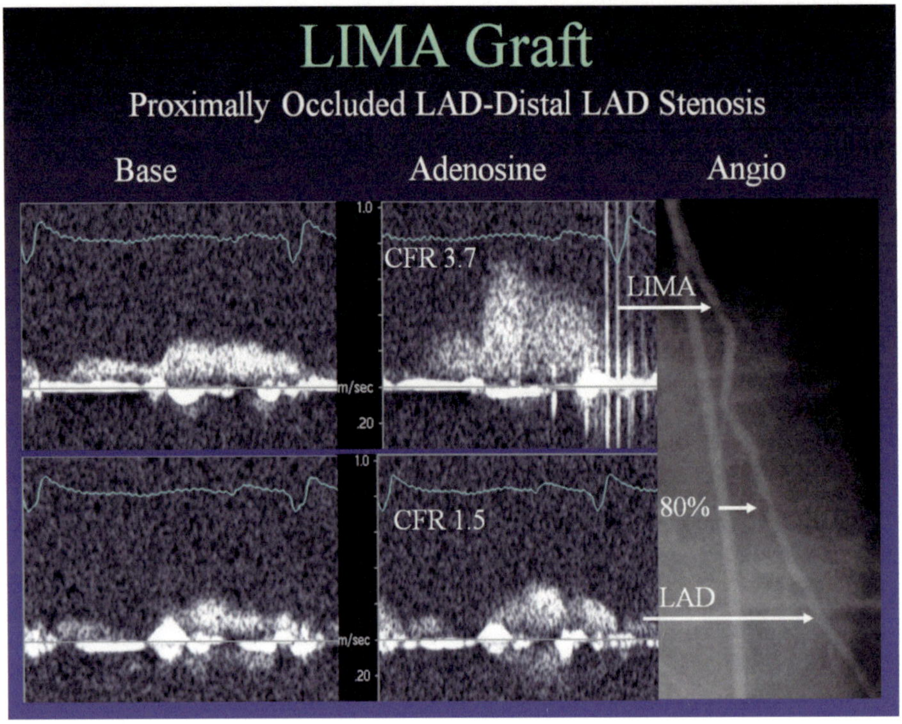

Fig. 19.

6. Coronary Flow Reserve and microcirculatory dysfunctions

High intraventricular pressure, determining compression on microcirculation, generates a CFR much greater in subepicardial layer, than in subendocardial. CFR, then, dissolves first in subendocardial layer, when problems occur[35] **(FIG 20)**. Whether an epicardial coronary stenosis is present or not, CFR reduction can be caused by any condition producing microcirculation impairment: for intrinsic (inflammations,, endothelial damages, etc.) or extrinsic reasons (extra-vascular compression). There are 3 main types of microvascular dysfunctions (MD):

- *MD with epicardial coronary obstruction:* atheromatous lesions are often related to microcirculation flow regulation impairment.
- *Inadequate revascularization:* after surgical or percutaneous revascularization procedures, tissue edema and increased blood levels of free radicals can greatly damage microcirculation functionality.
- *No angiographically significant lesions:* these are the cases of cardiac syndrome X (microvascular angina) or conditions related to several risk factors causing microvascular functionality damages, such as hypertension or diabetes mellitus.

A reduced TTE-CFR means microcirculation impairment only if the coronary angiography does not show any epicardial stenosis. Performing a TTE-CFR assessment combined with an echocardiographic stress test for the coronary flow estimation in the anterior descending artery and the regional wall motion study is possible to overcome such limitations. The resulting scenarios are[29]:

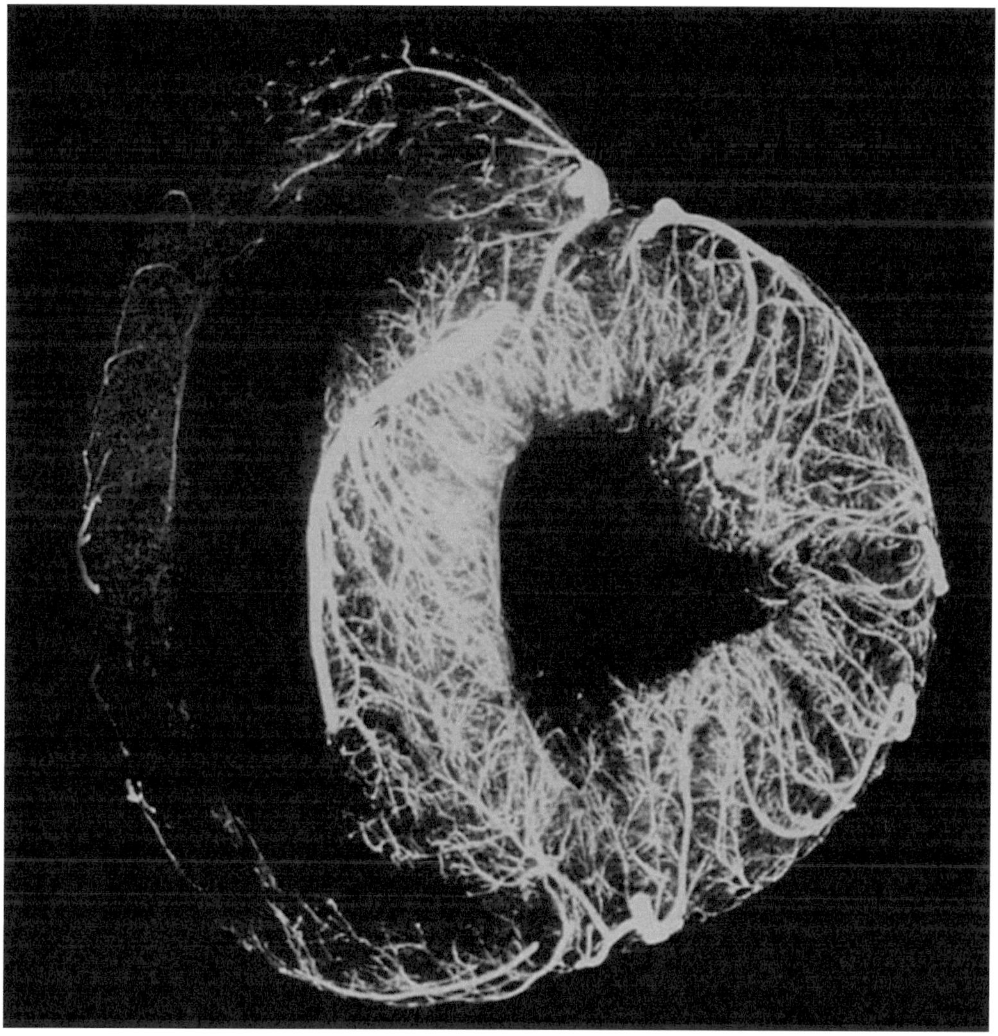

Fig. 20.

a. Normal TTE-CFR + Normal wall motion = no damage.
b. Reduced TTE-CFR + Impaired wall motion = epicardial coronary stenosis
c. Reduced TTE-CFR + Normal or increased wall motion = coronary microcirculation isolated dysfunction.
d. Normal TTE-CFR + impaired wall motion in locations far from the observed artery

In this last possibility, it's mandatory to perform TTE-CFR on right and circumflex coronary arteries too or to base any further decision only on the analysis of regional wall motion.

Microvascular dysfunction without angiographically assessed epicardial coronary stenoses knows various causes, such as hypertensive cardiomyopathy, diabetes mellitus, hypertrophic cardiomyopathy, idiopathic dilated cardiomyopathy, cardiac syndrome X. TTE-CFR reduction, in these conditions, is highly variable, but it may become wider than observed as an exclusive consequence of anterior descending artery stenoses[36]. Hypertensive cardiomyopathy is nowadays the most assessed in all these conditions, using TTE-CFR; many studies showed that coronary reserve is reduced even without a clear left ventricle hypertrophy: probably this happens because of microcirculatory remodeling[37]. Functional and morphological microcirculatory modifications are strictly joined and bioptic myocardial samples confirm this linkage. Endothelial dysfunction and extra-vascular compression are further possible causes. Concerning diabetes mellitus, especially for type 2, CFR reduction is insulin resistance[38] related, while hyperglycaemic concentrations play a background role. Microangiopathy in diabetes knows the same progression, both in coronary microcirculation and in retina[39]. CFR can be reduced in dilated cardiomyopathy, mostly for the ventricular shear stress, which characterises this condition[40]. Cardiac syndrome X may reduce CFR just like observable in epicardial coronary stenoses[41]: stress tests induce angina pectoris, ST segment depression and scintigraphically relevant myocardial perfusion defects. TTE-CFR test effectiveness and wall motion analysis (echographic stress test using the fast protocol of dipyridamole injection) are maximized if also a coronarographic assessment is performed as a cross-check for the presence of epicardial coronary stenoses. After a revascularization procedure, microcirculatory conditions are crucially important: many studies showed that microvascular damage after acute myocardial infarction reaches its peak 48 hours after reperfusion[42]. Then, performing a CFR assessment after that peak time, provides important information on the microcirculatory damage and is a predictor of left ventricle functional recovery. In Myocardial Contrast Echocardiography (MCE) the non-reflow extent, which is greater in patients with a reduced TTE-CFR (<2.5) than observable in patient with normal TTE-CFR (>2.5) and during the follow-up, the highest TTE-CFR values are related to the functional recovery, well indicated by the WMSI[43]. The CFR assessment does not help in differentiating microcirculatory dysfunction and epiacrdial stenoses when both problems are present, but in one case: in patients who underwent heart transplantation. TTE-CFR provides useful information on microcirculation and on the Cardiac Allograft Vasculopathy (CAV), a condition implying both epicardial coronary and microvasculation disease[44]. Angiograpghy usually underestimate the seriousness of the problem[44] and the Intravascular Ultrasound (IVUS) is the (invasive) gold standard examination to perform[45]. This is a micro- and macrovascular kind of damage and a reduced TTE-CFR allows a diagnosis of CAV if <2.7 (sensitivity 87%, specificity 82%)[46].

7. References

[1] Hozumi T, Yoshida K, Akasaka T, et al. "Noninvasive assessment of coronary flow velocity and coronary flow velocity reserve in the left anterior descending coronary artery by Doppler echocardiography: comparison with invasive technique". J Am Coll Cardiol 1998; 32: 1251-1260.

[2] Beanlands RS, Muzik O, Melon P, et al. "Noninvasive quantification of regional myocardial flow reserve in patients with coronary atherosclerosis using nitrogen-13 ammonia positron emission tomography. Determination of extent of altered vascular reactivity". J Am Coll Cardiol 1995; 26: 1465-1475.

[3] Barbato A, Arnadouse W, Aengevaeren GW, et al. "Validation of coronary flow reserve measurement by thermodiluition in clinical practice" Eur Heart J 2004; 25:219-223.

[4] De Bruyne B, Baudhuin T, Melin JA, et al. "Coronary flow reserve calculated from pressure measurement in humans. Validation with Positron Emission Tomography". Circulation 1994; 89: 1013-1022.

[5] Fearon WP, Balsam LB, Farouque HM, et al. "Novel index for invasively assessing the coronary microcirculation". Circulation 2003; 107: 3129-3132.

[6] Wilson RF, Laughlin DE, Ackell PH, et al. "Transluminal subselective measurement of coronary artery blood flow velocity and vasodilator reserve in humans". Circulation 1985; 72: 82-92.

[7] Youn HJ & Forster E. "Transesophageal echocardiography (TEE) in the evaluation of the coronary arteries". Cardiol Clin 2000; 18: 833-848.

[8] Yamagishi M, Yasu T, Ohara K, et al. "Detection of coronary blood flow associated with main left coronary artery stenosis by transesophageal Doppler color flowechocardiography". J Am Coll Cardiol 1991; 17: 87-93.

[9] Iliceto S, Marangelli V, Memmola C, et al. "Transesophageal Doppler echocardiography evaluation of coronary blood flow velocity in baseline conditions and during dipyridamole-induced coronary vasodilation". Circulation 1991; 83: 61-69.

[10] Redberg RF, Sobol Y, Chou TM, et al. "Adenosine-induced coronary vasodilation during transesophageal Doppler echocardiography. Rapid and safe measurement of coronary flow reserve ratio can predict significant left anterior descending stenosis". Circulation 1995; 92: 190-196.

[11] Paraskevaidis IA, Tsiapras D, Karavolias GK, et al. "Serial evaluation of coronary flow reserve by transesophageal Doppler Echocardiography after angioplasty of proximal left anterior descending left coronary artery: a 6-month follow-up study". Coron Artery Dis 2001; 12: 45-52.

[12] de Simone L, Caso P, Severino S, et al. "Reduction of coronary flow reserve non invasively determined by transthoracic Doppler echocardiography as a predictor of left anterior descending coronary artery stenosis". It Heart J 2000; 1: 234-239.

[13] Murata E, Hozumi T, Matsumura Y, et al. "Coronary flow velocity reserve measurement in three major coronary arteries using transthoracic Doppler echocardiography" Echocardiography 2006; 23: 279-286.

[14] Kaufmann PA, Jenni R. "Coronary flow reserve assessment from average peak velocity profiles alone must be judged with caution". J Am Coll Cardiol 2000; .35: 1363-1364.

[15] Reis ES, Holubkov R, Lee JS, et al. "Coronaty flow velocity response to adenosine characterizes coronary microvascular function in women with chest pain and no obstructive coronary artery disease". J Am Coll Cardiol. 1999; 33: 1469-1475.
[16] Gilgorova S, Agrusta M. "Pacing stress echocardiography". Cardiovasc Ultrasound 2005; 3: 36.
[17] Marcus M, Wright C, Doty D, et al. "Measurement of coronary velocity and reactive hyperemia in the coronary circulation in humans" Circ Res 1981; 49: 877-891.
[18] Picano E. "Stress echocardiography". Springer-Verlag, Heidelberg (Germany) 2003 (4th Edition).
[19] Picano E, Lattanzi F, Masini M, et al. "High dose dipyridamole echocardiography test in effort angina pectoris". J Am Coll Cardiol 1986; 8: 848-854.
[20] Dal Porto R, Faletra F, Picano E, et al. "Safety, feasibility and diagnostic accuracy of accelerated high-dose dipyridamole stress echocardiography". Am J Cardiol 2001; 87: 520-524.
[21] Dimitrow PP, Galderisi M, Rigo F. "The noninvasive documentation of coronary macrocirculation impairment: role of transthoracic echocardiography". Cardiovasc Ultrasound 2005; 3: 184.
[22] Iskandrian AS, Verani MS, Heo J. "Pharmacologic stress testing: mechanism of action, hemodynamic responses and results in detection of coronary artery disease". J Nucl Cardiol 1994; 1: 94-111.
[23] Rossen JD, Quillen JE, Lopez AG, et al. "Comparison of coronary vasodilation with intravenous dipyridamole and adenosine". J Am Coll Cardiol 1991; 18: 485-491.
[24] Caiati C, Montaldo C, Zedda N, et al. "Validation of a new, noninvasive method (contrast-enhanced transthoracic second Harmonic echo Doppler) for the evaluation of coronary flow reserve: comparison with intracoronary Doppler flow wire". J Am Coll Cardiol 1999; 34: 1193-1200.
[25] Voci P, Pizzuto F, Mariano E, et al. "Usefullness of coronary flow reserve measured by transthoracic coronary Doppler ultrasound to detect severe left anterior descending coronary artery stenosis". Am J Cardiol 2003; 92: 1320-1324.
[26] Warltier DC, Zyvoloski M, Gross GJ, et al. "redistribution of myocardial blood flow distal to a dynamic coronary arterial stenosis by sympathomimetic amines: comparison of dopamine, dobutamine and isoproterenol". Am J Cardiol 1981; 48: 269-279.
[27] Takeuchi M, miyazaki C, Yoshitani H, et al. "Assessment of coronary flow velocity with transthoracic Doppler echocardiography during dobutamine stress echocardiography". J Am Coll Cardiol 2001; 38: 117-123.
[28] Schächinger V, Britten MB, Zeiher AM, et al. "Prognostic impact of coronary vasodilator dysfunction on adverse long-term outcome of coronary heart disease". Circulation 2000; 101: 1899-1906.
[29] Galderisi M, D'Errico A. "Beta-blockers and coronary flow reserve: the importance of a vasodilatory action". Drugs 2008; 68: 579-590.
[30] Daimon M, Watanabe H, Yamagishi H, et al. "Physiologic assessment of coronary artery stenosis by coronary flow reserve measurements with transthoracic Doppler

echocardiography: comparison with exercise thallium-201 single-photon emission computed tomography. J Am Coll Cardiol 2001; 37: 1310-1315.

[31] Krzanowski M, Bodzon W, Dimitrow PP. "Imaging of all three coronary arteries by transthoracic echocardiography. An illustrated guide". Cardiovascular Ultrasound 2003, 1.

[32] Chamuleau SA, Tio RA, de Cock CC, et al. "Prognostic value of coronary blood flow velocity and myocardial perfusion in intermediate coronary narrowings and multivessel disease". J Am Coll Cardiol 2002; 39: 852-858.

[33] Ruscazio M, Montisci R, Colonna P, et al. "Detection of coronary restenosis after coronary angioplasty by contrast-enhanced transthoracic echocardiographic Doppler assessment of coronary flow velocity reserve". J Am Coll Cardiol 2002; 40: 896-903.

[34] Pizzuto F, Voci P, Mariano E, et al. "Evaluation of flow in the left anterior descending coronary artery but not in the left internal mammary artery graft predicts significant stenosis of the arterial conduit". J Am Coll Cardiol 2005; 45: 424-432.

[35] Dimitrow PP, Galderisi M, Rigo F. "The non-invasive documentation of coronary microcirculation impairment: role of transthoracic echocardiography". Cardiovasc Ultrasound 2005; 3: 184.

[36] Rigo F, Gherardi S, Galderisi M, Cortigiani L. "Coronary flow reserve evaluation in stress-echocardiography laboratory". J Cardiovasc Med 2006; 7: 472-479.

[37] Kozakova M, Galletta F, Gregorini L, et al. "Coronary vasodilator capacity and epicardial vessel remodeling in physiological and hypertensive hypertrophy". Hypertension 2000; 36: 343-349.

[38] Quinones MJ, Hernandez Pampaloni M, Schelbert H, et al. "Coronary vasomotor abnormalities in insulin-resistant individuals". Ann Intern Med 2004; 140: 700-708.

[39] Pop-Busui R, Kirkwood I, Schmid H, et al. "Sympathetic dysfunction in type I diabetes: association with impaired myocardial blood flow reserve and diastolic dysfunction". J Am Coll Cardiol 2004; 44: 2368-2374.

[40] Vanderheyden M, Bartunek J, Verstreken S, et al. "Non-invasive assessment of coronary flow reserve in idiopathic dilated cardiomyopathy: hemodynamic correlations". Eur J Echocardiogr 2005; 6: 47-53.

[41] Crea F, Lanza GA. "Angina pectoris and normal coronary arteries: cardiac Syndrome X". Heart 2004; 90: 457-463.

[42] Rochitte CE, Lima JA, Bluemke DA, et al. "Magnitude and time course of microvascular obstruction and tissue injury after acute myocardial infarction". Circulation 1998; 98: 1006-1014.

[43] Montisci R, Chen L, Ruscazio M, et al. "Noninvasive coronary flow reserve is correlated with microvascular integrity and myocardial viability after primary angioplasty in acute myocardial infarction". Heart 2006; 92: 1113-1118.

[44] Caforio AL, Tona F, Fortina AB, et al. "Immune and nonimmune predictors of cardiac allograft vasculopathy onset and severity: multivariate risk factor analysis and role of immunosuppression". Am J Transplant 2004; 4: 962-970.

[45] Rickenbacher PR, Pinto FJ, Lewis NP, et al. "Prognostic importance of intimal thickness as measured by intracoronary ultrasound after cardiac transplantation". Circulation 1995; 92: 3445-3552.

[46] Tona F, Caforio AL, Montisci R, et al. "Coronary flow reserve by contrast-enhanced echocardiography: a new noninvasive diagnostic tool for cardiac allograft vasculopathy". Am J Transplant 2006; 6 (5 Pt 1): 998-1003.

4

Coronary Microvascular Dysfunction in CAD: Consequences and Potential Therapeutic Applications

Alan N. Beneze[1], Jeffrey M. Gold[4] and Betsy B. Dokken[1,2,3]

[1]*University of Arizona College of Medicine*

[2]*University of Arizona Department of Medicine, Section of Endocrinology*

[3]*University of Arizona Sarver Heart Center*

[4]*Inpatient Physicians Consultants, Tucson, Arizona*

USA

1. Introduction

Substantial research and clinical effort has been directed toward the understanding, identification and management of coronary artery disease (CAD). As a result, the processes of cholesterol accumulation and inflammation that lead to large vessel occlusions have been fully elucidated. In contrast to those with CAD, many patients have symptoms of angina and reductions in coronary flow reserve despite normal coronary angiography of the large epicardial arteries. In this situation the vessels that limit flow to myocardium are the more distal epicardial prearterioles and intramyocardial arterioles – vessels typically too small to be directly visualized by conventional coronary angiography. These vessels comprise the coronary microcirculation. Coronary microvascular dysfunction (CMVD), in contrast to CAD, continues to be poorly understood and difficult to manage. In addition, the presence of CMVD can be a confounding factor in the management of patients with CAD.

2. Anatomy and physiology of the coronary microcirculation

The coronary arterial network is generally divided into three sequential morphological zones. The large epicardial coronary arteries decrease in diameter from 2-5 to 500 microns as they branch off of the aorta and travel distally along the epicardium. Distal to the large coronary arteries are epicardial pre-arterioles that decrease in diameter from 500 to 100 microns. Finally, the pre-arterioles give rise to intramyocardial arterioles that measure 100 microns or less in diameter. Coronary arterioles and pre-arterioles dilate and constrict in large part through feedback mechanisms in order to maintain a constant blood flow shear stress across the interior surface of the vessels (Camici & Crea, 2007).

Blood flow shear stress is the average laminar force per unit of cross sectional area of the vessel surface, applied parallel to the vessel wall. The interior surfaces of all blood vessels are lined with endothelial cells. Endothelial cells detect changes in blood flow shear stress and respond with signals to the surrounding smooth muscle cells to either relax in response to an increase in shear stress or contract in response to a decrease in shear stress. It remains unclear exactly how endothelial cells are able to detect and respond to these fluctuations in shear stress. Some studies have identified the protein caveolin-1 (CAV-1, which forms caveolae) as a receptor in this process (Traub & Berk, 1998). Other evidence suggests that endothelial cells respond to an increase in shear stress by activating endothelial nitric oxide synthase (eNOS) which in turn catalyzes the production and release of nitric oxide (NO), a potent vasodilator (Traub & Berk, 1998). The roles of CAV-1 and of eNOS are examples of many different pathways involved in the process of arteriolar dilatation. Arterioles (500 microns or less) located deep within the myocardium are exposed to a complex milieu of hormones and cytokines, some of which also perform roles essential to the fine auto-regulation of vasoconstriction and vasodilatation.

Normal function of the microcirculation is dependent on the production and bioavailability of nitric oxide (NO) (Traub & Berk, 1998). NO is produced in the endothelium by nitric oxide synthase (NOS). There are three isoforms of NOS; endothelial NOS (eNOS), inducible NOS (iNOS) and neuronal NOS (nNOS). NOS converts L-arginine into nitric oxide (NO), which diffuses into surrounding vascular smooth muscle cells (VSMC) and induces relaxation. Relaxation of VSMC is caused by the binding of NO to guanylyl cyclase and subsequent activation of the enzyme. Guanylyl cyclase catalyzes the dephosphorylation of GTP to produce cGMP, which is a second messenger for many cellular functions. Cyclic GMP induces smooth muscle relaxation by suppressing intracellular entry of calcium through voltage-gated calcium channels, by activating (via phosphorylation) ATP-dependent potassium channels, or by activating the enzyme myosin light chain phosphatase, which dephosphorylates myosin light chains and relaxes smooth muscle (Traub & Berk, 1998). Subsequently, vasodilation occurs and blood flow is increased. The bioavailability of NO is critical to normal vascular function.

3. Clinical presentation of coronary microvascular dysfunction

In addition to occlusion of a coronary artery, myocardial ischemia may be caused by resistance to coronary blood flow related to increased vascular tone. In the healthy individual, epicardial coronary arteries contribute minimal resistance to blood flow as long as they are free of occlusive disease (Maseri, Beltrame, & Shimokawa, 2009). The pre-arterioles contribute about 20% of the total resistance to blood flow (Maseri et al., 2009), and the remainder of the coronary microcirculation collectively accounts for 60%-80% of the total resistance to blood flow (John F. Beltrame, Crea, & Camici, 2009). Dysfunction of a single arteriole would not affect overall cardiac function. However, an abnormal increase in resistance to blood flow through an entire network of coronary arterioles could cause ischemia in a large segment of myocardium. In some cases, coronary microvascular dysfunction can cause ischemia to a similar degree as that caused by large epicardial coronary artery occlusions. Indeed, up to 30% of patients who present with angina and myocardial infarction have patent epicardial coronary arteries at the time of cardiac catheterization (Romeo, Rosano, Martuscelli, Lombardo, & Valente, 1993; Vesely & Dilsizian). In some cases, cardiac angiography is able to detect a "slow blood flow phenomenon" based on delayed opacification of the microcirculation (J. F. Beltrame, Limaye, & Horowitz, 2002; Tambe, Zimmerma.Ha, Demany, & Mascaren.E, 1972), but in general the use of cardiac angiography is limited to the observation of only those vessels that are 500 microns or larger in size (Vesely & Dilsizian). Most studies suggest that coronary microvascular dysfunction (CMVD) remains stable over time and is associated with a good overall prognosis in the majority of cases. Nonetheless, as many as 20-30% of patients with CMVD develop progressive symptoms of angina, sustain acute myocardial infarctions, and demonstrate reductions in cardiac function (G. A. Lanza & Crea, 2010). Some markers of ischemia in such patients include increased levels of plasma lactate and lipid peroxidase (both byproducts of anaerobic glucose metabolism), decreased oxygen saturation within the coronary sinus, and a shift in myocardial phosphate utilization on magnetic resonance spectroscopy (G. A. Lanza & Crea, 2010).

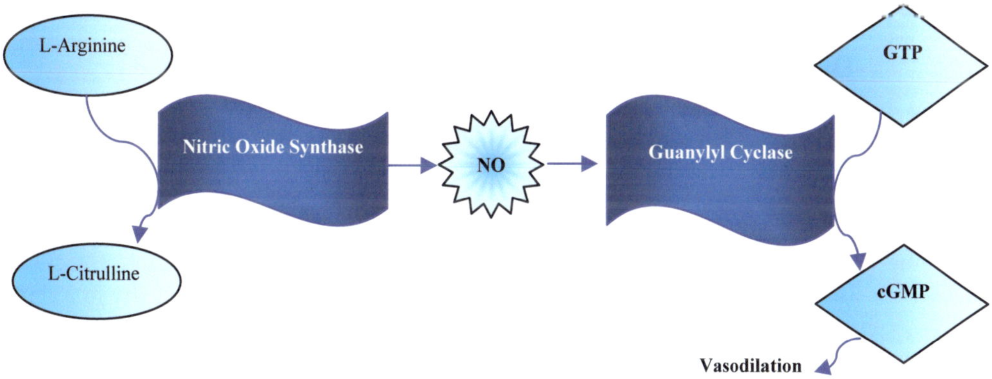

Fig. 1. Nitric oxide (NO) is produced in endothelial cells using L-arginine as a substrate. NO diffuses readily across plasma membranes to vascular smooth muscle cells. The synthesis of cyclic guanylyl monophosphate (cGMP) from guanylyl triphosphate (GTP) causes relaxation of vascular smooth muscle, and subsequent vasodilation.

4. Classification of coronary microvascular dysfunction

There are several broad categories of CMVD (Camici & Crea, 2007). The first category is classified as CMVD in the absence of obstructive large vessel CAD, based on the macroscopic findings at the time of coronary catheterization. The second category of microvascular dysfunction is defined as CMVD in the presence of cardiomyopathy. The third category is classified as CMVD in the presence of obstructive large vessel CAD. Clearly, in this subtype, the cardiac risk factors that induce the formation of occlusive disease within the large epicardial coronary arteries may also negatively impact blood flow through the small coronary arterioles.

The fourth category is classified as iatrogenic coronary microvascular dysfunction. This type of CMVD refers to the paradoxical "no re-flow phenomenon" associated with reperfusion injury. This occurs in the microcirculation, downstream of arteries recently made patent by thrombolysis, percutaneous angioplasty, stenting, or bypass grafting. This "no re-flow phenomenon" is identified based on persistent low blood flow (according to the TIMI flow scale (Antman et al., 1999)) after successful revascularization procedures. TIMI is an acronym for "thrombolysis in myocardial infarction" (Antman et al., 1999), and the flow scale measures the amount of time it takes (in seconds) for contrast dye to fill the length of a coronary artery during angiography (Camici & Crea, 2007).

One mechanism of reperfusion injury is distal embolization of plaque and thrombin in the small arterioles. Increased adrenergic tone following an acute cardiac event could cause vasoconstriction in the coronary microcirculation. However, in some cases, microvascular blood flow deficits have been measured in small vessels remote from the region of the infarct and revascularization (Gregorini et al., 1999), which are not explained by "no-reflow" or adrenergic stimulation. Moreover, microvascular reperfusion abnormalities can persist for as long as 3-6 months following the revascularization (John F. Beltrame et al., 2009). Myocardial ischemia initially causes a decrease in the level of intracellular ATP, a change from aerobic to anaerobic metabolism, a buildup of toxic byproducts of anaerobic metabolism, and a decrease in the pH. The restoration of oxygenated blood flow to recently ischemic tissue induces a cascade of toxic events. Some of these events might include, but are not limited to, abnormal leukocyte or platelet aggregation, complement activation, osmotic overloading of the mitochondria, and subsequent dysfunction of the microcirculation.

5. Cardiac Syndrome X

"Syndrome X" is the label used to describe an additional clinical phenomenon associated with CMVD. The label "syndrome X" typically refers to the presence of all of the following characteristics: angina or angina-like chest pain with exertion; ST- segment abnormalities during cardiac stress testing; absence of cardiac wall motion abnormalities during stress testing; and normal and patent coronary arteries without coronary artery vasospasm during cardiac catheterization (Bellamy et al., 1998). Therefore, "syndrome X" is a clustering of clinical signs and symptoms that indicate myocardial ischemia on exertion in the absence of evident coronary artery disease.

Most available evidence points to CMVD as the pathology responsible for "syndrome X". Zeiher et al (1995) found a suboptimal increase in coronary blood flow (CBF) in response to the endothelium-dependent vasodilator acetylcholine compared with an optimal increase in CBF in response to the endothelium-independent vasodilator papaverine, in patients with "syndrome X" (Zeiher, Krause, Schachinger, Minners, & Moser, 1995). In addition, a subsequent study of patients with "syndrome X" showed similar suboptimal CBF response to both endothelium-dependent and endothelium-independent vasodilators (Chauhan, Mullins, Taylor, Petch, & Schofield, 1997).

The central nervous system (CNS) has also been implicated in the process of microvascular angina, "syndrome X", and CMVD in general. Major CNS events such as massive strokes and subarachnoid hemorrhages sometimes lead to chest pain and diffuse ST- wave abnormalities on ECG thought to be induced in part by alterations in the autonomic adrenergic innervation of the coronary arteries (Kono et al., 1994). In one extreme but rare disease entity called "Stress-Related Cardiomyopathy" or Takotsubo (Japanese for "octopus trap") Disease, a single event of extreme physical or emotional stress by itself can induce cardiac ischemia characterized by ST- segment abnormalities on electrocardiogram (ECG) and segmental wall akinesis (typically the apical wall) on ECHO giving way to the "octopus trap" appearance of the heart muscle (Bybee & Prasad, 2008; Kume et al., 2005; Tsuchihashi et al., 2001). In addition, several cases of toxic pheochromocytoma have been observed to cause cardiac ischemia and ST- wave abnormalities (Shaw, Rafferty, & Tait, 1987; Yamanaka et al., 1994). Researchers have generally applied the terms "neurogenically-stunned myocardium" or "catecholamine myopathy" to these anectodal cases.

6. Measurement of coronary microvascular function

Investigators have been using a variety of direct and indirect methods to measure blood flow through the small coronary arterioles in order to facilitate the study of the coronary microcirculation. One direct method for measurement is the passage of a guide wire tipped with a thermistor probe and pressure sensor into the epicardial arteries to measure blood flow by thermodilution (Vesely & Dilsizian). Indirect methods of measurement have included transthoracic echocardiography with doppler flow analysis (TTE-DR), contrast stress echocardiography, thallium scintigraphy, positron emission tomography using ^{82}rubidium as a marker, and cardiovascular magnetic resonance (CMR) using gadolinium as a flow tracer. Many of these tests are expensive, time-consuming, expose patients to radioactivity, and provide limited information on the microvasculature. Still, the ultimate goal of each modality is to measure coronary perfusion based on several mathematic equations. Coronary blood flow (CBF) is the measurement of the amount of blood that passes through a cross section of the artery per unit of time. Coronary flow reserve (CFR) is a calculation of the ratio of maximally-stimulated CBF within a particular coronary artery to the CBF through the same artery at rest. Flow is maximized using physical or chemical stimuli to cause vasodilation. A ratio of less than 2 - 2.5 is considered abnormal (G. A. Lanza & Crea, 2010). Regional myocardial blood flow (MBF), which equals the amount of blood flow (milliliters/minute/gram) through a segment of myocardium, can also be measured (Vesely & Dilsizian). A normal resting MBF is usually 0.6 - 1.3 ml/min/g and should increase 3 - 4 fold during the peak response (Vesely & Dilsizian). In thallium scintigraphy, the injection of a vasodilator simulates an increase in cardiac stress by preferentially dilating normal vessels that in turn potentially divert blood flow from diseased vessels. A post-stress disparity in blood flow will appear in the form of an abnormal redistribution of thallium, the radioactive marker. Large vessel occlusions typically appear as segmental areas of decreased blood flow corresponding to the perfusion territories of one or more of the main epicardial coronary arteries with or without associated cardiac wall motion abnormalities. By comparison, microvascular disease often appears as patchy isolated areas of decreased blood flow, most often with no evidence of associated wall motion abnormalities (G. A. Lanza & Crea, 2010). All of these imaging modalities carry a certain margin of error, and, while they can be instrumental in locating a large coronary vessel occlusion, they often do not provide helpful information in cases of CMVD (Maseri et al., 2009).

7. Treatment

The various etiologies of CMVD as well as the lack of data from clinical trials preclude a definitive treatment regimen. As a result, multiple pharmacologic attempts have been made to limit CMVD induced morbidity and mortality. CMVD is typically treated similarly to coronary artery disease. Beta-blockers, nitrates and calcium channel blockers have long been used for CMVD, but only beta-blockers have shown beneficial effects in clinical trials. Additional agents such as angiotensin-converting enzyme inhibitors and angiotensin II receptor blockers have also been considered for persistent symptoms despite optimal anti-ischemic drug therapy. Alpha adrenergic antagonists, statins, estrogens, xanthine derivatives, adenosine and tricyclic antidepressants have also been investigated for treatment of CMVD-induced angina. Other experimental therapies include GLP-1, L-arginine, nicorandil, tetrahydrobiopterin and nitrite. This section will examine the evidence in support of the pharmacologic treatment of CMVD.

7.1 Anti-anginals

Beta blockers, nitrates and calcium channel blockers are the conventional anti-anginal drugs used most often for ischemic chest pain with associated ECG changes in the presence or absence of coronary artery lesions. There are no definitive trials indicating a superior anti-anginal therapy for the treatment of CMVD. However, beta blockers seem to be the most effective at decreasing the severity and frequency of chest pain and they are considered first line therapy. One randomized, double-blinded prospective trial found that beta blockers, but not calcium channel blockers or nitrates, significantly reduced chest pain episodes in patients diagnosed with cardiac "syndrome X" (Gaetano Antonio Lanza, Colonna, Pasceri, & Maseri, 1999). Similarly, in 16 patients with transient myocardial ischemia and normal coronary angiography randomized to treatment with propanolol, verapamil or placebo, those patients receiving propanolol had significantly fewer episodes of ischemic chest pain when compared to placebo (Bugiardini, Borghi, Biagetti, & Puddu, 1989).

Nitrates are frequently used to treat chest pain but their effectiveness in coronary microvascular dysfunction is unclear. Radice et al (1994) showed that exercise duration and time to 1-mm ST-segment depression in patients with CMVD improved with nitroglycerin administration, albeit significantly less than in patients with CAD (Radice, Giudici, Albertini, & Mannarini, 1994). Similarly, another study showed an improvement in time to angina and peak ST-segment depression with nitroglycerin administration (Bugiardini et al., 1993). However, approximately 50% of patients CMVD taking sublingual nitrates for chest pain experience minimal relief (J. Kaski et al., 1995) and exercise tolerance tests for patients with CMVD worsened with nitrate use (G. Lanza, Manzoli, Bia, Crea, & Maseri, 1994; Radice et al., 1996).

Similarly, calcium channel blockers (CCB) have limited effectiveness in the treatment of CMVD. A 4 week treatment with nisoldipine (a dihydropyridine CCB) significantly increased exercise duration and time to angina in patients with CMVD (Özçelik, Altun, & Özbay, 1999). Similarly, a 4-week trial of nifedipine or verapamil (a non-dihydropyridine CCB) showed a significant improvement in exercise tolerance and angina (Cannon, Watson, Rosing, & Epstein, 1985). Montorsi et al (1990) showed improvement in ST-segment depression during exercise in patients with CMVD treated with nifedipine for 4 weeks (Montorsi et al., 1990). In contrast, Lanza et al (1999) demonstrated that calcium channel blockers did not decrease the number of episodes of chest pain (Gaetano Antonio Lanza et al., 1999). In addition, a 7-day treatment with verapamil made no difference in the frequency of episodes of ST-segment depression, measured by continuous ECG monitoring over 2 days (Bugiardini et al., 1989).

7.2 Statins

The role of statins in the primary and secondary prevention of cardiovascular events has been well established, as has the improvement of endothelial function via non-cholesterol lowering effects (Rosenson & Tangney, 1998). Statins are beneficial in patients with CMVD and they are commonly used in patients with hypercholesterolemia. In a randomized, placebo-controlled study, pravastatin improved exercise duration and time to ST-segment depression in patients with CMVD (Kayikcioglu et al., 2003). Similar results were reported by Fabian et al (2004) using simvastatin (Fábián et al., 2004). Pizzi et al (2004) found that a 6-

month trial of atorvastatin and ramipril significantly improved exercise tolerance and symptoms of chest pain secondary to CMVD, possibly through the reduction of oxidative stress (Pizzi, Manfrini, Fontana, & Bugiardini, 2004).

7.3 Angiotensin converting enzyme inhibition

As mentioned above, angiotensin converting enzyme inhibitors (ACE-I) have been associated with improvement of chest pain and ECG-findings in patients with CMVD (Pizzi et al., 2004). Kaski et al (1994) found an increase in exercise time and time to ST segment depression in patients with reduced coronary flow taking enalapril (Juan Carlos Kaski, Rosano, Krzyzowska-Dickinson, Martuscelli, & Romeo, 1994). Evidence from Nalbantgil et al (1998) further supported these findings in patients with CMVD taking cilazapril (Nalbantgil et al., 1998). Long-term inhibition of ACE is associated with improved nitric oxide bioavailability (Chen, Hsu, Wu, Lin, & Chang, 2002), which may be one mechanism by which ACE-Is reduce episodes of chest pain in patients with CMVD.

7.4 Metformin

Metformin has been shown to have vasculoprotective properties and can improve endothelial function (Mather, Verma, & Anderson, 2001). These vascular effects have proven to be beneficial for patients with CMVD. In a randomized, double blinded, placebo controlled study, Jadhav et al (2006) found that metformin improved vascular function and decreased myocardial ischemia in non-diabetic women with chest pain and angiographically normal coronary arteries (Jadhav et al., 2006). This study found a significant reduction in the incidence of chest pain and ST-segment depression during exercise treadmill testing. Similarly, Kapinya et al (2008) conducted a retrospective, observational study investigating cardiac stress test results in patients with chest pain without cardiac biomarker rise. These investigators found that patients previously taking metformin had significantly less ischemia and infarction compared to patients previously taking insulin or insulin secretagogues (Kapinya, Nijjar, Stanek, & Amanullah, 2008).

7.5 Hormone replacement therapy/estrogen

The high proportion of peri- and post-menopausal women with CMVD raises questions about the lack of estrogen as a pathophysiologic cause of CMVD and its replacement as a potential therapy. Hormone replacement therapy has been shown to improve endothelial function (J C Kaski, 2006; Roque et al., 1998; Sitges et al., 2001) as well as decrease episodes of angina (Rosano et al., 1996) and increase exercise tolerance (Albertsson, Emanuelsson, & Milsom, 1996). However, the risk of breast cancer and thromboemoblic disease has limited the possibilities of hormone replacement therapy for CMVD (Committee, 2004; Investigators, 2002).

7.6 Other pharmacologic therapies

7.6.1 Imipramine

Imipramine, a tricyclic antidepressant, has been shown to improve chest pain symptoms but not quality of life in patients with CMVD (Cox, Hann, & Kaski, 1998). The hypothesized mechanism of this effect is not through vasoactive pathways, but through its visceral analgesic effects (Cannon et al., 1994). The American College of Cardiology recommends imipramine for treatment of CMVD in patients who have failed treatment with risk factor reduction, beta blockers, calcium channel blockers or nitrates (Wright et al., 2011).

7.6.2 L-arginine

L-arginine is a substrate for the production of NO by NOS (Palmer, Ashton, & Moncada, 1988). In patients with angina and normal coronary arteries, intravenous infusion of L-arginine restored nitric oxide activity and resulted in the improvement of endothelial function (Piatti et al., 2003). In addition, chronic L-arginine supplementation enhanced NO synthesis in diabetic animals (Kohli et al., 2004), and improved coronary microvascular endothelial function in humans (Lerman, Burnett, Higano, McKinley, & Holmes, 1998). These findings demonstrate a potential role for L-arginine in the treatment of CMVD.

7.6.3 Tetrahydrobiopterin

Tetrahydrobiopterin (BH_4) is a co-factor required for the production of NO from L-arginine and molecular oxygen (Scott-Burden, 1995), and BH_4 deficiency causes decreased NO production by diabetic coronary endothelium (Meininger et al., 2000). In addition, intracoronary BH_4 improved acetylcholine-induced microvascular dilator responses in patients with endothelial dysfunction *in vivo*. Thus, supplementation with BH_4 may be a novel therapeutic means to increase NO availability for patients with coronary microvascular disease (Setoguchi, Mohri, Shimokawa, & Takeshita, 2001).

7.6.4 Alpha antagonists

Alpha adrenergic antagonists decrease alpha-mediated vasoconstriction and have been hypothesized to improve CMVD symptoms. However, a study by Bøtker et al (1998) proved disappointing. Doxazosin did not increase exercise tolerance or time to ST-segment depression during exercise versus placebo (Bøtker, Sonne, Schmitz, & Nielsen, 1998).

7.6.5 Xanthine derivatives

Xanthine derivatives such as theophylline, bamiphylline and aminophylline have been used to reduce chest pain symptoms related to CMVD. Emdin et al (1989) found that aminophylline had a beneficial effect on exercise induced chest pain and ischemic ECG changes in patients with CMVD (Emdin, Picano, Lattanzi, & L'Abbate, 1989). The proposed mechanism for this is through the inhibition of pain transmission through adenosine receptor blockade. In addition, myocardial flow maldistribution (elicited by inconsistent adenosine release in the presence of increased coronary arteriolar resistance) may also have been prevented, but this was not measured directly (Emdin et al., 1989).

7.6.6 Nicorandil

Nicorandil (nicotinamide nitrate) is a hybrid between a nitrate and an activator of ATP-sensitive potassium channels. Its vasodilatory mechanisms include guanylyl cyclase activation and hyperpolarization (Akai et al., 1995) which preferentially relaxes VSMC in the microcirculation (Akai et al., 1995). Ito et al demonstrated preservation of microvascular integrity by intravenous nicorandil after coronary ischemia and reperfusion (Ito et al., 1999). Ikeda et al (1994) found that post-angiography treatment with nicorandil improved coronary microvascular function and was associated with earlier recovery of ST segment elevation and greater regional wall motion in the infarcted area after reperfusion (Ikeda et al., 2004). In addition, in a prospective study, patients with end-stage renal disease who were taking oral nicorandil prior to an ischemic coronary event had improved outcomes after revascularization (Ishii et al., 2007).

7.6.7 Nitrite

Until recently, nitrite was typically thought of as a biologically inactive metabolite of nitric oxide metabolism. However, more recent findings have determined that the generation of NO from the reduction of nitrite can occur *in vivo,* under a variety of physiologic and pathophysiologic conditions (Vitturi & Patel, 2011). Nitrite is cardioprotective after episodes of ischemia and reperfusion in a variety of experimental models, and clinical trials are underway to determine the vasculoprotective and cardioprotective actions of nitrite therapy in patients with cardiovascular disease (Calvert & Lefer, 2009).

7.6.8 Glucagon-like peptide-1 (GLP-1)

GLP-1 is an incretin hormone that regulates post-prandial metabolism and blood glucose concentration. GLP-1 is also biologically active in the cardiovascular system. GLP-1 improves endothelial function *in vivo* (Basu et al., 2007; T. Nystrom, 2008; Thomas Nystrom et al., 2004), attenuates the expression of pro-inflammatory cytokines (Liu, Hu, Simpson, & Dear, 2008) and adhesion molecules (Liu, Dear, Knudsen, & Simpson, 2009) in cultured endothelial cells, decreases inflammatory injury in intact endothelium (Dozier et al., 2009), and protects myocardium from ischemia/reperfusion injury in isolated heart models and *in vivo* (Ban et al., 2008; Bose, Mocanu, Carr, Brand, & Yellon, 2004, 2005; Bose, Mocanu, Carr, & Yellon, 2007; B. B. Dokken, Labonte, Davis-Gorman, & McDonagh, 2007; Huisamen, Genade, & Lochner, 2008; Sonne, Engstrom, & Treiman, 2008; Timmers et al., 2009). The mechanisms of GLP-1 in the vasculature are not well-understood, but preliminary findings suggest that it may decrease endothelial production of ROS (Bloomgarden; Brownlee, 2006) and enhance endothelium-dependent vasodilation through nitric oxide (NO) signaling (Ban et al., 2008; Basu et al., 2007; Tesauro et al., 2009). We recently reported that GLP-1 prevents coronary microcirculatory dysfunction in swine when administered after cardiac arrest and resuscitation (Betsy B Dokken et al., 2009). Endogenous GLP-1 is decreased in patients with type 2 diabetes, who incidentally are more likely to have CMVD. GLP-1-receptor agonists are currently FDA approved for the treatment of hyperglycemia in patients with type 2 diabetes. Substantial effort is currently underway to determine the mechanisms of the protective effects of GLP-1 and its related peptides.

In summary, the optimal therapy for CMVD is far from defined. In a recent study investigating the long-term prognoses of patient's with CMVD, Lamendola et al (2010) found that chest pain episodes remained unchanged in one-third of patients and worsened significantly in 14% despite treatment with either beta-blockers, calcium channel blockers, nitrates, ACE inhibitors or statins (Lamendola et al., 2010).

8. Conclusion

The coronary microcirculation modulates blood flow throughout the heart, and thus is of major importance in both health and disease. The presence of CMVD complicates the presentation and management of patients with CAD. Due to the multifactorial nature of CMVD and to the difficulty associated with accurately measuring its function, the coronary microcirculation has received limited attention. In order to determine appropriate strategies for the diagnosis and management of CMVD, the physiology, pathophysiology and pharmacology of the coronary microcirculation demands further investigation.

9. References

Akai, K., Wang, Y., Sato, K., Sekiguchi, N., Sugimura, A., Kumagai, T., et al. (1995). Vasodilatory Effect of Nicorandil on Coronary Arterial Microvessels: Its Dependency on Vessel Size and the Involvement of the ATP-Sensitive Potassium Channels. *Journal of Cardiovascular Pharmacology, 26*(4), 541-547.

Albertsson, P. A., Emanuelsson, H., & Milsom, I. (1996). Beneficial effect of treatment with transdermal estradiol-17-[beta] on exercise-induced angina and ST segment depression in syndrome X. *International Journal of Cardiology, 54*(1), 13-20.

Antman, E. M., Giugliano, R. P., Gibson, C. M., McCabe, C. H., Coussement, P., Kleiman, N. S., et al. (1999). Abciximab Facilitates the Rate and Extent of Thrombolysis : Results of the Thrombolysis In Myocardial Infarction (TIMI) 14 Trial. *Circulation, 99*(21), 2720-2732.

Ban, K., Noyan-Ashraf, M. H., Hoefer, J., Bolz, S. S., Drucker, D. J., & Husain, M. (2008). Cardioprotective and vasodilatory actions of glucagon-like peptide 1 receptor are mediated through both glucagon-like peptide 1 receptor-dependent and -independent pathways. *Circulation, 117*(18), 2340-2350.

Basu, A., Charkoudian, N., Schrage, W., Rizza, R. A., Basu, R., & Joyner, M. J. (2007). Beneficial effects of GLP-1 on endothelial function in humans: dampening by glyburide but not by glimepiride. *Am J Physiol Endocrinol Metab, 293*(5), E1289-1295.

Bellamy, M. F., Goodfellow, J., Tweddel, A. C., Dunstan, F. D. J., Lewis, M. J., & Henderson, A. H. (1998). Syndrome X and endothelial dysfunction. *Cardiovascular Research, 40*(2), 410-417.

Beltrame, J. F., Crea, F., & Camici, P. (2009). Advances in Coronary Microvascular Dysfunction. *Heart, Lung and Circulation, 18*(1), 19-27.

Beltrame, J. F., Limaye, S. B., & Horowitz, J. D. (2002). The Coronary Slow Flow Phenomenon: A New Coronary Microvascular Disorder. *Cardiology, 97*(4), 197-202.

Bloomgarden, Z. T. Incretin Concepts. *Diabetes Care, 33*(2), e20-e25.

Bose, A. K., Mocanu, M. M., Carr, R. D., Brand, C. L., & Yellon, D. M. (2004). *Myocardial infarct size attenuation by glucagon like peptide-1 (GLP-1) in both in vivo and in vitro rat heart.*

Bose, A. K., Mocanu, M. M., Carr, R. D., Brand, C. L., & Yellon, D. M. (2005). Glucagon-like peptide 1 can directly protect the heart against ischemia/reperfusion injury. *Diabetes, 54*(1), 146-151.

Bose, A. K., Mocanu, M. M., Carr, R. D., & Yellon, D. M. (2007). Myocardial ischaemia-reperfusion injury is attenuated by intact glucagon like peptide-1 (GLP-1) in the in vitro rat heart and may involve the p70s6K pathway. *Cardiovascular Drugs and Therapy, 21*(4), 253-256.

Bøtker, H. E., Sonne, H. S., Schmitz, O., & Nielsen, T. T. (1998). Effects of doxazosin on exercise-induced angina pectoris, ST-segment depression, and insulin sensitivity in patients with syndrome X. *The American Journal of Cardiology, 82*(11), 1352-1356.

Brownlee, M. (2006). GLP-1 (9-36) Methods and Compositions, *http://www.wipo.int/pctdb/en/wo.jsp?IA=WO2005060986* (Vol. Patent EP1701731).

Bugiardini, R., Borghi, A., Biagetti, L., & Puddu, P. (1989). Comparison of verapamil versus propranolol therapy in syndrome X. *The American Journal of Cardiology, 63*(5), 286-290.

Bugiardini, R., Borghi, A., Pozzati, A., Ottani, F., Morgagni, G. L., & Puddu, P. (1993). The paradox of nitrates in patients with angina pectoris and angiographically normal coronary arteries. *The American Journal of Cardiology, 72*(3), 343-347.

Bybee, K. A., & Prasad, A. (2008). Stress-Related Cardiomyopathy Syndromes. *Circulation, 118*(4), 397-409.

Calvert, J. W., & Lefer, D. J. (2009). Myocardial protection by nitrite. *Cardiovascular Research, 83*(2), 195-203.

Camici, P. G., & Crea, F. (2007). Coronary Microvascular Dysfunction. *N Engl J Med, 356*(8), 830-840.

Cannon, R. O., Quyyumi, A. A., Mincemoyer, R., Stine, A. M., Gracely, R. H., Smith, W. B., et al. (1994). Imipramine in Patients with Chest Pain Despite Normal Coronary Angiograms. *New England Journal of Medicine, 330*(20), 1411-1417.

Cannon, R. O., Watson, R. M., Rosing, D. R., & Epstein, S. E. (1985). Efficacy of calcium channel blocker therapy for angina pectoris resulting from small-vessel coronary artery disease and abnormal vasodilator reserve. *The American Journal of Cardiology, 56*(4), 242-246.

Chauhan, A., Mullins, P. A., Taylor, G., Petch, M. C., & Schofield, P. M. (1997). Both endothelium-dependent and endothelium-independent function is impaired in patients with angina pectoris and normal coronary angiograms. *European Heart Journal, 18*(1), 60-68.

Chen, J.-W., Hsu, N.-W., Wu, T.-C., Lin, S.-J., & Chang, M.-S. (2002). Long-term angiotensin-converting enzyme inhibition reduces plasma asymmetric dimethylarginine and improves endothelial nitric oxide bioavailability and coronary microvascular function in patients with syndrome X. *The American Journal of Cardiology, 90*(9), 974-982.

The Women's Health Initiative Steering Committee (2004). Effects of Conjugated Equine Estrogen in Postmenopausal Women With Hysterectomy. *JAMA: The Journal of the American Medical Association, 291*(14), 1701-1712.

Cox, I. D., Hann, C. M., & Kaski, J. C. (1998). Low dose imipramine improves chest pain but not quality of life in patients with angina and normal coronary angiograms. *European Heart Journal, 19*(2), 250-254.

Dokken, B. B., Huebner, K., Rogers, D. C., Allen, D., Teachey, M. K., Panchal, A. R., et al. (2009). Abstract P87: Glucagon-like Peptide-1 Attenuates Post-resuscitation Myocardial Microcirculatory Dysfunction in a Swine Model of Prolonged Ventricular Fibrillation. *Circulation, 120*(18_MeetingAbstracts), S1459-c-1460.

Dokken, B. B., Labonte, L. R., Davis-Gorman, G., & McDonagh, P. F. (2007). *Postconditioning with GLP-1 in vivo decreases myocardial infarct size in rats.*

Dozier, K. C., Cureton, E. L., Kwan, R. O., Curran, B., Sadjadi, J., & Victorino, G. P. (2009). Glucagon-like peptide-1 protects mesenteric endothelium from injury during inflammation. *Peptides, 30*(9), 1735-1741.

Emdin, M., Picano, E., Lattanzi, F., & L'Abbate, A. (1989). Improved exercise capacity with acute aminophylline administration in patients with syndrome X. *J Am Coll Cardiol, 14*(6), 1450-1453.

Fábián, E., Varga, A., Picano, E., Vajo, Z., Rónaszéki, A., & Csanády, M. (2004). Effect of simvastatin on endothelial function in cardiac syndrome X patients. *The American Journal of Cardiology, 94*(5), 652-655.

Gregorini, L., Marco, J., KozÃ kovÃ , M., Palombo, C., Anguissola, G. B., Marco, I., et al. (1999). Alpha-Adrenergic Blockade Improves Recovery of Myocardial Perfusion and Function After Coronary Stenting in Patients With Acute Myocardial Infarction. *Circulation, 99*(4), 482-490.

Huisamen, B., Genade, S., & Lochner, A. (2008). Signalling pathways activated by glucagon-like peptide-1 (7-36) amide in the rat heart and their role in protection against ischaemia. *Cardiovascular Journal of Africa, 19*(2), 77-83.

Ikeda, N., Yasu, T., Kubo, N., Hashimoto, S., Tsuruya, Y., Fujii, M., et al. (2004). Nicorandil versus isosorbide dinitrate as adjunctive treatment to direct balloon angioplasty in acute myocardial infarction. *Heart, 90*(2), 181-185.

Investigators, W. G. f. t. W. s. H. I. (2002). Risks and Benefits of Estrogen Plus Progestin in Healthy Postmenopausal Women. *JAMA: The Journal of the American Medical Association, 288*(3), 321-333.

Ishii, H., Toriyama, T., Aoyama, T., Takahashi, H., Yamada, S., Kasuga, H., et al. (2007). Efficacy of oral nicorandil in patients with end-stage renal disease: A retrospective chart review after coronary angioplasty in japanese patients receiving hemodialysis. *Clinical Therapeutics, 29*(1), 110-122.

Ito, H., Taniyama, Y., Iwakura, K., Nishikawa, N., Masuyama, T., Kuzuya, T., et al. (1999). Intravenous nicorandil can preserve microvascular integrity and myocardial viability in patients with reperfused anterior wall myocardial infarction. *Journal of the American College of Cardiology, 33*(3), 654-660.

Jadhav, S., Ferrell, W., Greer, I. A., Petrie, J. R., Cobbe, S. M., & Sattar, N. (2006). Effects of Metformin on Microvascular Function and Exercise Tolerance in Women With Angina and Normal Coronary Arteries: A Randomized, Double-Blind, Placebo-Controlled Study. *J Am Coll Cardiol, 48*(5), 956-963.

Kapinya, K., Nijjar, P. S., Stanek, M., & Amanullah, A. (2008). Insulin-sensitizing antihyperglycaemic medications are associated with better outcome in patients with diabetes undergoing cardiac stress testing. *Internal Medicine Journal, 38*(4), 259-264.

Kaski, J., Rosano, G., Collins, P., Nihoyannopoulos, P., Maseri, A., & Poole-Wilson, P. (1995). Cardiac syndrome X: clinical characteristics and left ventricular function. Long-term follow-up study. *J Am Coll Cardiol, 25*(4), 807-814.

Kaski, J. C. (2006). Cardiac syndrome X in women: the role of oestrogen deficiency. *Heart, 92*(suppl 3), iii5-iii9.

Kaski, J. C., Rosano, G. M. C., Krzyzowska-Dickinson, K., Martuscelli, E., & Romeo, F. (1994). "Syndrome X" as a consequence of acute myocardial infarction. *The American Journal of Cardiology, 74*(5), 494-495.

Kayikcioglu, M., Payzin, S., Yavuzgil, O., Kultursay, H., Can, L. H., & Soydan, I. (2003). Benefits of statin treatment in cardiac syndrome-X. *European Heart Journal, 24*(22), 1999-2005.

Kohli, R., Meininger, C. J., Haynes, T. E., Yan, W., Self, J. T., & Wu, G. (2004). Dietary L-Arginine Supplementation Enhances Endothelial Nitric Oxide Synthesis in Streptozotocin-Induced Diabetic Rats. *J. Nutr., 134*(3), 600-608.

Kono, T., Morita, H., Kuroiwa, T., Onaka, K., Takatsuka, H., & Fujiwara, A. (1994). Left-ventricular wall-motion abnormalities in patients with subarachnoid hemmhorage: Neurogenic stunned myocardium. *Journal of the American College of Cardiology, 24*(3), 636-640.

Kume, T., Akasaka, T., Kawamoto, T., Yoshitani, H., Watanabe, N., Neishi, Y., et al. (2005). Assessment of coronary microcirculation in patients with takotsubo-like left ventricular dysfunction. *Circulation Journal, 69*(8), 934-939.

Lamendola, P., Lanza, G. A., Spinelli, A., Sgueglia, G. A., Di Monaco, A., Barone, L., et al. (2010). Long-term prognosis of patients with cardiac syndrome X. *International Journal of Cardiology, 140*(2), 197-199.

Lanza, G., Manzoli, A., Bia, E., Crea, F., & Maseri, A. (1994). Acute effects of nitrates on exercise testing in patients with syndrome X. Clinical and pathophysiological implications. *Circulation, 90*(6), 2695-2700.

Lanza, G. A., Colonna, G., Pasceri, V., & Maseri, A. (1999). Atenolol versus amlodipine versus isosorbide-5-mononitrate on anginal symptoms in syndrome X. *The American Journal of Cardiology, 84*(7), 854-856.

Lanza, G. A., & Crea, F. (2010). Primary Coronary Microvascular Dysfunction Clinical Presentation, Pathophysiology, and Management. *Circulation, 121*(21), 2317-2325.

Lerman, A., Burnett, J. C., Higano, S. T., McKinley, L. J., & Holmes, D. R. (1998). Long-term L-Arginine Supplementation Improves Small-Vessel Coronary Endothelial Function in Humans. *Circulation, 97*(21), 2123-2128.

Liu, H., Dear, A., Knudsen, L., & Simpson, R. (2009). A long-acting GLP-1 analogue attenuates induction of PAI-1 and vascular adhesion molecules. *J Endocrinol, 201*, 59-66.

Liu, H., Hu, Y., Simpson, R. W., & Dear, A. E. (2008). Glucagon-like peptide-1 attenuates tumour necrosis factor-{alpha}-mediated induction of plasmogen activator inhibitor-1 expression. *J Endocrinol, 196*(1), 57-65.

Maseri, A., Beltrame, J. F., & Shimokawa, H. (2009). Role of Coronary Vasoconstriction in Ischemic Heart Disease and Search for Novel Therapeutic Targets (vol 73, pg 399, 2009). *Circulation Journal, 73*(4), 783-783.

Mather, K. J., Verma, S., & Anderson, T. J. (2001). Improved endothelial function with metformin in type 2 diabetes mellitus. *J Am Coll Cardiol, 37*(5), 1344-1350.

Meininger, C. J., Marinos, R. S., Hatakeyama, K., Martinez-Zaguilan, R., Rojas, J. D., Kelly, K. A., et al. (2000). Impaired nitric oxide production in coronary endothelial cells of the spontaneously diabetic BB rat is due to tetrahydrobiopterin deficiency. *Biochemical Journal, 349*, 353-356.

Montorsi, P., Cozzi, S., Loaldi, A., Fabbiocchi, F., Polese, A., De Cesare, N., et al. (1990). Acute coronary vasomotor effects of nifedipine and therapeutic correlates in syndrome X. *The American Journal of Cardiology, 66*(3), 302-307.

Nalbantgil, I., Önder, R., Altintig, A., Nalbantgil, S., Kilicciogl u, B., Boydak, B., et al. (1998). Therapeutic Benefits of Cilazapril in Patients with Syndrome X. *Cardiology, 89*(2), 130-133.

Nystrom, T. (2008). The potential beneficial role of glucagon-like peptide-1 in endothelial dysfunction and heart failure associated with insulin resistance. *Hormone and Metabolic Research, 40*(9), 593-606.

Nystrom, T., Gutniak, M. K., Zhang, Q., Zhang, F., Holst, J. J., Ahren, B., et al. (2004). Effects of glucagon-like peptide-1 on endothelial function in type 2 diabetes patients with stable coronary artery disease. *Am J Physiol Endocrinol Metab, 287*(6), E1209-1215.

Özçelik, F., Altun, A., & Özbay, G. (1999). Antianginal and anti-ischemic effects of nisoldipine and ramipril in patients with syndrome X. *Clinical Cardiology, 22*(5), 361-365.

Palmer, R. M. J., Ashton, D. S., & Moncada, S. (1988). Vascular endothelial cells synthesize nitric oxide from L-arginine. *Nature, 333*(6174), 664-666.

Piatti, P., Fragasso, G., Monti, L. D., Setola, E., Lucotti, P., Fermo, I., et al. (2003). Acute Intravenous l-Arginine Infusion Decreases Endothelin-1 Levels and Improves Endothelial Function in Patients With Angina Pectoris and Normal Coronary Arteriograms. *Circulation, 107*(3), 429-436.

Pizzi, C., Manfrini, O., Fontana, F., & Bugiardini, R. (2004). Angiotensin-Converting Enzyme Inhibitors and 3-Hydroxy-3-Methylglutaryl Coenzyme A Reductase in Cardiac Syndrome X. *Circulation, 109*(1), 53-58.

Radice, M., Giudici, V., Albertini, A., & Mannarini, A. (1994). Usefulness of changes in exercise tolerance induced by nitroglycerin in identifying patients with syndrome X. *American Heart Journal, 127*(3), 531-535.

Radice, M., Giudici, V., Pusineri, E., Breghi, L., Nicoli, T., Peci, P., et al. (1996). Different effects of acute administration of aminophylline and nitroglycerin on exercise capacity in patients with syndrome X. *The American Journal of Cardiology, 78*(1), 88-90.

Romeo, F., Rosano, G. M. C., Martuscelli, E., Lombardo, L., & Valente, A. (1993). Long-term follow-up of patients initially diagnosed with syndrome-X. *American Journal of Cardiology, 71*(8), 669-673.

Roque, M., Heras, M., Roig, E., Masotti, M., Rigol, M., Betriu, A., et al. (1998). Short-term effects of transdermal estrogen replacement therapy on coronary vascular reactivity in postmenopausal women with angina pectoris and normal results on coronary angiograms. *J Am Coll Cardiol, 31*(1), 139-143.

Rosano, G., Peters, N., Lefroy, D., Lindsay, D., Sarrel, P., Collins, P., et al. (1996). 17-beta-Estradiol therapy lessens angina in postmenopausal women with syndrome X. *J Am Coll Cardiol, 28*(6), 1500-1505.

Rosenson, R. S., & Tangney, C. C. (1998). Antiatherothrombotic Properties of Statins. *JAMA: The Journal of the American Medical Association, 279*(20), 1643-1650.

Scott-Burden, T. (1995). Regulation of Nitric Oxide Production by Tetrahydrobiopterin. *Circulation, 91*(1), 248-250.

Setoguchi, S., Mohri, M., Shimokawa, H., & Takeshita, A. (2001). Tetrahydrobiopterin improves endothelial dysfunction in coronary microcirculation in patients without epicardial coronary artery disease. *Journal of the American College of Cardiology, 38*(2), 493-498.

Shaw, T. R. D., Rafferty, P., & Tait, G. W. (1987). Transient shock and myocardial impairment caused by pheochromocytoma crisis *British Heart Journal, 57*(2), 194-198.

Sitges, M., Heras, M., Roig, E., Duran, M., Masotti, M., Zurbano, M. J., et al. (2001). Acute and mid-term combined hormone replacement therapy improves endothelial function in post-menopausal women with angina and angiographically normal coronary arteries. *European Heart Journal, 22*(22), 2116-2124.

Sonne, D. P., Engstrom, T., & Treiman, M. (2008). Protective effects of GLP-1 analogues exendin-4 and GLP-1(9-36) amide against ischemia-reperfusion injury in rat heart. *Regulatory Peptides, 146*(1-3), 243-249.

Tambe, A. A., Zimmerma.Ha, Demany, M. A., & Mascaren.E. (1972). Angina-pectoris and slow flow velocity of dye in coronary arteries-a new angiographic finding. *American Heart Journal, 84*(1), 66-&.

Tesauro, M., Schinzari, F., Rovella, V., Mores, N., Pitocco, D., Ghirlanda, G., et al. (2009). Abstract 5147: GLP-1 Improves Insulin-Stimulated Nitric Oxide-Dependent Vasodilator Responsiveness in Patients With Metabolic Syndrome. *Circulation, 120* (MeetingAbstracts), S1060-d-1061.

Timmers, L., Henriques, J. P. S., de Kleijn, D. P. V., DeVries, J. H., Kemperman, H., Steendijk, P., et al. (2009). Exenatide Reduces Infarct Size and Improves Cardiac Function in a Porcine Model of Ischemia and Reperfusion Injury. *Journal of the American College of Cardiology, 53*(6), 501-510.

Traub, O., & Berk, B. C. (1998). Laminar shear stress - Mechanisms by which endothelial cells transduce an atheroprotective force. *Arteriosclerosis Thrombosis and Vascular Biology, 18*(5), 677-685.

Tsuchihashi, K., Ueshima, K., Uchida, T., Oh-mura, N., Kimura, K., Owa, M., et al. (2001). Transient left ventricular apical ballooning without coronary artery stenosis: A novel heart syndrome mimicking acute myocardial infarction. *Journal of the American College of Cardiology, 38*(1), 11-18.

Vesely, M., & Dilsizian, V. Microvascular Angina: Assessment of Coronary Blood Flow, Flow Reserve, and Metabolism. *Current Cardiology Reports, 13*(2), 151-158.

Vitturi, D. A., & Patel, R. P. (2011). Current perspectives and challenges in understanding the role of nitrite as an integral player in nitric oxide biology and therapy. *Free Radical Biology and Medicine, 51*(4), 805-812.

Wright, R. S., Anderson, J. L., Adams, C. D., Bridges, C. R., Casey, D. E., Jr, Ettinger, S. M., et al. (2011). 2011 ACCF/AHA Focused Update Incorporated Into the ACC/AHA 2007 Guidelines for the Management of Patients With Unstable Angina/Non-ST-Elevation Myocardial Infarction: A Report of the American College of Cardiology Foundation/American Heart Association Task Force on Practice Guidelines. *J Am Coll Cardiol, 57*(19), e215-367.

Yamanaka, O., Yasumasa, F., Nakamura, T., Ohno, A., Endo, Y., Yoshimi, K., et al. (1994). Myocardial stunning-like phenomenon during a crisis of pheochromocytoma *Japanese Circulation Journal-English Edition, 58*(9), 737-742.

Zeiher, A. M., Krause, T., Schachinger, V., Minners, J., & Moser, E. (1995). Impaired endothelium-dependent vasodilation of coronary resistance vessels is associated with exercise-induced myocardial ischemia. *Circulation, 91*(9), 2345-2352.

5

Coronary Artery Disease and Pregnancy

Titia P.E. Ruys[1], Mark R. Johnson[2] and Jolien W. Roos-Hesselink[1]
[1]*Department of Cardiology, Thorax centre, Erasmus Medical Centre, Rotterdam,*
[2]*Academic Department of Obstetrics and Gynaecology, Imperial College London, Chelsea and Westminster Hospital, London,*
[1]*The Netherlands*
[2]*UK*

1. Introduction

Although an acute coronary syndrome (ACS) in women of childbearing age is rare, consequences are considerable, especially in pregnant women. In this chapter we will give an overview of the current literature regarding pregnancy and ACS. Acute coronary syndrome prior to pregnancy, acute coronary syndrome in the antepartum, peripartum and post partum period and heart failure during pregnancy will be described using patient cases, followed by an overview of literature and recommendations. Epidemiology, pathophysiology, counselling, use of medication, treatment possibilities, delivery, maternal and fetal outcome will be discussed.

2. Epidemiology

Acute coronary syndrome is rare in women of childbearing age (16 to 45 years of age). During these years pregnancy has shown to increase the risk of ACS three- to fourfold. (James et al., 2006) Between 1991-2000 the overall incidence of pregnancy related acute coronary syndrome was reported 2,7 per 100.000 deliveries. (Ladner et al., 2005) A decade later James published on risk factors of ACS during pregnancy in a population based study in the United States, he reported an incidence of 6,2 per 100.000 deliveries between 2000-2002. (James et al., 2006) The higher incidence can be explained by three causes: First of all with the improved diagnostic tests, especially troponin assessment, more women with acute chest pain have been diagnosed with ACS; secondly, an increase of known cardiovascular risk factors is seen in the pregnant population; and finally, maternal age increased in the western world. (Ventura., 2004)

Cardiovascular risk factors specific for ACS during pregnancy are very similar to the risk factors of non-pregnant patients. The main risk factors for ACS in women are smoking, lipid metabolism disorders, hypertension and diabetes. But in pregnant patients also thrombophilia and anaemia are risk factors for ACS. In the last decades lifestyle has changed in the western world. (Ogden et al., 2006) As a consequence of high calorie intake and little exercise the incidence of obesity and diabetes has increased drastically. (Cecchine et al., 2010)

In addition to cardiovascular risk factors, a few obstetric risk factors have been discovered. The most important being multiparity, but also a history of preeclampsia, post-partum haemorrhage, transfusions and post-partum infections are risk factors for ACS during pregnancy. (Ladner et al., 2005) In addition, obstetric complications may elevate the risk of developing ACS later in life. Still birth, preeclampsia and recurrent miscarriage are a risk factor for ACS later in life in the general population. Endothelial dysfunction is hypothesised to be the link between hypertension in the pregnancy and cardiovascular disease later in life. (Pina, 2011)

Maternal age is one of the most important risk factor for ACS during pregnancy. Over the age of 30 women have an odds ratio of 9.5. This is even higher in women over 40, with an odds ratio of 31.6. (James et al., 2006) There is a continuing trend of childbearing at older ages, caused by carrier choices of highly educated women. The advances in reproductive technology enable many older women to conceive, leading to more women with a high risk for ACS during pregnancy. Therefore it may be expected that the incidence of ACS during pregnancy will increase further in the coming years.

3. Changes during pregnancy

Knowledge of the normal physiological changes during pregnancy, labour and the postpartum period is essential for doctors looking after pregnant women with heart disease. In the following section we will give an overview of the most important physiological changes in pregnancy.

The majority of the cardiovascular changes occur in the first twenty weeks of gestation. The first hemodynamic change is a decline in total peripheral vascular resistance (TPVR) of 40-70%. The decline in TPVR is a response to circulating gestational hormones. The drop in TPVR results in a relatively underfilled vascular state reflected by a fall in blood pressure. The blood volume increases with 1-1,5 litre (30-50%) as a response to the low blood pressure. The increase in plasma volume is relatively higher than the increase in red blood cells resulting in a physiological haemodilution. The combined changes result in a fifty percent increase in circulating blood volume during pregnancy. (Robson et al., 1989)

Cardiac afterload decreases with the fall in TPVR and cardiac preload increases with the rise of blood volume. These changes result in an increase in cardiac output of 30-50% from the 20th week of gestation as shown in figure 1. During pregnancy heart rate increases by 10-20 beats per minute, this mainly happens in the third trimester. Pregnancy is associated with changes in cardiac structure secondary to the increase in cardiac output, with left ventricular dimensions increasing from between 10-30%; ejection fraction and fractional shortening also increase. (Hunter & Robson, 1992)

The vascular system changes with the increase in stroke volume. Arterial stiffness decreases during the first trimester, but slightly rises from the second trimester and vascular distensibility is increased. (Ulusoy et al., 2006) These changes are partially mediated by gestational hormones, for example estrogen has favourable effects on the endothelium and vascular smooth muscle cells and increases vasodilatation (Mendelsohn & Karas, 1999), but progestins reduce estradiol-induced endothelium-mediated vascular relaxation. (Skafar et al., 1997)

Delivery increases the stroke volume by 20%, which contributes to the 25% increase in cardiac output. This is initiated by the greater maternal oxygen consumption caused by the increase in uterine contractions in combination with maternal stress and pain, which in turn stimulates higher epinephrine levels.

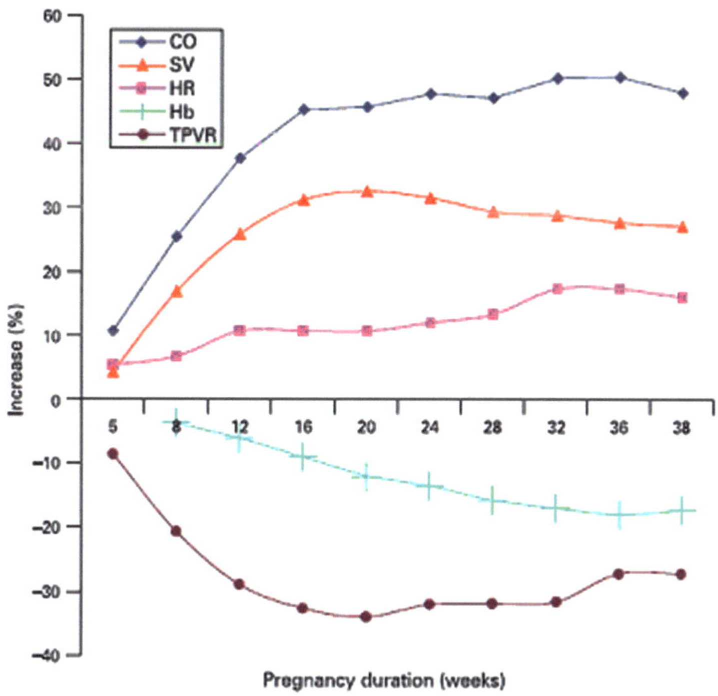

Fig. 1. Hemodynamic changes in the normal pregnancy: CO cardiac output, SV stroke volume, HR heart rate, Hb haemoglobin concentration and TPVR total peripheral vascular resistance. Reproduced from: "Karamermer Y, Roos-Hesselink JW. Pregnancy and adult congenital heart disease. Expert Rev Cardiovasc Ther 2007; 5: 859-869" with permission of Expert Reviews Ltd .

Major hemodynamic changes also occur during the puerperium, (from birth until 6 to 8 weeks after delivery). Decompression of the inferior cava and the return of uterine blood to the circulation (auto-transfusion) cause a period of overfilling. In women with impaired cardiac function this may result in cardiac decompensation. All gestational hemodynamic changes return to prepregnancy levels 3-12 months after pregnancy.

Pregnancy is a hypercoagulable state, probably an evolutionary adaptation to reduce the risk of severe haemorrhage after labour. There is a decrease in releasable tissue plasminogen activator (tPA), an increase in fast-acting tPA inhibitor and an increase in factors V, VII, VIII, IX, X, XII and von Willebrand factor. (Fletcher et al., 1979) Protein S is increased throughout pregnancy, while increased resistance to activated protein C is only seen during the second and third trimesters. (Coolman et al., 2006) The hypercoagulable state is partially reversed by haemodilution and the activation of the fibrinolytic system. During delivery the placenta and myometrium release tPA inhibitors further increasing the hypercoagulable state (Yoshima et al., 1992); but by around 6 weeks after pregnancy the coagulation and fibrinolytic systems return to normal.

In summary pregnancy is a hypercoagulable state and an increase of 30-50% in cardiac output is seen as a result of decrease of vascular resistance and increased blood volume, stroke volume and heart rate.

4. Medication during pregnancy

The food and drug administration (FDA) made a classification system for the use of drugs in pregnant women:

Category A: Adequate and well-controlled studies have failed to demonstrate a risk to the fetus in the first trimester of pregnancy (and there is no evidence of risk in later trimesters).

Category B: Animal reproduction studies have failed to demonstrate a risk to the fetus and there are no adequate and well-controlled studies in pregnant women.

Category C: Animal reproduction studies have shown an adverse effect on the fetus and there are no adequate and well-controlled studies in humans, but potential benefits may warrant use of the drug in pregnant women despite potential risks.

Category D: There is positive evidence of human fetal risk based on adverse reaction data from investigational or marketing experience or studies in humans, but potential benefits may warrant use of the drug in pregnant women despite potential risks.

Category X: Studies in animals or humans have demonstrated fetal abnormalities and/or there is positive evidence of human fetal risk based on adverse reaction data from investigational or marketing experience, and the risks involved in use of the drug in pregnant women clearly outweigh potential benefits.

In table 1 an oversight is given on the safety during pregnancy and breast feeding of drugs which are commonly prescribed by cardiologist.

Medication	**Indication**	**FDA**	**Safe during pregnancy**	**Extra information**	**Safe during breast feeding**	**Extra information**
Atenolol	Hypertension, Arrhythmias,	D	Yes	IUGR and premature birth	No	A case report of adverse effects
Other beta blockers	Hypertension, Arrhythmias, Marfan disease ACS	C	Yes	Low birth weight, hypoglycemia and bradycardia in the fetus	Yes	Careful monitoring of the neonatal heart rate
ACE inhibitors	Hypertension, Heart failure	D	No	High incidence fetal death and fetotoxic effect: renal failure, renal dysplasia	Yes	Traces are detected in breast milk, fetal monitoring is advisable

ARB	Hypertension, Heart failure	D	No	High incidence fetal death and fetal anuria	No data	
Spironolactone	Hypertension, Heart failure	D	No	Potential anti-androgenic effects on the developing male fetus	Yes	
Thiazide diuretics	Hypertension, Heart failure	C	No	Hypovolemia can lead to reduced uterine perfusion	Yes	May suppress lactation
Loop diuretics	Hypertension, Heart failure	C	Yes	Hypovolemia can lead to reduced uterine perfusion	Yes	
Digoxin	Arrhythmias	C	Yes	No reports of congenital defects	Yes	Neonatal heart rate should be monitored after delivery
Nitrates	Hypertension, Angina	B	Yes	Careful titration is advised to avoid maternal hypotension	No data	
Calcium channel antagonists	Hypertension, Preeclampsia	C	Yes	Diltiazem: an increase in major birth defects have been reported	Yes	Excreted in breast milk
Statins	Lipid disorders	X	No	Animal studies demonstrated increased skeletal abnormalities, fetal and neonatal mortality	No	Probably appears in breast milk, there are some concerns with disruption of infant lipid metabolism
Aspirin	ACS, Arrhythmias	C	Yes	Low dose aspirin is safe	Yes	No adverse effects have been reported in low dose
Clopidogrel	ACS	B	No data	The benefits of using clopidogrel in some high risk pregnancies may outweigh the potential fetal risks	No	
LMWH and UFH	Arrhythmias Diminished ventricular function Thrombosis	C	Yes	Factor Xa should by measured to monitor the therapeutic levels of LMWH, which may fluctuate during pregnancy	Yes	

Table 1. Medication. ACE: Angiotensin-converting enzyme inhibitors. ARB: Angiotentin receptor antagonists.

5. Pre-existing coronary disease

A 39 year old woman was seen at the out patient clinic of a referral hospital for counselling. Three month earlier she had suffered a non ST elevation myocardial infarction (NSTEMI). On coronary angiogram (CAG) a thrombotic occlusion of an atherosclerotic lesion of the left coronary artery was seen and treated with a drug eluting stent. She had never been pregnant, had recently stopped smoking, was a non diabetic and normotensive. Her family history did not reveal any cardiovascular disease. Her left ventricular function was assessed with echocardiography and the estimated ejection fraction was 48%. She was prescribed aspirin, clopidogrel, simvastatine, perindopril and nifedipine.

5.1 Counselling prior to pregnancy

Ideally all women of reproductive age with cardiac disease should undergo thorough evaluation before becoming pregnant. This evaluation should focus on identifying and quantifying risk to the mother and the unborn child. During pre pregnancy counselling life expectancy and ethical aspects of parenthood should also be discussed. An exercise test and echocardiogram should be performed. Risk stratification is made to inform the patient of possible complications during pregnancy. The influence of pregnancy on the cardiac condition has to be considered, but also the cardiac condition may influence pregnancy outcome, especially the incidence of hypertension, preeclampsia, arrhythmias and thrombotic complications may be higher.

Low dose aspirin, beta blockade and nitrates should be continued during pregnancy. The safety of clopidogrel is unknown. In individual cases with recent drug eluting stent placement, continuation should be considered. ACE inhibitors and ARBs should be stopped in all patients or in the pre-conception clinic or immediately when pregnancy is diagnosed. Generally, statins should be stopped, however, in an individual patient with very high cholesterol, continuation may be considered.

5.2 Recurrence rate

Only limited data on recurrence risks have been published. Badui et al described 18 women in the literature with previous ACS, the mothers were 1 or 2 years after ACS and none of these patients had a recurrent ACS. (Badui & Enciso, 1996) One of the reasons for this lack of data is the fact that many women are advised against pregnancy after ACS. Doctors advise against pregnancy for a number of reasons, first it is suggested that the hypercoagulable state of pregnancy raises the chance of recurrence of thrombotic obstruction of the coronary arteries. Second the increase in left ventricular mass and heart rate lead to a high cardiac oxygen demand. The increased cardiac oxygen demand can lead to relative coronary flow mismatch in patients with pre-existing coronary artery disease. Finally, fear of complications may make them conservative.

The first patient was advised to wait for at least 3 more months before trying to become pregnant to make sure that she was cardiovascularly stable. Before conception perindopril, statin and clopidogrel are advised to be discontinued until after delivery. If pregnancy occurred, then the plan was made for outpatient review at 6, 12, 20 and 32 weeks of gestation.

5.3 Impaired left ventricular function

A 41 year old patient presented to the out patient department of a referral hospital with a desire for pregnancy. She had not been pregnant before. One year earlier she had suffered from a STEMI, CAG at that time revealed atherosclerosis and thrombosis of the LAD and she was treated with thrombosuction and a drug-eluting stent. Six month after the ACS her left ventricular function was measured with echocardiography, ejection fraction was 35 %.

In 2000 Siu published predictors of cardiac events, mainly heart failure and arrhythmias. Prior cardiac events, left ventricular outflow obstruction, NYHA class > II, cyanosis and systemic ventricular dysfunction (ejection fraction >40%) were predictor for adverse maternal outcome. If one predictor was present, cardiac event rate was 27%. (Siu et al., 2001) However, the patient population consisted of patients with congenital or valvular disease and a diminished systemic ventricular function was mainly found in patients with transposition of the great arteries after atrial repair. To use these results to predict cardiac events in ischemic cardiomyopathy patients is at least questionable.

Generally women are advised against pregnancy if they have a left ventricular dysfunction with an ejection fraction under 40% and have a dilated left ventricle. (Prebitero et al., 2009) In a study on pregnancy in patients with dilated cardiomyopathy, an OR of 43 was found for moderate or severe left ventricular dysfunction and 39% of the pregnancies where complicated. (Grewal et al., 2009) Risk factors for adverse events were moderate (EF 30%-44%) or severe (EF<30%) ventricular dysfunction and NYHA class III or IV at baseline or prior cardiac event. Compared with non-pregnant patients with dilated cardiomyopathy, pregnant patients needed more medication and adverse cardiac events were more common. Pregnancy seemed to have a negative impact on the short-term clinical course for women with dilated cardiomyopathy. (Grewal et al., 2010) We need similar data for women with ischemic left ventricular dysfunction.

In case of heart failure during pregnancy diuretics are considered to be first choice, but diuretics could result in hypovolemia, leading to reduced uterine perfusion and so should be used with caution. Nitrates can be used safely and digoxin can be considered, especially if the patients has atrial fibrillation. Such patients should be treated in hospital and bed rest is advisable.

In the study of Grewal et al, the neonatal complication rate was high, especially in women with severe dilated cardiomyopathy, suggesting that in the context of severe left ventricular dysfunction, the heart may not be able perfuse the utero-placental circulation sufficiently. Therefore, regular growth scans to indentify fetal growth restriction and frequent review in a combined clinic with an obstetrician and cardiologist is advised. (Signore et al., 2010)

The second patient was informed about the high maternal and fetal risks associated with pregnancy in women with impaired left ventricular function as well as the lack of information on the recurrence rates of ACS during pregnancy. She decided not to take the risk.

5.4 Delivery

Planning delivery should be done in a multidisciplinary team consisting of an obstetrician, anaesthesiologist and cardiologist. The patient should be informed about the considerations prior to delivery, since patients preference has to be taken into account. Timing of delivery is individualized, according to the cardiac and obstetric status of the mother and fetal well being. In patients with heart failure delivery at 34 weeks can be considered to allow early optimisation of treatment modalities for the mother.

The mode of delivery depends on the maternal hemodynamic situation and obstetric factors. Women with adequate cardiac output may tolerate induction of labour and vaginal delivery. Vaginal delivery can lead to fluctuations in blood pressure, especially in prolonged labour. Assisted vaginal delivery (by vacuum or forceps extraction) is recommended in some women to avoid excessive maternal efforts and prolonged labour. (Roth & Elkayam, 2008) Adequate pain relief is very important, but epidural anaesthesia is contraindicated when the patient is on antithrombotic or anticoagulant treatment.

During caesarean section blood pressure can be controlled, stress and pain can be relieved and a stable environment can be created. However, caesarean section has been associated with a higher risk of venous thrombo-embolism, infection and peripartum haemorrhage. In some cases general anaesthesia will be necessary with some risk of complication. (Deneux-Tharax et al., 2006) In addition, blood loss during caesarean section has been shown to be greater than during vaginal delivery.

5.5 Post partum period

The volume shifts caused by auto-transfusion can be dangerous in patients with diminished left ventricular function. Close monitoring on a medium care unit may be advisable for the first 3 days after delivery. Early recognition of heart failure and immediate treatment with diuretics can be achieved by close monitoring of the patients and measurement of the central venous pressure. Some cardiologists advise prophylaxic diuretics in patients with severe systemic ventricular dysfunction. Ideally monitoring should be done in a unit with neonatal care, since early bonding of mother and child is very important. In patients with normal ventricular function after ACS prior to pregnancy close monitoring in-hospital for at least three days after delivery is advisable. The main risk during this period consists of thrombo-embolic events cause by the hypercoagulable state of pregnancy exacerbated by even higher tPA inhibitor levels immediately after delivery.

5.6 Breast feeding

The effects of breast feeding on maternal cardiovascular function are caused by circulating hormones. High levels of oxytocin circulate through the body. In the study of Mezzacappa cardiac output during breastfeeding was found to be higher than in bottle feeding mothers. They describe a decrease in heart rate and a slight increase in systolic blood pressure during the first minutes of breast feeding. (Mezzacappa et al., 2001) Light et al described a lower blood pressure in breast feeding mothers one hour after breast feeding. (Light et al., 2000) In the first weeks of breast feeding, women produce around 800 millilitres of milk daily. With the production of breast milk large volume shifts take place, these may cause a problem in patients with reduced left ventricular function.

The fluctuations in blood pressure may be harmful in severely symptomatic patients and bottle feeding should be considered. Lactation is also associated with a risk of bacteraemia secondary to mastitis.

6. Angina in the pregnant patient

A 41 year old patient presented to the emergency department with acute chest pain. There was a myocardial infarction at young age in her family history. She was 18 weeks pregnant with her first child. She did not take any alcohol or medication during pregnancy. But she was continuing smoking during pregnancy. She had a blood pressure of 135/85mmHg, a pulse of 95 beats per minute and auscultation of the chest revealed normal breath sounds without rales. The ECG was normal. Transthoracic echocardiography revealed no wall abnormalities. Troponine levels were normal. During exercise testing she performed 92% of expected and during testing a down sloping ST depression of 2-3 mm was found in lead II, III and aVf.

6.1 Signs and symptoms

Evaluating chest pain in pregnant women can be challenging, since chest pain in pregnancy is common and can be caused by various conditions. Most often chest pain is caused by gastro-oesophageal reflux which is benign in most cases. Chest pain should never be ignored as it may also represent possible life threatening disease such as pericarditis, myocarditis, aortic dissection, hypertensive crisis, pulmonary thrombo-embolism or acute coronary syndrome. Urgent complete cardiac review is always appropriate if a pregnant woman presents with chest pain.

Physical examination can be misleading, hypotension and tachycardia are physiological responses to normal pregnancy (as describe in sub-chapter 3). In this case normal lung examination and oxygen saturation made pneumonic disease less likely, but pulmonary thrombo-embolism remained a possibility. Measuring blood pressure in both arms is important since aortic dissection is a part of the differential diagnosis.

6.2 Diagnostic testing

Criteria for ACS in pregnancy are the same as in non pregnant women, consisting of a combination of symptoms, ECG changes and positive cardiac markers. Normal diagnostic tests can be used in pregnancy, but outcome has to be evaluated against normal pregnancy values, since abnormal values can be normal in pregnancy. Table (2) gives a brief summary of the changes most often seen in diagnostic tests.

Diagnostic test	Effect of normal pregnancy
Electrocardiogram	Left axis deviation and Q waves in lead III and aVF, inverted T waves in lead III
Exercise test	Decreased exercise tolerance
Echocardiogram	Increase in left ventricular mass, mild mitral regurgitation
Serum creatinine kinase	Elevated during labour
Troponin	Not affected during normal pregnancy

Table 2. The changes in diagnostic tests in normal pregnancy.

The electrocardiogram (ECG) changes as a result of the upward shift of the diaphragm with the growing uterus. A left axis deviation with Q waves in lead III and aVF is seen in the third trimester. T waves can be inverted in lead III, V1 and V2. In case of a caesarean section with general anaesthesia ST depression is seen often. (Prebitero et al., 2009)

The use of echocardiography is safe in pregnancy because echocardiography does not involve radiation. Detection of wall motion abnormalities can be used as a sign of possible acute coronary syndrome. In normal patients exercise tests are used to confirm the diagnosis of coronary artery disease or after ACS to establish exercise capacity and exclude residual ischemia. In pregnancy it is advisable to use submaximal exercise (<70% of the maximum predicted heart rate) testing, since fetal bradycardia and absence of body movement have been described after heavy maternal exercise. (Elkayam et al., 1998) There is no evidence of increased risk of spontaneous abortion after exercise testing.

Biomarkers are used in the cardiological practice to confirm the diagnosis of acute coronary syndrome. During labour elevated creatinine kinase (CK) and CK MB are found due to uterine contractions. These levels normalize during the second day after labour. (Poh & Lee, 2010) Troponine I is not elevated in normal pregnancy, as a result troponin I is the recommended biomarker in pregnancy. However, troponin I serum levels can be elevated in patients with pre-eclampsia and hypertensive crisis. It is not totally clear whether this is a sign of cardiac ischemia in these partients.

Chest radiography is only used in pregnancy during emergency medical conditions. If proper shielding of the abdomen is used radiation of chest radiography is considered relatively safe (especially in the third trimester). (Hirshfeld et al., 2005)

6.3 Treatment choices in patients with chest pain

The choice of treatment is dependent on the diagnosis and the presence of ECG changes. In patients without any ECG changes, other causes of chest pain should be considered; troponin should be measured in all patients. In women with ACS, conservative treatment (bed)rest, nitrates and beta blockers is advised. In NSTEMI patients a careful assessment should be made. Troponin levels, hemodynamic state and relief of pain determine whether the patient should have a coronary angiogram. A coronary angiogram will reveal the origin of the problem, eg dissection, thrombus. But a conservative treatment may be best in the majority of patients. STEMI patients need immediate treatment and PCI as first choice treatment should be performed as soon as possible.

In patients with angina catherization should be considered. If proper shielding of the abdomen is used, radiation dose is low. An interventional procedure may result in a fetal exposure of <1 rad. Termination of pregnancy is generally not recommended, although it may be considered when the fetal radiation dose exceeds 10 rad. (Roth & Elkayam, 2008)

The patient became pain free after the use of nitroglycerine and was treated with beta blockade. Further pregnancy was uneventful and she delivered a healthy baby boy at 39 weeks after spontaneous vaginal delivery.

7. Acute coronary syndrome during the first or second trimester of pregnancy

A 38 year old patient came to the emergency department with acute chest pain. She was 25 weeks pregnant with her second child. The first pregnancy was complicated by preeclampsia. She has no dyspnoea, syncope, cough or fever. She did not smoke nor use any alcohol or medication during pregnancy. She had a blood pressure of 100/60mmHg, a pulse of 105 beats per minute and was tachypnoeic at 24 breath per minute. Oxygen saturation by pulse oximetry was 99%. Auscultation of the chest revealed normal breath sounds without rales. The heart sounds were normal, no murmur or gallop was heard. Abdominal examination did not reveal any abnormalities and there was no oedema.

The results of the ECG were consistent with STEMI of the anterior wall with ST elevation in V1-V3 and ST depression in lead II, III and aVF. Transthoracic echocardiography revealed a dyskenetic left anterior wall. The patient underwent coronary angiography three hours after onset of complaints and revealed a thrombotic obstruction of the left main artery with TIMI flow grade 1.

7.1 Cause of ACS

ACS in pregnancy has other causes than in the non-pregnant state. In the review of Roth and Elkayam only 40% (41 of the 103 patients) was caused by coronary artery stenosis. (Roth & Elkayam, 2008) Other causes were thrombus in 8%, coronary artery dissection in 27%, vascular spasm in 2% and normal coronary arteries were found in 13% of the patients. (Roth & Elkayam, 2008) ACS has been noted to occur more often in the anterior wall. (Iadanzo et al., 2007)

Coronary dissection is very rare in the non-pregnant population, but more frequently seen in pregnancy (27%) especially in patients with ACS in the peripartum period (50%). Excess of progesterone is thought to be one of the causes of coronary dissection, since it causes biochemical changes of collagen in the coronary vessel wall and weakens the media. The impact of increased blood volume and cardiac output may cause extra wall stress which is hypothesised to be an additional factor (Roth & Elkayam, 2008) also autoimmune conditions, such as systemic lupus erythromatosis and anti-phospolipid-antibody syndrome, have been linked to coronary artery dissection. (Nallamonthu et al., 2005)

Normal coronary artery morphology is found in 13% of patients, perhaps caused by transient coronary spasm or thrombus. Vascular spasm was found in 2% of the case reports described by Roth. (Roth & Elkayam, 2008) Spasm might be caused by enhanced vascular reactivity to angiotensin II, norepinephrine and endothelial dysfunction. (Nisell et al., 1985) Vascular spasm in combination with the hypercoagulable state of pregnancy may cause coronary thrombus leading to acute coronary syndrome. Patients who continue to smoke during pregnancy have an increased risk of coronary artery thrombosis due to enhanced platelet aggregability in smokers.

7.2 Treatment

When tests have confirmed the diagnosis of acute coronary syndrome, it is important to make a treatment plan and inform the patient about maternal and fetal risks of all possible treatment options.

There is only limited information available on PCI during pregnancy. Nowadays pregnancy is not a contraindication for PCI and since PCI is the primary treatment for non-pregnant STEMI patients, more and more cases of stenting during pregnancy are published. With PCI as a treatment modality during pregnancy mortality of ACS has dropped. James described PCI in 135 patients (of which 127 were with stenting), but no information on outcome was published. In the first review of Roth and Elkayam in 1996 only 3 of the 125 patients had PCI. (Roth & Elkayam, 1996) Whereas in their second review 38 patients had a PCI, all with bare metal stenting. In this review 92 patients had a coronary angiogram (of which 43 were postpartum). After PCI one patient needed CABG because of extensive coronary dissection. (Roth & Elkayam, 2008)

The preference for bare metal stenting is caused by the requirement of dual anti-platelet treatment around the delivery and the lack of experience. The use of drug eluting stents has been described in 2 case reports. One patient with STEMI at 27 weeks of gestation received a drug eluting stent, she delivered a healthy child by elective caesarean section at 35 weeks. Antiplatelet therapy was continued during delivery. However, post partum she had a haemoglobin drop of 5 g/dL and needed a blood transfusion. (Al-Aqeedi & Al-Nabti, 2008)

Since pregnant women are excluded from most clinical trials no randomised controlled trials have been preformed on thrombolytic therapy, PCI or CABG in the pregnancy. However, thrombotic therapy is considered to be relatively contraindicated in patient with acute coronary syndrome because of bleeding complications. In stroke, pulmonary embolism and mechanical heart valve thrombosis there is some clinical experience with several strategies such as tPA, urokinase and streptokinase. This medication does not cross the utero-placental barrier. (Leohardt et al., 2006) Maternal and fetal outcomes were favourable, but complications, as maternal haemorrhage, fetal loss, abruption placenta, preterm delivery and post partum haemorrhage have been reported in up to 10% and maternal mortality was 1.2 %. (Turrentine et al., 1995) The risk of haemorrhage is highest in the peripartum period (Murugappan et al,. 2006) and given the high incidence of coronary dissection in pregnancy, the use of thrombolytic therapy could lead to haemorrhage and further progression of the dissection. Thrombolytic therapy should be considered in case of thrombosis and possibly when primary PCI is not available. (Roth & Elkayam, 2008)

Very limited data is available on coronary artery bypass grafting (CABG) during pregnancy, no conclusion on safety for the mother or the unborn child can be made. In normal non-pregnant patients with ACS CABG is used when multiple vessels or the left main coronary artery are involved. (Nallamonthu et al., 2005) In the data by James 61 women underwent CABG, but there was no specific data on outcome in these patients. In the case study of Roth and Elkayam 10 patients were described who underwent CABG, of which were 7 due to coronary artery dissection, (Roth & Elkayam, 2008) in these cases one fetal death and one late maternal death were reported. (Garvey, 1998) Large differences in maternal mortality rates were found for ACS in pregnant women in the last decades, ranging from 5,1%(James et al., 2006) to 38%. (Koul et al., 2001) The decline in mortality rate could be explained by the detection of ACS in less severely ill patients as well as improvement in treatment options in the last decades. (Roth & Elkayam, 2008)

7.3 Delivery

Delivery should be postponed if possible for at least 2 or 3 weeks after the ACS to allow adequate healing. (Prebitero et al., 2009) Anti-platelet therapy should be continued in case of recent stent implantation, low dose aspirin is also advisable in patient with other forms of coronary artery disease, but doctors should be aware of a higher risk of post partum haemorrhage. Vaginal delivery with shortened second stage of labour and adequate pain relief can be safe. Caesarean section is the preferred mode of delivery in patients with cardiac instability.

7.4 Post partum period

Close monitoring on a medium care unit may be advisable for the first 3 days after delivery. With anticoagulant and anti-platelet therapy given during pregnancy, special attention should be paid to major haemorrhage. Ideally monitoring should be done in a unit with neonatal monitoring.

In our patient thrombosuction was performed and a bare metal stent was inserted. She was treated with heparin for 24 hours and received aspirin, beta blockade and nitrates during the remainder of the pregnancy. Clopidogrel was not given during pregnancy. She delivered 12 weeks later at 37 weeks by the assisted vaginal route. Epidural pain medication was given to limit pain and stress. A healthy girl (3045 gram) was born. After delivery she was treated with a statin and an ACE inhibitor.

8. Acute coronary syndrome in the third trimester

A 34 year old patient presented to the emergency department with acute chest pain. She was 36 weeks pregnant. The results of the ECG were consistent with acute myocardial infarction of the anterior wall. The patient underwent cardiac catheterisation two hours after onset of symptoms, coronary angiogram revealed a coronary artery dissection of the left anterior descending artery.

8.1 ACS in the third trimester

Coronary artery disease in the peripartum period differs from ACS in the antepartum period in terms of coronary abnormality, cause, treatment options and mortality rate. Coronary dissection was the primary cause of coronary artery disease in the peripartum period (50%) and more commonly in post-partum period (34%) compared to antepartum period (11%). This is probably the result of hormonal changes and the stress on the walls of the coronary arteries during labour. In some cases an association with the administration of the medicine terbutaline (a medicine used to stop early uterine contractions) was found.

The mortality rate in patients with ACS in the peripartum period is 18% versus 9% in the antepartum and postpartum period. (Roth & Elkayam, 2008) This was also shown in the study of Ladner, who reprted a mortality rate of 19% in the peripartum period. No specific cause for the high maternal mortality in the peripartum period was given. Different causes for high mortality rates could be hypothesized. The symptoms could be misinterpreted during delivery and both patient delay as well as doctor delay could lead to late recognition of ACS. A second reason could be the complication and mortality rate is relatively higher in patients with coronary artery dissection compared to coronary arthrosclerosis. (Basso et al., 1996) A third reason is that major haemorrhage may result from anti-thrombotic therapy. And finally, cardiac failure after delivery caused by autotransfusion with stressing the injured myocytes could lead to maternal death. Moran et al described myocardial ischemia in normal patients during elective caesarean section. By using Holter monitoring and analysis of troponin I he showed ischemic changes in 8% of the patients and 81% had ST segment changes. None of these patients needed any form of treatment. This study showed that even normal healthy women experience ECG changes which may reflect some myocardial ischemia during caesarean section. (Moran et al., 2001)

8.2 Treatment in peripartum period

Treatment options are limited in the peripartum period, since anticoagulation and antithrombotic therapy should be discontinued 24 hours prior to delivery to avoid major bleeding complications. PCI is the treatment of choice in patients with STEMI. As pregnant patients have a substantial higher chance of coronary dissection and a high maternal mortality, PCI should be preformed in a larger referral centre with cardiothoracic surgery standby.

8.3 Delivery and postpartum period

Caesarean section prior to CAG is a possible strategy in patients with ACS diagnosed after 32 to 34 weeks of gestation. (Hameed & Sklansky, 2007) At this point fetal outcome is generally good and maternal benefit is high because of reduced stress during the last weeks of pregnancy and the use of antithrombotic therapy after PCI. Close monitoring on a medium care unit may be advisable for the first 3 days after delivery.

It is very important to consider ACS in peripartum patients with acute chest pain. Early recognition and diagnosis can save lives. A healthy baby girl was born at 39 weeks. The patient stayed in the hospital until 3 days after delivery.

9. Acute coronary syndrome in the postpartum period

After delivery of a healthy girl, a 31 year old patient was treated with bromocriptine to suppress lactation. Four days after delivery she presented to the emergency department with acute severe chest pain. The ECG showed an acute anterior myocardial infarction with ST elevation in V1-V3. Coronary angiography revealed a dissection of the left anterior descending artery and she was treated with bare metal stenting. She remained in the hospital for 3 more days and was treated with betacblockade, aspirin and clopidogrel.

9.1 Post partum ACS

Coronary dissection was found in 34% of the coronary angiograms and this was the most frequent cause of ACS in the postpartum period as it was in the peripartum period. Postpartum, some cases of ACS are associated with the administration of medicine. There are nineteen cases reported of ACS after the administration of bromocriptine, which is used to suppress lactation. Bromocriptine has dopaminergic agonist properties and may have vasopastic effects which can lead to thrombus formation. (Hopp et al., 1996) This medication has been taken off the market as a lactation suppressant because of these reports. The second medicine associated with ACS is ergotamine, which is commonly used to prevent post partum haemorrhage by stimulating uterine contractions. Ergot derivatives are known to reduce the capacity of the intravascular lumen by 15-20% in normal coronary arteries. Eight cases of postpartum myocardial infarction have been described. (Eom, 2005) It is important to consider ACS as a possible complication before administration of this medicine in high risk patients (high age and cardiovascular risk factors).

9.2 Treatment post partum ACS

After delivery the treatment options are greater. Only maternal health determines the treatment, as is usual in "normal" cardiac patients PCI is the treatment of choice. Drug eluting stents can be used now. However, the uterine vascular bed has to be considered a large wound until one week after delivery.

Bromocriptin, ergotamine and terbutaline have been associated with post partum ACS.

10. Neonatal outcome

Neonatal outcome is strongly correlated with maternal outcome. In the first report of Roth and Elkayam 16 fetal deaths in 125 pregnancies (13%) were reported, of which 10 (62%) associated with maternal death. (Roth & Elkayam, 1996) In the second report only a 9% fetal death rate was reported, of which two were elective terminations because of potential drug teratogenicity. (Roth & Elkayam, 2008) Ladner et al described low birth weight and prematurity in patients with antenatal ACS and a 10% fetal death rate was reported in patients with intrapartum ACS. (Ladner et al., 2005)

Fetal mortality is high in cardiac surgery during pregnancy with rates as high as 30% (Parry & Westaby, 1996). Factors which predicted an adverse fetal outcome were severity of maternal illness, total operative time, emergency surgery, reoperation, advanced maternal age and gestational age. (Barth, 2009)

During cardiopulmonary bypass, continuous fetal monitoring should be performed. The fetal heart rate can be used as an indicator of placental perfusion to guide bypass pump flow. (Chandrasekhar et al., 2009) Uterine monitoring is essential to allow early control of these contractions as they are associated with significant fetal loss. (Parry & Westaby, 1996) Deleterious effects on the fetus are thought to be related to hypotension, hypothermia, embolic complications and inadequate placental flow. Caesarean delivery prior to CABG or PCI can be considered from 28 weeks of gestation. (Barth, 2009)

Fetal mortality in PCI compared to CABG is low. Proper shielding of the abdomen is essential in fetal protection. (Roth & Elkayam, 2008) Where chest radiography is considered relatively safe (especially in the third trimester). Cardiac catherization and intervention procedures may result higher fetal exposure with some chance of fetal abnormalities, especially when used in the first trimester.

11. Conclusion

Acute coronary syndrome in women of childbearing age is rare, but pregnancy has shown to increase the risk of ACS 3- to 4-fold. (James et al., 2006) The overall incidence of pregnancy related acute coronary syndrome was reported between 2.7 and 6.2 per 100,000 deliveries and seems to have been increased in the last decade. Maternal age is one of the most important risk factor for ACS during pregnancy. Mortality rate has declined over the last decades from 19% in 1922-1994 to 5,1% in 2001-2002, probably as a result of improvement in treatment modalities.

Evaluating chest pain in pregnant woman can be challenging, since chest pain in pregnancy is common and may be caused by benign as well as life threatening diseases. Physical examination and diagnostic tests can be misleading, since normal pregnancy changes the results of these tests. Coronary artery disease in pregnancy has different causes than seen in non-pregnant women, artherosclerosis is less frequently found, whereas thrombus, dissection, spasm and normal coronary arteries are more often reported. In table 3 an overview is given of the management and outcome in the different patient groups.

Not all medication is safe during pregnancy, fetal and maternal risks have to be taken into account when medication is given. Pregnancy is not a contraindication for PCI anymore and this is probably the main reason maternal mortality has fallen recently. Very limited data is

Patient group	Counselling	First treatment choice	Maternal outcome	Fetal outcome
Previous ACS	Check medication	Medication	No data	No data
ACS and impaired LV function	Risk stratification	Medication	No data, high risk	No data
ACS antepartum	Not applicable	PCI	9 % mortality	11 % mortality
ACS peripartum	Not applicable	PCI	18 % mortality	5 % mortality
ACS postpartum	Not applicable	PCI	9 % mortality	No fetal mortality

Table 3 Oversight of different patient groups in ACS in pregnancy.

available on CABG during pregnancy, and it should only be considered when all other therapeutic options have failed. Neonatal outcome is strongly correlated with maternal outcome; reported mortality was highest in the peripartum period.

The delivery should be planned by a multidisciplinary team consisting of an obstetrician, anaesthesiologist and cardiologist. Women with adequate cardiac output may tolerate induction of labour and vaginal delivery, but it is possible to create a potentially more stable environment during a caesarean section in high risk patients. Close monitoring in-hospital for at least one week after delivery is advised for patients with ACS in pregnancy.

12. References

Al-Aqeedi, R. & Al-Nabti, A. (2008). Drug-eluting stent implantation for acute myocardial infarction during pregnancy with use of glycoprotein IIb/IIIa inhibitor, aspirin and clopidogrel. *J Invasive Cardiol,* Vol. 20, No. 5, (May 2008), pp. e146-149, ISSN1557-2501

Badui, E. & Enciso, R. (1996). Acute myocardial infarction during pregnancy and puerperium: a review. *Angiology,* Vol. 47, No. 8, (August 1996), pp. 739-756, ISSN 0003-3197

Barth, W. (2009). Cardiac surgery in pregnancy. *Clin Obstet Gynecol,* Vol. 52, No. 4, (December 2009), pp. 630-46, ISSN 1532-5520

Basso, C.; Morgagni, G.; & Thiene, G. (1996) Spontaneous coronary artery dissection: a neglected cause of acute myocardial ischaemia and sudden death. *Heart,* Vol. 75, No. 5, (May 1996), pp. 451-454, ISSN 1355-6037

Bonow, R.; Carabello, B. & Chatterjee, K.; et al. (2008). Focused update incorporated into the ACC/AHA 2006 guidelines for the management of patients with valvular heart disease: a report of the American College of Cardiology/American Heart Association Task Force on Practice Guidelines (Writing Committee to Revise the 1998 Guidelines for the Management of Patients With Valvular Heart Disease): endorsed by the Society of Cardiovascular Anesthesiologists, Society for Cardiovascular Angiography and Interventions, and Society of Thoracic Surgeons. *Circulation,* Vol. 118, No. 15, (October 2008), pp. e523-661, ISSN 1524-4539

Butters, L.; Kennedy, S. & Rubin, P. (1990). Atenolol in essential hypertension during pregnancy. *BMJ*, Vol. 301, No. 6752, (September 1990), pp 87-89, ISSN 0959-8138

Caton, A.; Bell, E. & Druschel, C.; et al. (2009). Antihypertensive medication use during pregnancy and the risk of cardiovascular malformations. *Hypertension*, Vol. 54, No.1, (July 2009), pp. 63-70, ISSN 1524-4563

Cecchini, M.; Sassi, F. & Chisholm, D.; et al. (2010). Tackling of unhealthy diets, physical inactivity, and obesity: health effects and cost-effectiveness. *Lancet*, Vol. 376, No. 9754, (November 2010), pp. 1775-1784, ISSN 1474-547X

Chandrasekhar. S.; Cook, C. & Collard, C. (2009). Cardiac surgery in the parturient. *Anesth Analg*, Vol. 108, No. 3, (March 2009), pp. 777-785, ISSN 1526-7598

Clark, S.; Belfort, M. & Hankins, G.; et al. (2008) Maternal death in the 21st century: causes, prevention, and relationship to cesarean delivery. *Am J Obstet Gynecol*, Vol. 199, No. 1, (July 2008), pp. e1-5, ISSN 1097-6868

CLASP. (1994). CLASP: a randomised trial of low-dose aspirin for the prevention and treatment of pre-eclampsia among 9364 pregnant women. CLASP (Collaborative Low-dose Aspirin Study in Pregnancy) Collaborative Group. *Lancet*, Vol. 343, No. 8898, (March 1994), pp. 619-629, ISSN 0140-6736

Coolman, M.; de Groot, C. & Steegers-Theunissen, R. et al. (2006). Concentrations of plasminogen activators and their inhibitors in blood preconceptionally, during and after pregnancy. *Eur J Obstet Gynecol Reprod Biol*, Vol. 128, No. 1-2, (September-October 2006), pp. 22-28, ISSN 0301-2115

Deneux-Tharaux, C.; Carmona, E. & Breart, G.; et al. (2006). Postpartum maternal mortality and cesarean delivery. *Obstet Gynecol*, Vol. 108, No. 3, (September 2006), pp. 541-548, ISSN 0029-7844

Elkayam, U. &, Gleicher, N. (1998). Hemodynamics and cardiac function during normal pregnancy and the puerperium. *Cardiac Problems in Pregnancy*. Wiley-Liss. ISBN 0-471-16358-9 New York, United States of America

Eom, M.; Lee, J.; Chung, J. & Lee, H. (2005). An autopsy case of postpartum acute myocardial infarction associated with postpartum ergot alkaloids administration in old-aged pregnant women. *Yonsei Med J*, Vol. 46, No. 6, (December 2005), pp.866-869, ISSN 0513-5796

Fletcher, A.; Alkjaersig, N. & Burstein R. (1979). The influence of pregnancy upon blood coagulation and plasma fibrinolytic enzyme function. *Am J Obstet Gynecol*, Vol. 134, No. 7, (August 1979), pp. 743-751, ISSN 0002-9378

Garvey. P.; Elovitz, M. & Landsberger. E. (1998). Aortic dissection and myocardial infarction in a pregnant patient with Turner syndrome. *Obstet Gynecol*, Vol. 91, No 5, (May 1998), pp. 864, ISSN 0029-7844

Gibson, P. & Rosene-Montella, K. (2001). Drugs in pregnancy. Anticoagulants. *Best Pract Res Clin Obstet Gynaecol*, Vol. 15, No. 6, (December 2001), pp. 847-861, ISSN 1521-6934

Grewal, J.; Siu, S. & Sermer, M.; et al. (2009). Pregnancy outcomes in women with dilated cardiomyopathy. *J Am Coll Cardiol*, Vol. 55, No. 1, (December 2009), pp. 45-52, ISSN 1558-3597

Hameed, A. & Sklansky, M. (2007). Pregnancy: maternal and fetal heart disease. *Curr Probl Cardiol*, Vol. 32, No. 8, (August 2007), pp.419-494, ISSN 0146-2806

Hirshfeld, J.; Balter, S. & Lindsay, B.; et al. (2005). ACCF/AHA/HRS/SCAI clinical competence statement on physician knowledge to optimize patient safety and image quality in fluoroscopically guided invasive cardiovascular procedures: a report of the American College of Cardiology Foundation/American Heart Association/American College of Physicians Task Force on Clinical Competence and Training. *Circulation*, Vol. 111, No. 4, (February 2005), pp. 511-532, ISSN 1524-4539

Hopp, L.; Haider, B. & Iffy, L. (1996). Myocardial infarction postpartum in patients taking bromocriptine for the prevention of breast engorgement. *Int J Cardiol*, Vol. 57, No. 3, (December 1996), pp. 227-232, ISSN 0167-5273

Hunter, S. & Robson, S. (1992). Adaptation of the maternal heart in pregnancy. *Br Heart J*, Vol. 68, No. 6, (December 1992), pp. 540-543, ISSN 0007-0769

Iadanza, A.; Del Pasqua, A. & Favilli, R.; et al. (2007). Acute ST elevation myocardial infarction in pregnancy due to coronary vasospasm: a case report and review of literature. *Int J Cardiol*, Vol. 115, No. 1, (January 2007), pp. 81-85, ISSN 1874-1754

James, A.; Jamison, M. & Myers, E.; et al. (2006). Acute myocardial infarction in pregnancy: a United States population-based study. *Circulation*, Vol. 113, No. 12, (March 2006), pp. 1564-1571, ISSN 1524-4539

Joglar, J. & Page, R. Treatment of cardiac arrhythmias during pregnancy: safety considerations. *Drug Saf*, Vol. 20, No. 1, (January 1999), pp. 85-94, ISSN 0114-5916

Karamermer, Y. & Roos-Hesselink, J. (2007). Pregnancy and adult congenital heart disease. *Expert Rev Cardiovasc Ther*, Vol. 5, No. 5, (September 2007), pp. 859-869, ISSN 1744-8344

Karthikeyan, V.; Ferner, R. & Beevers, D.; et al. (2011). Are angiotensin-converting enzyme inhibitors and angiotensin receptor blockers safe in pregnancy: a report of ninety-one pregnancies. *J Hypertens*, Vol. 29, No. 2, (February 2011), pp, 396-399, ISSN 1473-5598

Koul, A.; Hollander, G. & Shani, J.; et al. (2001). Coronary artery dissection during pregnancy and the postpartum period: two case reports and review of literature. *Catheter Cardiovasc Interv*, Vol. 52, No. 1, (January 2001), pp. 88-94, ISSN 1522-1946

Ladner, H.; Danielsen, B. & Gilbert, W. (2005). Acute myocardial infarction in pregnancy and the puerperium: a population-based study. *Obstet Gynecol*, Vol. 105, No. 3, (March 2005), pp. 480-484, ISSN 0029-7844

Leonhardt, G.; Gaul, C. & Schleussner, E.; et al. (2006) Thrombolytic therapy in pregnancy. *J Thromb Thrombolysis*, Vol. 21, No. 3, (June 2006), pp. 271-276, ISSN 0929-5305

Liggins, G. & Howie, R. (1972). A controlled trial of antepartum glucocorticoid treatment for prevention of the respiratory distress syndrome in premature infants. *Pediatrics*, Vol. 50, No. 4, (October 1972), pp. 515-525, ISSN 0031-4005

Light, K.; Smith, T. & Amico, J.; et al. (2000) Oxytocin responsivity in mothers of infants: a preliminary study of relationships with blood pressure during laboratory stress and normal ambulatory activity. *Health Psychol*, Vol. 19, No. 6, (November 2000), pp. 560-567, ISSN 0278-6133

Lydakis, C.; Lip, G.; Beevers, M. & Beevers, D. (1999).Atenolol and fetal growth in pregnancies complicated by hypertension. *Am J Hypertens*, Vol. 12, No. 6, (June 1999), pp. 541-547, ISSN 0895-7061

Manders, M.; Sonder, G.; Mulder, E. & Visser, G. (1997). The effects of maternal exercise on fetal heart rate and movement patterns. *Early Hum Dev*, Vol. 48, No. 3, (May 1997), pp. 237-247, ISSN 0378-3782

Mendelsohn, M. & Karas, R. (1999) The protective effects of estrogen on the cardiovascular system. *N Engl J Med*, Vol. 340, No. 23, (June 1999) pp. 1801-1811, ISSN 0028-4793

Mezzacappa, E.; Kelsey, R.; Myers, M. & Katkin, E. (2001). Breast-feeding and maternal cardiovascular function. *Psychophysiology*, Vol. 38, No. 6, (November 2001), pp. 988-997, ISSN 0048-5772

Moran, C.; Ni Bhuinneain, M. & Gardiner, J.; et al. (2001). Myocardial ischaemia in normal patients undergoing elective Caesarean section: a peripartum assessment. *Anaesthesia*, Vol. 56, No. 11, (November 2001), pp. 1051-1058, ISSN 0003-2409

Murugappan, A.; Coplin, W. & Wechsler, L.; et al. (2005). Thrombolytic therapy of acute ischemic stroke during pregnancy. *Neurology*, Vol. 66, No. 5, (March 2006), pp. 768-770, ISSN 1526-632X

Nallamothu, B.; Saint, M.; Saint, S. & Mukherjee, D. (2005). Clinical problem-solving. Double jeopardy. *N Engl J Med*, Vol. 353, No. 1, (July 2005), pp. 75-80, ISSN 1533-4406

Newstead-Angel, J. & Gibson, P. (2009). Cardiac drug use in pregnancy: safety, effectiveness and obstetric implications. *Expert Rev Cardiovasc Ther*, Vol. 7, No. 12, (December 2009), pp. 1569-1580, ISSN 1744-8344

Nisell, H.; Hjemdahl, P. & Linde, B. (1985). Cardiovascular responses to circulating catecholamines in normal pregnancy and in pregnancy-induced hypertension. *Clin Physiol*, Vol. 5, No. 5, (October 1985), pp. 479-493, ISSN 0144-5979

Ogden, C.; Carroll, M. & Flegal, K.; et al. (2006). Prevalence of overweight and obesity in the United States, 1999-2004. *JAMA*, Vol. 295, No. 13, (April 2006), pp. 1549-1555, ISSN 1538-3598

Parry, A. & Westaby, S. (1996). Cardiopulmonary bypass during pregnancy. *Ann Thorac Surg*, Vol. 61, No. 6, (June 1996), 1865-1869, ISSN 0003-4975

Pierre-Louis, B.; Singh, P. & Frishman, W. (2008). Acute inferior wall myocardial infarction and percutaneous coronary intervention of the right coronary during active labor: a clinical report and review of the literature. *Cardiol Rev*, Vol. 16, No. 5, (September-October 2008), pp. 260-268, ISSN 1538-4683

Pina, I. Cardiovascular disease in women: challenge of the middle years. *Cardiol Rev*, Vol. 19, No. 2. (March 2011), pp. 71-75, ISSN 1538-4683

Poh, C. & Lee, C. (2010)Acute myocardial infarction in pregnant women. *Ann Acad Med Singapore*, Vol. 39, No. 3, (March 2010), pp. 247-253, ISSN 0304-4602

Pollack, P.; Shields, K. & Stepanavage, M.; et al. (2005). Pregnancy outcomes after maternal exposure to simvastatin and lovastatin. *Birth Defects Res A Clin Mol Teratol*, Vol. 73, No. 11, (November 2005), pp.888-896, ISSN 1542-0752

Presbitero, P.; Boccuzzi, G.; Groot, C. & Roos-Hesselink, J. (2009). Chapter 33 Pregnancy and Heart Disease, *ESC Textbook of Cardiovascular Medicine*, Blackwell publishing, Inc. ISBN 1-4051-2695-7, Massachusetts, United States of America

Quan, A. (2006). Fetopathy associated with exposure to angiotensin converting enzyme inhibitors and angiotensin receptor antagonists. *Early Hum Dev*, Vol. 82, No. 1, (January 2006), pp. 23-28, ISSN 0378-3782

Robson, S.; Hunter, S.; Boys, R. & Dunlop, W. (1989). Serial study of factors influencing changes in cardiac output during human pregnancy. *Am J Physiol*, Vol. 256, No. 4, (April 1989), pp. 1060-1065, ISSN 0002-9513

Roth, A. & Elkayam, U. (1996).Acute myocardial infarction associated with pregnancy. *Ann Intern Med*, Vol. 125, No. 9, (November 1996), pp. 751-762, ISSN 0003-4819

Roth, A. & Elkayam, U. (2008). Acute myocardial infarction associated with pregnancy. J *Am Coll Cardiol*, Vol. 52, No. 3, (July 2008), pp. 171-180, ISSN 1558-3597

Signore, C.; Spong, C. & Freeman, R. (28 October 2010). Overview of fetal assessment, in Up to date, 1 July 2011, Available from *www.utdol.com*

Siu, S.; Sermer, M. & Morton, B.; et al. (2001). Prospective multicenter study of pregnancy outcomes in women with heart disease. *Circulation*, Vol. 104, No. 5, (July 2001), pp. 515-521, ISSN 1524-4539

Skafar, D.; Xu, R. & Sowers, J.; et al. (1997). Clinical review 91: Female sex hormones and cardiovascular disease in women. *J Clin Endocrinol Metab*, Vol. 82, No. 12, (December 1997), pp. 3913-3918, ISSN 0021-972X

Turrentine, M.; Braems, G. & Ramirez, M. (1995). Use of thrombolytics for the treatment of thromboembolic disease during pregnancy. *Obstet Gynecol Surv*, Vol. 50, No. 7, (July 1995), pp. 534-41, ISSN 0029-7828

Ulusoy, R.; Demiralp, E. & Kucukarslan, N.; et al. (2006). Aortic elastic properties in young pregnant women. *Heart Vessels*, Vol. 21, No. 1, (Januari 2006), pp. 38-41, ISSN 0910-8327

Ventura, S.; Abma, J.; Mosher, W. & Henshaw, S. (2004). Estimated pregnancy rates for the United States, 1990-2000: an update. *Natl Vital Stat Rep*, Vol. 52, No. 23, (June 2004), pp. 1-9, ISSN 1551-8922

von Dadelszen, P.; Ornstein, M. & Magee, L.; et al. (2000). Fall in mean arterial pressure and fetal growth restriction in pregnancy hypertension: a meta-analysis. *Lancet*, Vol. 355, No. 9198, (January 2000), pp. 87-92, ISSN 0140-6736

Yoshimura, T.; Ito, M.; Nakamura, T. & Okamura, H. (1992). The influence of labor on thrombotic and fibrinolytic systems. *Eur J Obstet Gynecol Reprod Biol*, Vol. 44, No. 3, (May 1992), pp. 195-199, ISSN 0301-2115

Part 2

Coronary Artery Disease Diagnostics

6

Cardiovascular Biomarkers for the Detection of Cardiovascular Disease

David C. Gaze
Dept of Chemical Pathology Clinical Blood Sciences,
St George's Healthcare NHS Trust, London,
UK

1. Introduction

Cardiovascular disease (CVD) is the leading cause of death in the Western World. Evidence from post mortem studies demonstrated the presence of atheromatous lesions in coronary arteries in children (Stary 2000). It is often thought of as a disease associated with a modern sedentary lifestyle and a lipid abundant diet Recently Allam and colleagues (Allam *et al.* 2011) have imaged fifty two ancient Egyptian mummies using multi slice computer tomography and identified atherosclerotic lesions (arterial wall calcification) in 45% of cases with calcification sites located in the aorta, coronary carotid, iliac and femoral arteries as well as in peripheral arteries.

1.1 Cardiovascular epidemiology

The incidence of CVD is higher than for any cancer or other non-CVD condition. CVD caused 29% of global deaths in 2004. It is predicted that by 2030 23 million people will die from a CVD. Data from the USA suggests that CVD was responsible for 34% of deaths in 2006 and over 151,000 Americans who died were <65 years old. The incidence of CVD is declining in the Western World even though rates of lifestyle associated risk factors such as obesity smoking and type II diabetes mellitus are increasing. The decline is in part due to advances in therapeutic and invasive intervention. In creating better outcomes for those with acute cardiac conditions, patients develop heart failure which requires longer term treatment and monitoring and may in fact be a greater health burden than the acute events themselves.

1.2 Cardiovascular pathophysiology

The blood vessels (figure 1) of the cardiovascular system are comprised of three layers, the tunica intima (endothelium), tunica media (concentric smooth muscle) and tunica adventia (longitudinal collagen fibres). The three layers are analogous to the endo-, myo- and epicardium of the heart respectively.

Plaque formation (atherogenesis) is initiated with damage to the endothelium. Cholesterol rich low density lipoprotein (LDL) particles enter the intimal layer via the LDL receptor protein (Brown and Goldstein 1979), a mosaic cell surface protein that recognizes

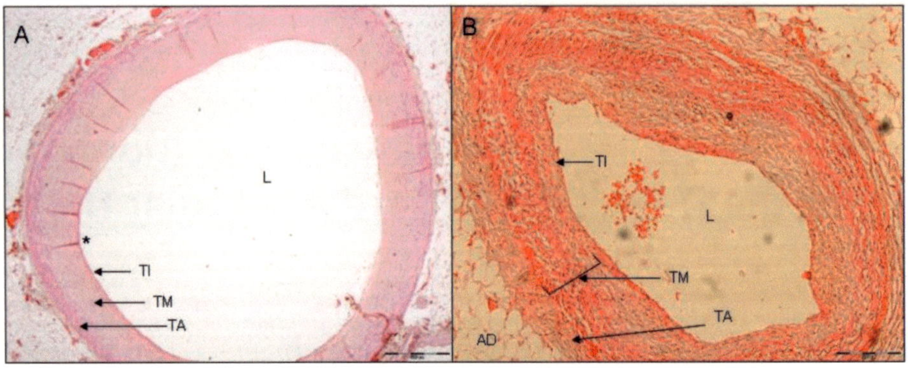

Fig. 1. A) Low powered haematoxylin and eosin (H&E) histological photomicrograph of a normal human artery (x40). B) Medium powered view (x200). AD, adipocytes; L, lumen; *, processing artefact; TI, tunica intima; TM, tunica media; TA, tunica adventia.

apolipoprotein B100 embedded in the LDL particle. It also recognizes apolipoprotein E found in chylomicrons and very low density lipoprotein remnants, or intermediate density lipoprotein. Macrophage cells accumulate oxidized lipid independently of the LDL receptor by endocytosis. This results in formation of juvenile raised fatty streaks within the endothelium. The macrophage release their lipid content and cytokines into the intima Cytokines stimulate intimal thickening by smooth muscle cell proliferation, which then secrete collagen, causing fibrosis (figure 2). The lesion appears raised and yellow.

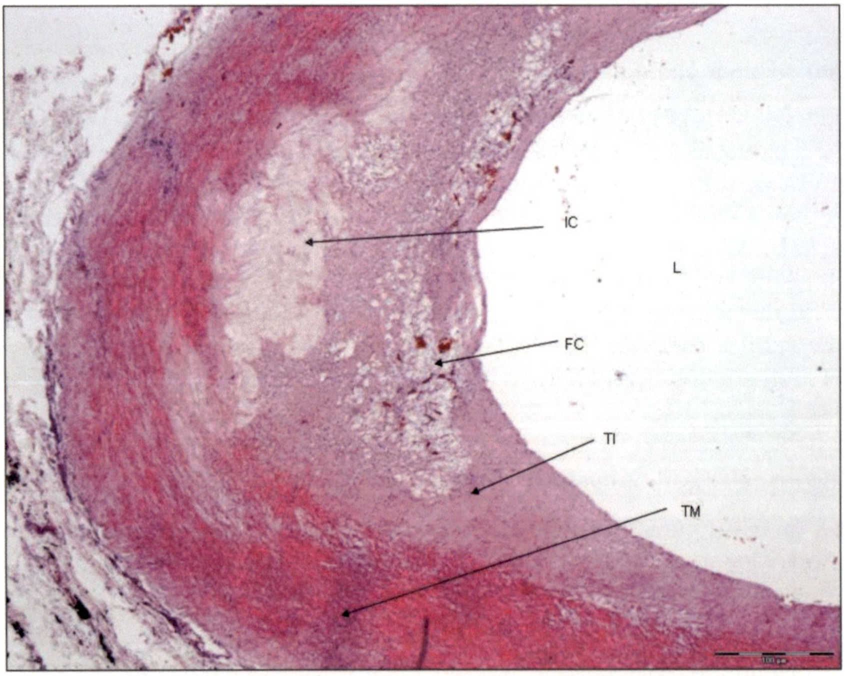

Fig. 2. Medium powered H&E histological micrograph of an intimal lesion (x200). FC, foam cell infiltrate; IC, intimal calcification; L, lumen; TI, tunica intima; TM, tunica media.

As the lesion develops, the medial layer of the vessel wall atrophies and the elastic lamina becomes disrupted. Collagen forms a fibrous cap over the lesion that appears hard and white (known as a fibrolipid plaque). The plaque contains macrophage laden with lipid (foam cells) as well as extracellular or 'free' lipid within the lesion. The endothelium is now in a fragile state. Ulceration of the cap occurs at weak points such as the shoulder region, near the endothelial lining. Rupture to the cap can cause turbulent blood flow in the lumen. The exposed lipid core causes aggregation of platelets and development of a thrombosis. This lesion grows due to further platelet aggregation and is responsible for narrowing of the lumen of the artery resulting in localized ischemia. Distal embolization of a piece of such thrombus may travel downstream and can completely occlude smaller arteries.

The symptomatic part of the continuum is known as the acute coronary syndrome (ACS) which is due to the rupture/erosion of the plaque. This produces, depending on the plaque size, vascular anatomy and presence of collateral vessels, a mismatch between the supply and demand for oxygen. A net reduction in supply compared to the demand results in ischemia. Tissue hypoxia proceeds resulting in inadequate blood/oxygen perfusion. If blood flow is not re-established, cardiac cell necrosis will occur. Post AMI survival results in remodelling processes in the myocardium and the development of cardiac failure.

2. Cardiovascular biomarkers

Cardiac biomarkers have played an important role in the diagnosis and management of patients with CVD since the 1950's (Gaze and Collinson 2005). The challenge has been the identification of a cardiospecific biomarker. A number of biomarkers are available which can be used for diagnosis and management of patients with CVD (figure 3). Many are not clinically measured due to cost and lack of an evidence base.

The cardiovascular biomarkers essentially fall into three categories. Those that identify patients at risk of atherosclerosis; those associated with plaque destabilisation and those which indicate rupture of the plaque and the detection of necrosis and cardiac insufficiency.

2.1 Plaque formation biomarkers

2.1.1 Cholesterol and lipid fractions

Cholesterol and lipoproteins such as oxidized low density lipoprotein (LDL), small dense LDL and intermediate density lipoprotein are atherogenic. The laboratory repertoire common for the determination of plaque development and progression include the measurement of cholesterol, triglycerides, high density lipoprotein (HDL) and calculation of LDL (Friedewald *et al.* 1972). Increasingly apolipoprotein-AI and lipoprotein B100 are measured. Direct measurement methods of LDL better reveal individuals at risk of CVD but are less often promoted due to the higher cost. A joint consensus statement by the American Diabetes Association and American College of Cardiology stated that direct LDL particle measurement by nuclear magnetic resonance (NMR) is superior to calculated LDL for assessing individual risk of CVD (Brunzell *et al.* 2008). Other lipid components such as small dense LDL and intermediate density lipoprotein which are particularly atherogenic can be measured but this is not common practice. Lipoprotein (a) contains a central core of LDL which is covalently bonded to a polypeptide chain of apolipoprotein a. This peptide shares sequence homology with plasminogen and has been proposed as a mechanism linking plaque rupture and the development of thrombosis.

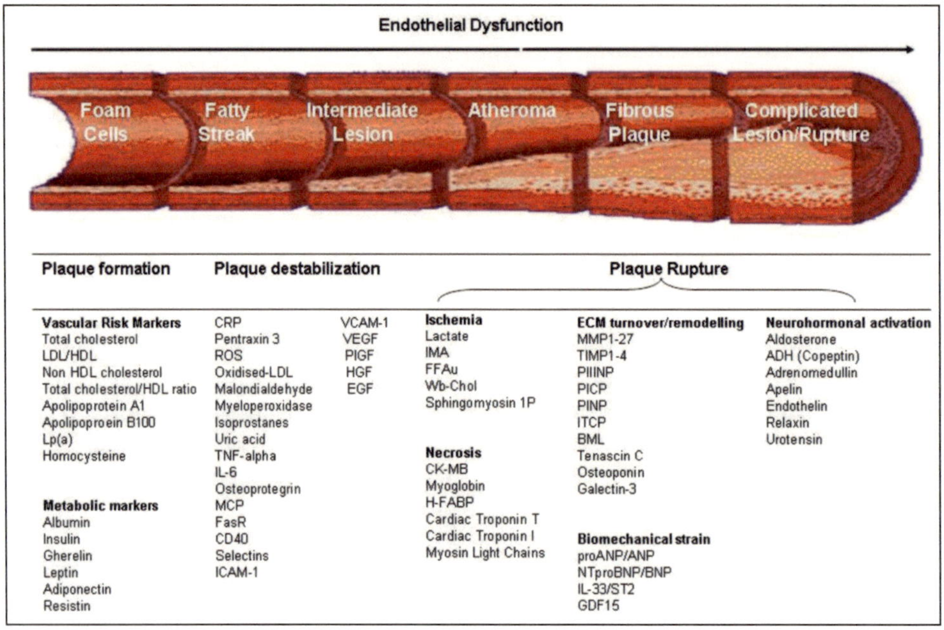

Fig. 3. Cardiovascular biomarkers for the assessment of cardiovascular disease. ADH, antidiuretic hormone; BML, basement membrane laminin; CRP, c-reactive protein; CD-40, cluster of differentiation-40; CK-MB, creatine kinase MB; EGF, epidermal growth factor; FFAu, unbound free fatty acid; GDF-15, growth differentiation factor 15; HDL, high densitiy lipoprotein; HGF, hepatic growth factor; ICAM-1, intracellular adhesion molecule 1; ICTP, type I collagen telopeptide, IL-6, interleukin 6; IL-33, interleukin 33; IMA, ischemia modified albumin; LDL, low densitiy lipoprotein; Lp(a), lipoprotein a; MCP, monocytes chemoattractant factor; MMP1 to 27, matrix metalloproteinase 1 to 27; PIIINP, procollagen III aminopropeptide; PICP, procollagen type I carboxy-terminal peptide; PINP, procollagen type I amino-terminal peptide; TIMP1 to 4, tissue inhibitors of matrix metalloproteinase 1 to 4; TNF-alpha, tumour necrosis factor alpha; VCAM-1, vascular cell adhesion molecule 1; VEGF, vascular endothelial growth factor; VLDL, very low density lipoprotein.

The biggest single cause of plaque initiation and inflammation is modified and oxidized LDL; however plaque development, progression and destabilisation are multifactorial. A number of assays exist for modified and oxidized LDL however they have not made the transition to automated immunoassay analysers. A large number of studies have been performed using oxidized LDL, however when this is translated to routine clinical use in the general chest pain population, the diagnostic and prognostic efficiency of the marker is questionable (Gaze *et al.* 2006b).

2.1.2 Homocysteine

Homocysteine is a sulphur containing amino acid (2-amino-4-sulfanylbutanoic acid, $C_4H_9NO_2S$), closely related to cysteine but with an additional methylene (CH_2) group. Homocysteine is not derived from dietary sources but rather it is biosynthesized from methionine (figure 4). Homocysteine can be recycled back to methionine or converted to cysteine catalysed by cystathionine β-synthase with pyridoxine (vitamin B_6) as a cofactor.

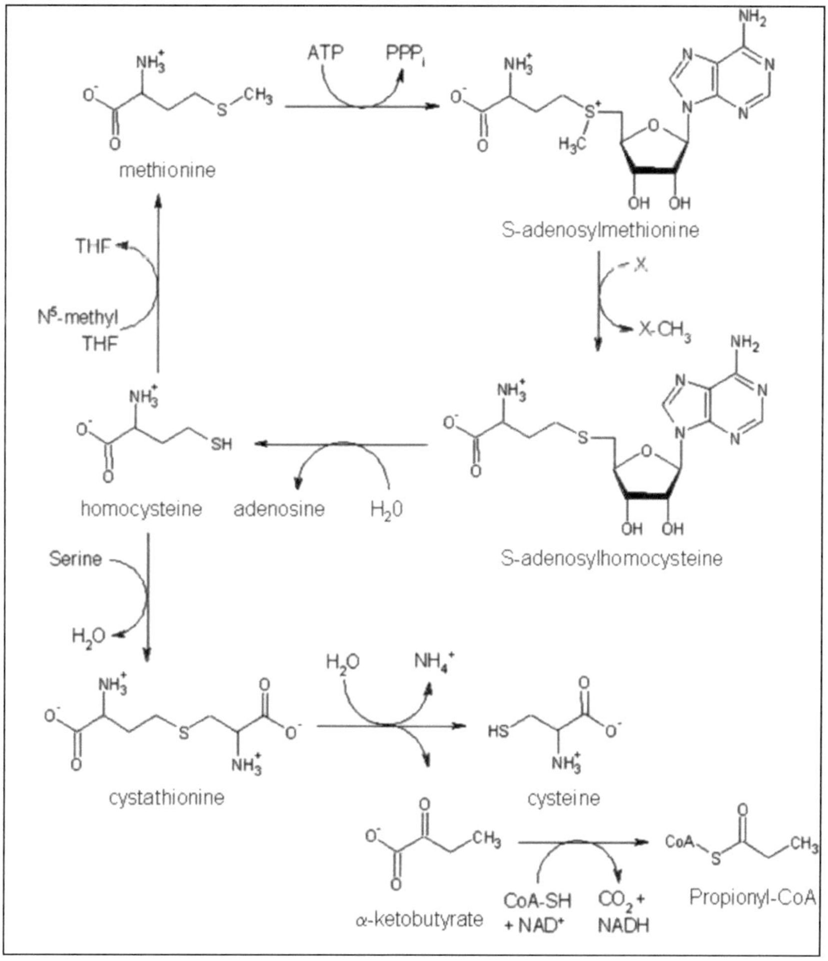

Fig. 4. Metabolism of Homocysteine. Homocysteine is biosynthesised by demethylation of dietary acquired methionine. Methionine receives adenosine triphosphate (ATP) to give S-adenosylmethionine (SAM), catalysed by S-adenosylmethionine synthetase. SAM transfers a methyl group to X (phospholipid, protein, myelin, catecholamine, polysaccharides, creatine, carnitine, DNA, RNA) to form X-CH_3. The adenosine is hydrolysed to give homocysteine which can be converted back to methionine via tetrahydrofolate (THF) or converted to the amino acid cysteine.

Homocysteine is biosynthesised by demethylation of dietary methionine. Methionine receives adenosine triphosphate (ATP) to give S-adenosylmethionine (SAM), catalysed by S-adenosylmethionine synthetase (EC 2.5.1.6). SAM transfers a methyl group to X-(phospholipid, protein, myelin, catecholamine, polysaccharides, creatine, carnitine, DNA, RNA) to form X-CH_3. The adenosine is hydrolysed to give homocysteine which can be converted back to methionine via tetrahydrofolate (THF) or converted to cysteine. Methionine salvage utilises N5-methyl tetrahydrofolate as the methyl donor and vitamin-B12 (cobalamin) associated enzyme tetrahydrofolate methyltransferase (EC 2.1.1.13).

Deficiencies in folic acid (vitamin B_9), pyridoxine (vitamin B_6) or cobalamin (Vitamin B_{12}) can give rise to a high plasma homocysteine. Homocysteineaemia is associated with disruptive damage to the endothelium. *In vitro* studies have demonstrated that homocysteine can induce direct damage to endothelial cells, increase platelet activity, increase collagen synthesis, smooth muscle cell proliferation and has pro-coagulant effects.

The Norwegian Vitamin Trial (NORVIT, clinicalTrials.gov # NCT00266487) was a large study of approximately 5000 post AMI subjects who were treated to reduce plasma homocysteine concentrations (Bonaa *et al.* 2006). Patients were randomised to receive one of four daily treatment regimens; 0.8 mg folic acid, 0.4 mg vitamin B_{12} and 40 mg vitamin B_6; 0.8 mg folic acid and 0.4 mg vitamin B_{12}; 40 mg of vitamin B_6 or finally a placebo. Patients were followed for a median of 40 months for recurrent AMI, stroke and sudden cardiac death. Overall, plasma homocysteine concentrations fell by 27% on patients taking folic acid and vitamin B_{12}. Risk ratio for the primary end-points was 1.08 (95%CI 0.93-1.25). Treatment with vitamin B6 showed similar results with no benefit with regard the primary end point. Patients who received the polypharmacy of folic acid, vitamin B12 and vitamin B6 were actually at increased risk of a cardiac event. Conversely in the HOPE-2 study, reduction of homocysteine by polypharmacy reduced the risk of stroke by 25% (Lonn *et al.* 2006). Homocysteine is elevated in patients with chronic kidney disease (CKD). In the renal HOPE-2 study (Mann *et al.* 2008) 307 patients with CKD (eGFR <60 ml/min) at high risk of CVD were randomised to folic acid and B vitamin polypharmacy and a further 312 received placebo for 5 years. The treated group showed a reduction in mean homocysteine from 15.9 μmol/L to 11.9 μmol/L (p=<0.001) but did not reduce in the placebo group. Treatment with polypharmacy to reduce plasma homocysteine in CKD patients did not reduce the risk of cardiovascular death, recurrent AMI or stroke.

2.2 Plaque destabilisation biomarkers

Endothelial injury results in chemotactic recruitment of mononuclear cells within the plaque. Interleukin-6 (IL-6) concentrations are increased in patients with established CVD as well as those who have an acute coronary syndrome. Kinetically, IL-6 rises and falls rapidly but produces an acute phase response. This in turn initiates the production of acute phase reactants such as C-reactive protein (CRP) and serum amyloid A protein.

2.2.1 C-reactive protein

C-reactive protein (CRP) is a hepatically derived pentraxin of 23KDa released from the liver during an acute phase response. Physiologically CRP resembles antibody and binds to phosphocholine expressed on the surface of necrotic or dying cells and some bacteria. CRP activates the complement system via the C1Q complex. The primary use of CRP is as a marker of infection, during which concentrations can be 100-fold higher than the limits of normal. CRP rises in response to an increase in plasma IL-6 produced by macrophages. CRP has a long plasma half-life and is now understood to be a mediator as well as a marker of atherothrombotic disease (Ridker 2003). In CVD patients, values are typically in the range 0-3 mg/L. Due to the development of sensitive assays, which can accurately report below 5 mg/L, highly sensitive CRP has been demonstrated to be a strong predictor of future cardiovascular events. Sensitive CRP has demonstrated better predictive power for adverse cardiac events than low density lipoprotein (LDL) cholesterol (Ridker 2003). A large number of studies have demonstrated that CRP is related to the risk of subsequent cardiac events in both patients with and without pre-existing CVD.

Plasma CRP concentrations of <1, 1 to 3, and >3mg/L correspond to low, moderate, and high-risk groups for future cardiovascular events respectively. Individuals with low LDL (<130 mg/dL; 3.37 mmol/L) cholesterol but high plasma CRP levels (>3mg/L) represent a high-risk group often missed in clinical practice. The addition of CRP to standard cholesterol evaluation may provide an improvement to global risk prediction and monitoring compliance with preventive intervention. Currently CRP is used as a risk predictor for primary prevention intervention. The use of aspirin is associated with a reduction in CRP concentrations and subsequent lower CVD event rate. The use of statin therapy (3-hydroxy-3-methy;-glutaryl-CoA (HMG-CoA) reductase inhibitors, EC 1.1.1.88) for hypercholesterolaemia is also associated with a reduction in serum CRP; suggesting statins themselves also exert a direct anti-inflammatory effect.

Whilst IL-6 may be a more sensitive marker for CVD prediction, it is less readily available in clinical chemistry laboratories as a routine assay and is harder to measure due to analyte stability and storage conditions.

2.2.2 Lipoprotein-associated phospholipase A2

Lipoprotein-associated phospholipase A2 (Lp-PLA_2) or platelet-activating factor (PAF) acetylhydrolase (EC 3.1.1.47) is a 45kDa intracellular phospholipase which hydrolyzes phospholipids in cellular membranes. It catalyses the degradation of PAF to inactive products by the hydrolysis of an acetyl group at position sn-2, resulting in the production of LYSO-PAF and acetate. It is encoded by the PLA22G gene at loci 6p21.2-p12 and consists of 441 amino acid residues. Attached to LDL, it is responsible for the hydrolysis of oxidised phospholipid in the LDL molecule. Less than 20% of Lp-PLA_2 is associated with HDL. Using immunohistochemical staining with monoclonal antibodies, it has been demonstrated that juvenile plaques show less staining for Lp-PLA_2 than rupture-prone or ruptured plaques (Kolodgie *et al.* 2006). In patients with cardiovascular metabolic syndrome, modification of Lp-PLA_2 through treatment of obesity, hyperlipidaemia and diabetes mellitus (Lp-PLA_2 is independent of insulin resistance), who would otherwise be at intermediate risk of a future cardiac event has shown promise. In a large meta analysis of over 79,000 participants (from 32 prospective studies) Lp-PLA_2 activity and mass demonstrate associations with CVD akin to the risk associated with non-HDL cholesterol or systolic blood pressure(Thompson *et al.* 2010). Lp-PLA_2 is a potential therapeutic target for CVD.

2.2.3 Myeloperoxidase

Myeloperoxidase (MPO) is a 144 KDa (144,000 Dalton) peroxidase enzyme (EC 1.11.1.7) present in abundance in neutrophil granulocytes and stored in azurophilic granules. The gene locus for MPO is 17q23.1. MPO is comprised of two 15 KDa light chains and two variable weighted glycosylated heavy chains which bind haem pigment responsible for the green colour in puss and mucus. The enzyme catalyses the conversion of chloride cosubstrate with hydrogen peroxide to chlorinating oxidants such as hypochlorous acid (hypochlorite).

MPO is a sensitive predictor of AMI. Patients with unstable plaques have higher macrophage and neutrophil counts than patients with stable coronary artery disease. MPO degrades the collagen layer of the atheroma making the lesion susceptible to erosion or rupture. MPO is a risk factor for long term mortality. A study of 885 patients receiving coronary angiography have been studied and followed for 13 years for cardiac mortality. MPO independently predicted coronary artery disease. The addition of CRP measurement improved risk prediction. Patients with elevated MPO or CRP had a 5-fold risk of cardiac mortality compared to a 4 fold risk of cardiac mortality if both markers were elevated (Heslop *et al.* 2010).

2.3 Plaque rupture

The classical view of plaque rupture is an increasingly outwardly growing plaque reducing the luminal space and thus limiting blood flow. It is now known that 80% of plaques that cause an ACS event are actually not flow limiting stenoses. Markers of coagulation are raised in the ACS patient and these include prothrombin fragment 1 and 2 and factor VIIa. Thrombin/antithrombin complex is often elevated and associated with increased plasma cardiac troponin. Inflammatory cells contribute to plaque rupture. Foam cells derived from macrophages congregate in the shoulder region of the vulnerable plaque. At this time, the foam cells express matrix metalloproteinase enzymes (MMPs). These proteolytic enzymes can inactivate zymogens (proMMP) enzymes as well as angiotensin II. A number of MMPs are synthesised and released by macrophage. These include interstitial collegnase (MMP-1), gelatinase enzymes (MMP-2 and MMP-9) and stromelysin (MMP-3). MMP-1 expression is increased by oxidised LDL interferon- gamma (IFN-γ), IL-1 and tumour necrosis factor alpha (TNF-α) (Rajavashisth *et al.* 1999).

2.4 Chest pain

Chest pain admissions are resource intensive and account for a large proportion of emergency care finances. >11 million patients with chest pain present annually to the emergency department in the USA. A final diagnosis of ST segment elevation myocardial infarction (STEMI); conferring the highest risk occurs in only 3% of chest pain presentations (Pope *et al.* 2000). Similar data are given for the UK. 700,000 annual patient attendances in England and Wales are due to chest pain and it is responsible for one quarter of hospital admissions (Goodacre *et al.* 2005). Patients demonstrating STEMI benefit from immediate pharmacological thrombolytic therapy or percutaneous coronary intervention with or without stent placement in order to establish coronary reperfusion. A large proportion of the remaining 97% of chest pain admissions do not have a final diagnosis of ACS (Storrow and Gibler 2000). Biomarkers are especially important in identifying those patients without classical electrocardiographic (ECG) changes who may have a non ST segment elevation myocardial infarction (NSTEMI).

2.5 Biomarkers of cardiac ischemia

The detection of cardiac ischemia prior to myocardial infarction is both a major diagnostic and therapeutic challenge. Detection of cardiac ischaemia prior to necrosis is a potential therapeutic (pharmacological or invasive) target to limit or prevent cellular necrosis. There is currently no gold-standard test for ischemia and currently the only method of detection in routine clinical use is to observe ST segment changes on the ECG. Historically serum lactate measurements were used however lactate has an extremely low cardiac specificity. Candidate markers including whole blood choline and unbound free fatty acids have been proposed however only ischemia modified albumin (IMA®) has taken the translational step from a basic science investigation into an FDA and CE marked commercial assay.

2.5.1 Whole blood choline

Choline is a product of phosphodiesteric cleavage of membrane phospholipids such as phosphatidylcholine and sphingomyelin; catalysed by phospholipase D (EC 3.1.4.4). Physiologically choline provides cell structural integrity, is the precursor for acetylcholine production and a source of methyl groups that participate in the S-adenosylmethionine synthesis pathway.

Whole blood (WBCHO) and plasma choline concentrations increase after stimulation of phospholipase D and the activation of coronary plaque cell surface receptors or ischemia. Phospholipase D activation in coronary plaques causes stimulation of macrophage by oxidised LDL, secretion of MMP and activation of platelets. WHBCO can be measured by high performance liquid chromatography coupled to mass spectrometry (HPLC-MS). In a study of over 300 patients with suspected ACS, WBCHO measured at admission was a significant predictor of cardiac death, cardiac arrest, arrhythmia, heart failure or the need for percutaneous coronary intervention at 30 day follow up (Danne *et al.* 2003). The predictive power was enhanced by the addition of either cTnT or cTnI and served not as a marker of myocardial cell necrosis but identified patients at high risk with unstable angina. WBCHO is therefore a better predictive tool than plasma choline for early risk stratification in patients who are cardiac troponin negative on admission. The current detection methodology using HPLC-MS is not suitable for urgent clinical use.

2.5.2 Unbound free fatty acids

Free fatty acids are produced from the breakdown of triglyceride. The majority of free fatty acids (FFA) circulate bound to albumin with a very small percentage appearing as the unbound free fatty acid (FFAu) form (Richieri and Kleinfeld 1995). The circulating level of FFA is limited to the availability of the albumin binding sites. The mechanism of FFAu release is not fully understood however increased catecholamines following cardiac ischemia may activate FFA release following lipolysis in adipocytes. FFAu are 14-fold higher post PCI, compared to pre procedural concentrations and were higher in those with associated ischemic ST segment changes on the ECG (Kleinfeld *et al.* 1996). An assay using recombinant fatty acid binding protein bound to a fluorescent tag (ADIFAB) (Richieri *et al.* 1999;Richieri *et al.* 1992) has been developed and a second generation assay using a fluorescent molecular probe (ADIFAB2) and a portable reader makes this a potential early marker for the point of care setting. Whilst this marker shows promise in the early phase of ischemia induced ACS, further trials are required to evaluate the diagnosis and prognostic value of FFAu in the chest pain population.

2.5.3 Ischemia modified albumin

A reduction in oxygen supply versus demand causes localized acidosis and the generation of free radicals. Copper and zinc ions, normally bound to proteins in the plasma are released from protein binding sites to circulate in the free form (Chevion *et al.* 1993;Cobbe and Poole-Wilson 1980;McCord 1985). The N-terminus of albumin binds transition metals such as, Co^{2+}, Ni^{2+} and Cu^{2+} ions (Sadler *et al.* 1994). The N-terminus however, is susceptible to biochemical alteration (Chan *et al.* 1995). Following a period of ischemia, a reduction in the ability of albumin to bind cobalt is apparent. This is the basis of the albumin cobalt-binding test (ACB® test) for IMA (figure 5) (Bar-Or *et al.* 2001). The assay measures the ability of albumin to bind a known amount of free cobalt added to the sample. Dithiothreitol (DTT) is added which binds the remaining unbound cobalt. The colorimetric change is read spectrophotometrically.

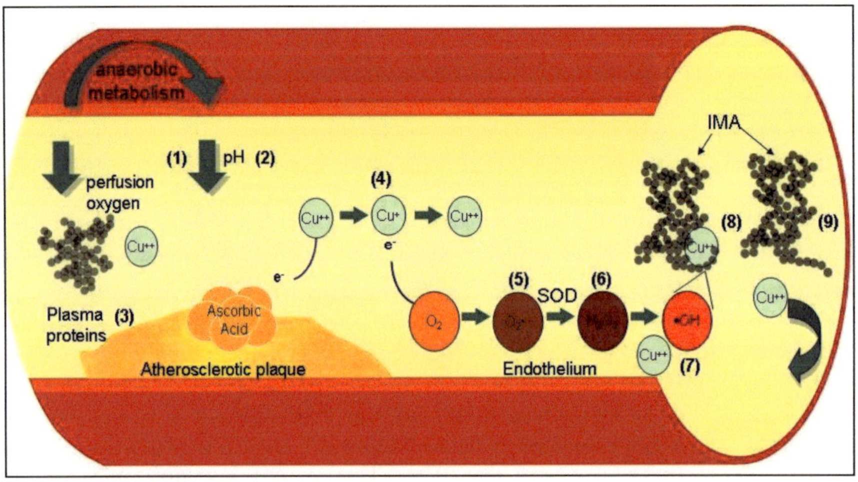

Fig. 5. Mechanism of Ischemia Modified Albumin generation: Reduced blood flow results in tissue hypoxia[1] resulting in a lower pH[2]. Cu^{++} is released from plasma proteins[3]. In the presence of ascorbic acid, Cu^{++} is converted to Cu^{+}[4]. Cu^{+} reacts with O_2 to form $O_2^{\bullet -}$[5]. Superoxide dismutase (SOD) dismutates the $O2^{\bullet -}$, forming H_2O_2[6]. Normally, H_2O_2 is harmlessly degraded to H_2O and O_2 by catalase. However, in the presence of metals such as copper or iron, H_2O_2 undergoes the Fenton reaction, forming OH• radicals[7]. Free Cu^{++} is scavenged by HSA, where it binds tightly to the N-terminus. OH• are highly reactive capable of damaging nucleic acids, lipids and proteins, including albumin. One site of damage is the N-terminus, where OH• alter the amino acids[8]. Altered albumin is incapable of binding Cu^{++}. Bound copper is released from the albumin[9], where it may be taken up again by the N-terminus of another albumin in a chain reaction which repeats the process of albumin binding and OH• formation.

Kinetically there is a rapid increase in serum IMA. In an angioplasty model, IMA values decreased at 6 hours post inflation and returned to baseline by 24 hours (Bar-Or *et al.* 2001;Sinha *et al.* 2006). The magnitude of IMA elevation correlates with the number and frequency of balloon inflations (Quiles *et al.* 2003), the presence of collateral vessels (Garrido *et al.* 2004), the need for revascularisation (Dusek *et al.* 2006) and is parallel to the transmyocardial lactate gradient (Sinha *et al.* 2006). The half-life of human albumin is 19-20 days. A truncated modified form would remain in the circulation following production for a number of days. The rapid reduction in IMA following the ischemic event suggests the modification is transient and reversible. IMA alone has a diagnostic sensitivity of 82% with

46% specificity if measured in the first three hours of presentation to the ED (Sinha *et al.* 2004). The combination of a positive ECG, cTnT (>0.05 μg/L) and IMA however demonstrated a 95% sensitivity for diagnosis of ACS. In a study of 538 patients admitted to a chest pain evaluation unit, admission measurement of IMA plus cTnT had 100% sensitivity for prediction of a final diagnosis of AMI (Collinson *et al.* 2006). IMA however lacks specificity for cardiac tissue and elevations can occur in a number of non-ACS conditions including autoimmune diseases, cancers, hepatic cirrhosis, haemorrhagic stroke, renal disease, peripheral vascular disease and polytrauma.

Elevated IMA and cTnT on admission predicts 20% of major adverse cardiac events. IMA appear to work best in conjunction with other tests such as cTn or the ECG. One year follow up of 208 patients presenting to the emergency department with chest pain demonstrated a survival disadvantage in those patients with a serum IMA at admission greater than the median concentration of the population group (Consuegra-Sanchez *et al.* 2008). There were 17 vs 9 (p=0.08) episodes of angina, 21 vs 10 combined endpoints (p=0.03) and 12 vs 4 12 month all-cause mortality (p=0.03) in the IMA positive group compared to the IMA negative group.

Although the assay has been cleared for *in vitro* diagnostic use, two problems remain to be resolved with IMA. First is the mechanism by which IMA is generated and the relationship to the underlying pathophysiological mechanisms during ischemia. The second is the assay format; Very low albumin (Zapico-Muniz *et al.* 2004;Gaze *et al.* 2006a) and the presence of co-existing lactic acidosis affect assay performance. Finally samples need to be analysed within a STAT fashion due to the instability of IMA (Gaze 2009).

2.6 Biomarkers of cardiomyocyte necrosis

2.6.1 Cardiac troponins

Markers of cardiac cell necrosis can be split into those located in the cytoplasm of the cell and those that form the structural apparatus which control muscle contraction. The cytosolic component contains myoglobin, LD, CK, CKMB as well as fatty acid binding protein (FABP). The structural compartment consists of the troponin proteins troponin T and troponin I (figure 6). Troponins have tissue specific isoforms. Cardiac troponin T (cTnT) and cardiac troponin I (cTnI) and are expressed uniquely in myocardial cells, whilst predominantly structural both cardiac troponins (cTn) have a small unbound cytosolic fraction (between 6% and 8% for cTnT and 2.8%-8.3% for cTnI).

The measurement of cardiac troponin is now considered the "Gold Standard" test for myocardial necrosis and the globally accepted ESC/ACCF/AHA/WHF universal definition of AMI has been widely adopted (Thygesen *et al.* 2007). The success of the measurement of troponin is due to the analytical and clinical sensitivity and specificity of the assays and the large evidence base for outcome prediction.

The sensitivity of any biochemical test is dependant on its ability to discriminate between the normal and abnormal state. A test that is elevated in all patients with a condition and is normal in all controls will have a sensitivity of 100%. Sensitivity is influenced by the background level of signal in the normal state and is referred to as noise. This in turn is compared to the change of signal in the abnormal state, known as the signal to noise ratio. It

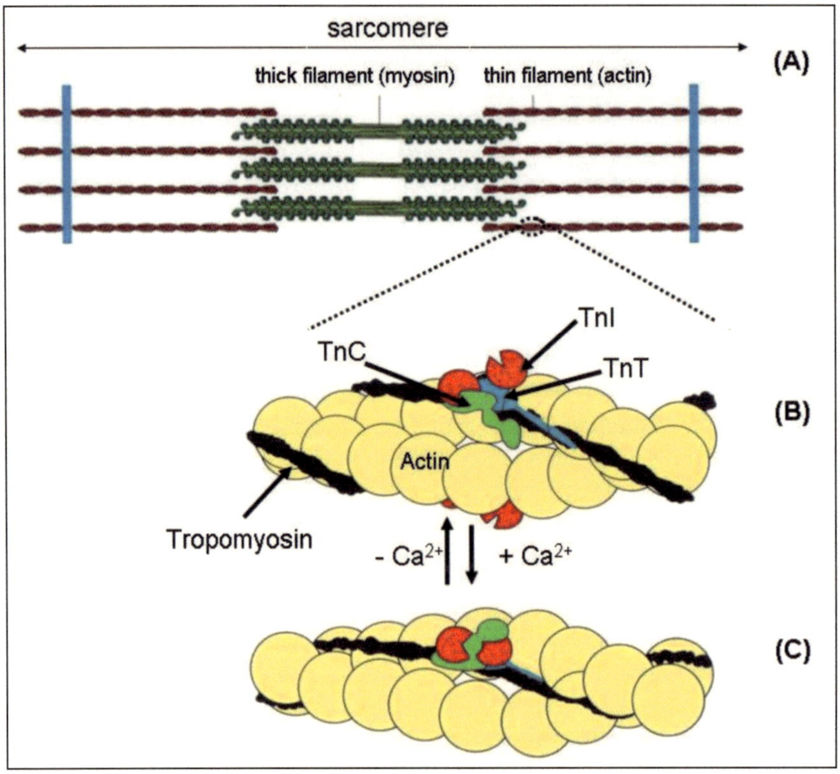

Fig. 6. (A) Anatomy of the sarcomere. (B) Structure of the troponin-tropomyosin complex. Composed of three proteins, troponin T (TnT, 39.7 kDa), which binds tropomyosin, troponin C the Ca^{2+} binding element (TnC, 18 kDa) and troponin I, the Mg^{2+} dependent ATPase inhibitor (TnI, 22.5 kDa), shown in the resting state. (C) During muscle contraction, Ca^{2+} is released from the t-tubules, and bind TnC, leading to a conformational change in the complex

was presumed that the circulating concentration of cTn in apparently healthy people was absolute zero, due to the intracellular location of the proteins. With the advent of more sensitive immunoassay methods the current commercial cTn assays demonstrate a background level in the circulation that appears to be determined by the detection limit of the assay. Although there may be a background level of cTn in the circulation, this is undetectable in the majority of cases by the assays currently commercially available. Elevation occurs only where there is myocardial damage. The combination of low background noise with cardiospecificity means that although in absolute terms the amount of cTn released is less than the amount of CKMB, the ability to detect it is much greater, and the signal to noise ratio is much higher. Using cTn specific assay, it has been demonstrated that elevations of the cardiac isoform do not occur where there is pure skeletal muscle trauma. In a study of 696 apparently healthy individuals aged 18-84 years, of which 45% were male, two commercial cTnI assays have demonstrated a gender difference, with a higher upper limit of normal in males. The other five cTnI assays and the cTnT assay tested did not demonstrate a gender difference. In the same population, CKMB mass was significantly higher in males compared to females (Apple *et al.* 2003).

Clinical studies of cTn have concentrated on the diagnostic and prognostic utility of the assays. Initial studies showed that cTnT could be detected in a significant proportion of patients who were classed as having unstable angina using the conventional World Health Organisation (WHO) criteria for myocardial infarction. In these studies, both short term and long term follow up showed that an elevated troponin was associated with an increased risk of cardiac event (Hamm *et al.* 1992).

Determination of cTn is by immunoassay. For both cTnT and cTnI, several generations of assay have existed and have been comprehensively reviewed (Collinson *et al.* 2001a). The measurement technology utilising electrochemiliuminesence for cTnT is supplied by one manufacturer (Roche Diagnostics) due to patent restrictions on the antibodies selected for the assay. Measurement of cTnI however is available on a range of immunoassay platforms from different manufacturers. Due to a lack of assay standardisation both for a common calibrator and for antibody selection, comparison between cTnI methods is often problematic. Despite this, a similar series of studies for the different cTnI methods has shown that cTnI elevation predicts adverse cardiac events in patients with unstable angina (Antman *et al.* 1996;Galvani *et al.* 1997;Collinson *et al.* 2001b). The use of cTnT and cTnI determinations results in approximately reclassification of 33% of unstable angina patients into patients who have suffered an AMI.

A number of manufactures have reformulated their assays or introduced high sensitive cTn with the aim of meeting the analytical requirements suggested in the universal definition of AMI. The introduction of such assays provides challenges both in terms of the analytical performance and validation/interpretation procedures for the laboratory and the relevance in the clinical setting. Many of these assays can now demonstrate a normal distribution of detectable cTn concentrations within a reference population (Collinson *et al.* 2009a) (Apple *et al.* 2010;Mingels *et al.* 2009) allowing more robust calculation of the 99th percentile concentration to define normality. These assays also allow the calculation of the biological variability of cardiac troponin (Wu *et al.* 2009).

The introduction of high sensitivity cTn assays will affect the clinical interpretation results. There will be a greater number of positives outside the remit of ACS, but within the ACS population, it may be possible to diagnose AMI earlier. Using the Centaur TnI-Ultra a 99th percentile of 0.039 μg/L (39ng/L) has been obtained from a population of 309 (41% male) apparently healthy individuals highly screened for cardiac risk factors. These included no history of vascular disease, diabetes mellitus, hypertension, or heavy alcohol intake, no cardiac medication, no renal failure (eGFR >60 mL/min/1.73 m^2), no significant cardiac disease on echocardiography, with a left ventricular ejection fraction of >50% (Collinson *et al.* 2009b). Within the reference population, cTnI was completely undetectable in 25 subjects and considered negative in 53%. There was no correlation between cTnI and age and there were no significant differences between gender (Collinson *et al.* 2009b). Using the same population, the researchers have defined the 99th percentile of the hs-cTnT assay (Roche Diagnostics) to be 15.5 ng/L and 42 ng/L for the Beckman Coulter enhanced AccuTnI assay. Of note are the differences between the numbers of detectable cTn by assay within the same reference population. Detectable concentrations were achieve in 58% of samples when measured using the hs-cTnT assay, 68% using the TnI-Ultra and 98% using the Access AccuTnI.

The prognostic value of the AccuTnI assay has been demonstrated in the Orbofiban in Patients with Unstable Coronary Syndromes (OPUS)-Thrombolysis in Myocardial Infarction (TIMI) 16 (OPUS-TIMI 16) clinical trial (Morrow *et al.* 2003). A cut point of $\geq$0.04 μg/L ($\geq$40 ng/L) was an independent predictor of the 30-day risk of death (odds ratio, OR), 4.1; (95%CI 1.2-13.8), death and AMI (OR, 3.4; 95%CI, 1.8-6.7), and death, MI, or ; 95% confidence interval, 95%CI) need for urgent revascularisation (OR, 2.3; 95%CI, 1.5-3.6) and was also associated with risk of death or development of a further AMI at 10 months.

Using the TnI-Ultra compared to the previous Centaur assay, Melanson and colleagues (Melanson *et al.* 2007) compared the rates of positivity obtained between the two assays over a 24 hour period in 103 patients who presented initially with a negative cTnI but converted to cTnI positive. TnI-Ultra was positive before cTnI in 66(64.1%) of cases demonstrating superior sensitivity. Furthermore, a single admission cTn measurement using hs-cTnI may be a useful rule-out test irrespective of the length of chest pain (Keller *et al.* 2009). Reichlin and colleagues also demonstrated excellent diagnostic performance of sensitive cTn assays at presentation (Reichlin *et al.* 2009).

It has been postulated that sensitive cTn, given the detection in asymptomatic healthy people without a history of cardiovascular disease; may be of value in identifying subjects at long term risk of ACS, i.e. cTn may have a role in primary prevention (Apple 2011). In a large community cohort of adults > 65 years; baseline and delta change in serial hs-cTnT measurements are associated with heart failure and cardiac death (deFilippi *et al.* 2010). Further, the use of N-terminal pro-b-type natriuretic peptide (NTproBNP) nor high sensitive CRP added to the risk assessment. In a second cohort of >3500 subjects aged 30-65 years recruited to the Dallas Heart Study, demonstrable hs-cTnT occurred in 25% of subjects; with higher rates in men compared to women (37% vs 13%) respectively. (de Lemos *et al.* 2010). There was separation in rates of positivity in those aged <40 and >60 years of age. Elevated hs-cTnT was associated with structural heart disease (left ventricular hypertrophy and left ventricular systolic dysfunction) and chronic kidney disease. The overall cardiovascular burden as measured by hs-cTnT in primary care may indicate end organ cardiac damage.

2.7 Heart failure

Survival rates following AMI are increasing, primarily due to a combination of early diagnosis and a rapid therapeutic or invasive intervention to open occlusions and to salvage myocardial tissue. Patients with some degree of damaged myocardium however further develop cardiac failure. Cardiac failure is a pathophysiological state in which an abnormality of cardiac function is responsible for the failure of the heart to pump blood at a rate commensurate with the requirements of the metabolising tissues. Cardiac failure affects 0.4-2% of the population and the age adjusted mortality due to cardiac failure is increasing (Remme and Swedberg 2001). There is a 50% survival rate four years after diagnosis (Cowie and Zaphiriou 2002). Currently, the clinical diagnostic methodologies available are inadequate due to poor sensitivity and specificity. There is heavy reliance on the identification of heart failure from symptoms, ECG changes and/or chest x-ray diagnosis. The 'gold standard' for diagnosis of cardiac failure is currently cardiac imaging technology including echocardiography or magnetic resonance imaging; however these are often expensive and not always routinely available. A blood borne marker of cardiac dysfunction is therefore highly desirable.

B type natriuretic peptide (BNP) is a hormone secreted predominantly by ventricular wall myocytes in response to increased ventricular stretch. It is not stored following production, but is under constant renewal by transcription and translation of mRNA. A prohormone proBNP is produced within the myocyte. This prohormone is cleaved by the enzyme corin to give the active portion of the molecule, B type natriuretic peptide (BNP) and the N terminal portion of the hormone, NTproBNP. Both are available as routine biomarker assay tests on a range of immunoassay platforms. The half-life of the active BNP is short (20 minutes) compared to that of the NTproBNP (120 minutes).

Measurements of NTproBNP and BNP are used in the diagnosis of suspected acute or chronic cardiac failure. It has been demonstrated that the measurement of BNP/NTproBNP allows exclusion with a high certainty of left ventricular systolic dysfunction (LVSD) in patients presenting to primary care with symptoms suggestive of heart failure, mainly shortness of breath (McDonagh *et al.* 2008;Cowie *et al.* 1997;Zaphiriou *et al.* 2005). It has been suggested, therefore, that BNP/NTproBNP measurement should be used as the "gold standard" test for the detection of ventricular dysfunction. In a prospective randomised trial of diagnosis based on BNP with conventional clinical diagnosis in 452 patients, the diagnostic pathway including BNP produced reduction in hospital stay; stay in intensive care and lower cost but with equivalent mortality (Mueller *et al.* 2004).

The role of BNP/NTproBNP in patients presenting with ACS however remains more uncertain. Studies have shown that measurement of NTproBNP/BNP on admission in both selected and unselected suspected ACS patients can be used to predict outcome. A study of 2525 patients enrolled in a clinical trial (OPUS-TIMI 16) with a mixed population of ST segment elevation MI (STEMI), non ST segment elevation MI (NSTEMI) and unstable angina pectoris (UAP) showed that quartiles of BNP concentrations were predictive of survival. There was a 9% mortality rate in the highest quartile compared with less than 1% in the lowest quartile at 10 months follow up. The population was dichotomised into those with BNP above or below the cut point of 80pg/L. An elevated BNP $\geq$80pg/mL showed a significantly greater risk of death, heart failure or MI both at 30 days and at 10 months (de Lemos *et al.* 2001). In a study of 666 patients admitted with AMI, BNP and NTproBNP were measured 24-96 hours from symptom onset. Subsequent death or heart failure was predicted by BNP/NTproBNP levels even when ejection fraction exceeded 40% (Richards *et al.* 2003). BNP/NTproBNP measurements have been combined with other biomarkers including CRP and cTn (Sabatine *et al.* 2002) or cTn alone (Jernberg *et al.* 2002) Measurements of BNP/NTproBNP provide additive information under these circumstances with the worst prognosis seen when the greatest number of biomarkers are elevated.

3. Conclusion

There are a number of cardiovascular biomarkers that aid the clinician in the identification of the risk of developing cardiovascular disease. Many are specialised tests and are not offered in the routine clinical chemistry laboratory. A large evidence base exists for those that are commonly measured as markers of the acute coronary syndrome. Biomarkers should be used in an algorithm along with the clinical signs and the results of other diagnostic modalities such as the ECG, stress test or echocardiography.

Any novel cardiac biomarker should prove clinically useful and cost effective with the ultimate aim of altering patient management and reduce mortality. The cardiac troponins are the most successful of the candidate markers and have influenced an alteration to the definition of acute myocardial infarction. The B type natriuretic peptide has a large evidence base for the diagnosis and more importantly the monitoring of heart failure. A reliable marker of cardiac ischemia remains to be demonstrated and is the focus of current research studies.

4. References

Allam, A. H., Thompson, R. C., Wann, L. S., Miyamoto, M. I., El-Halim Nur El-Din, El Maksoud, G. A., Al Tohamy, S. M., Badr, I., Rahman Amer, H. A., Sutherland, M. L., Sutherland, J. D., and Thomas, G. S. (2011). Atherosclerosis in Ancient Egyptian Mummies The Horus Study. *JACC.Cardiovasc.Imaging*.

Antman, E. M., Tanasijevic, M. J., Thompson, B., Schactman, M., McCabe, C. H., Cannon, C. P., Fischer, G. A., Fung, A. Y., Thompson, C., Wybenga, D., and Braunwald, E. (1996). Cardiac-specific troponin I levels to predict the risk of mortality in patients with acute coronary syndromes. *N.Engl.J Med.* 335, 1342-1349.

Apple, F. S. (2011). High-sensitivity cardiac troponin for screening large populations of healthy people: is there risk? *Clin.Chem.* 57, 537-539.

Apple, F. S., Quist, H. E., Doyle, P. J., Otto, A. P., and Murakami, M. M. (2003). Plasma 99th percentile reference limits for cardiac troponin and creatine kinase MB mass for use with European Society of Cardiology/American College of Cardiology consensus recommendations. *Clin.Chem.* 49, 1331-1336.

Apple, F. S., Simpson, P. A., and Murakami, M. M. (2010). Defining the serum 99th percentile in a normal reference population measured by a high-sensitivity cardiac troponin I assay. *Clin.Biochem.* 43, 1034-1036.

Bar-Or, D., Winkler, J. V., Vanbenthuysen, K., Harris, L., Lau, E., and Hetzel, F. W. (2001). Reduced albumin-cobalt binding with transient myocardial ischemia after elective percutaneous transluminal coronary angioplasty: a preliminary comparison to creatine kinase-MB, myoglobin, and troponin I. *Am.Heart J* 141, 985-991.

Bonaa, K. H., Njolstad, I., Ueland, P. M., Schirmer, H., Tverdal, A., Steigen, T., Wang, H., Nordrehaug, J. E., Arnesen, E., and Rasmussen, K. (2006). Homocysteine lowering and cardiovascular events after acute myocardial infarction. *N.Engl.J.Med.* 354, 1578-1588.

Brown, M. S. and Goldstein, J. L. (1979). Receptor-mediated endocytosis: insights from the lipoprotein receptor system. *Proc.Natl.Acad.Sci.U.S.A* 76, 3330-3337.

Brunzell, J. D., Davidson, M., Furberg, C. D., Goldberg, R. B., Howard, B. V., Stein, J. H., and Witztum, J. L. (2008). Lipoprotein management in patients with cardiometabolic risk: consensus conference report from the American Diabetes Association and the American College of Cardiology Foundation. *J.Am.Coll.Cardiol.* 51, 1512-1524.

Chan, B., Dodsworth, N., Woodrow, J., Tucker, A., and Harris, R. (1995). Site-specific N-terminal auto-degradation of human serum albumin. *Eur.J.Biochem.* 227, 524-528.

Chevion, M., Jiang, Y., Har-El, R., Berenshtein, E., Uretzky, G., and Kitrossky, N. (1993). Copper and iron are mobilized following myocardial ischemia: possible predictive criteria for tissue injury. *Proc.Natl.Acad.Sci.U.S.A* 90, 1102-1106.

Cobbe, S. M. and Poole-Wilson, P. A. (1980). The time of onset and severity of acidosis in myocardial ischaemia. *J.Mol.Cell Cardiol.* 12, 745-760.

Collinson, P. O., Boa, F. G., and Gaze, D. C. (2001a). Measurement of cardiac troponins. *Ann.Clin.Biochem.* 38, 423-449.

Collinson, P. O., Clifford-Mobley, O., Gaze, D., Boa, F., and Senior, R. (2009a). Assay imprecision and 99th-percentile reference value of a high-sensitivity cardiac troponin I assay. *Clin.Chem.* 55, 1433-1434.

Collinson, P. O., Clifford-Mobley, O., Gaze, D., Boa, F., and Senior, R. (2009b). Assay imprecision and 99th-percentile reference value of a high-sensitivity cardiac troponin I assay. *Clin.Chem.* 55, 1433-1434.

Collinson, P. O., Gaze, D. C., Bainbridge, K., Morris, F., Morris, B., Price, A., and Goodacre, S. (2006). Utility of admission cardiac troponin and "Ischemia Modified Albumin" measurements for rapid evaluation and rule out of suspected acute myocardial infarction in the emergency department. *Emerg.Med.J.* 23, 256-261.

Collinson, P. O., Wiggins, N., and Gaze, D. C. (2001b). Clinical evaluation of the ACS:180 cardiac troponin I assay. *Ann.Clin.Biochem.* 38, 509-519.

Consuegra-Sanchez, L., Bouzas-Mosquera, A., Sinha, M. K., Collinson, P. O., Gaze, D. C., and Kaski, J. C. (2008). Ischemia-modified albumin predicts short-term outcome and 1-year mortality in patients attending the emergency department for acute ischemic chest pain. *Heart Vessels* 23, 174-180.

Cowie, M. R., Struthers, A. D., Wood, D. A., Coats, A. J., Thompson, S. G., Poole-Wilson, P. A., and Sutton, G. C. (1997). Value of natriuretic peptides in assessment of patients with possible new heart failure in primary care. *Lancet* 350, 1349-1353.

Cowie, M. R. and Zaphiriou, A. (2002). Management of chronic heart failure. *BMJ* 325, 422-425.

Danne, O., Mockel, M., Lueders, C., Mugge, C., Zschunke, G. A., Lufft, H., Muller, C., and Frei, U. (2003). Prognostic implications of elevated whole blood choline levels in acute coronary syndromes. *Am.J.Cardiol.* 91, 1060-1067.

de Lemos, J. A., Drazner, M. H., Omland, T., Ayers, C. R., Khera, A., Rohatgi, A., Hashim, I., Berry, J. D., Das, S. R., Morrow, D. A., and McGuire, D. K. (2010). Association of troponin T detected with a highly sensitive assay and cardiac structure and mortality risk in the general population. *JAMA* 304, 2503-2512.

de Lemos, J. A., Morrow, D. A., Bentley, J. H., Omland, T., Sabatine, M. S., McCabe, C. H., Hall, C., Cannon, C. P., and Braunwald, E. (2001). The prognostic value of B-type natriuretic peptide in patients with acute coronary syndromes. *N.Engl.J.Med.* 345, 1014-1021.

deFilippi, C. R., de Lemos, J. A., Christenson, R. H., Gottdiener, J. S., Kop, W. J., Zhan, M., and Seliger, S. L. (2010). Association of serial measures of cardiac troponin T using a sensitive assay with incident heart failure and cardiovascular mortality in older adults. *JAMA* 304, 2494-2502.

Dusek, J., St'asek, J., Tichy, M., Bis, J., Gregor, J., Vojacek, J., Masin, V., Polansky, P., Brtko, M., and Cernohorsky, D. (2006). Prognostic significance of ischemia modified albumin after percutaneous coronary intervention. *Clin.Chim.Acta* 367, 77-80.

Friedewald, W. T., Levy, R. I., and Fredrickson, D. S. (1972). Estimation of the concentration of low-density lipoprotein cholesterol in plasma, without use of the preparative ultracentrifuge. *Clin.Chem.* 18, 499-502.

Galvani, M., Ottani, F., Ferrini, D., Ladenson, J. H., Destro, A., Baccos, D., Rusticali, F., and Jaffe, A. S. (1997). Prognostic influence of elevated values of cardiac troponin I in patients with unstable angina. *Circulation* 95, 2053-2059.

Garrido, I. P., Roy, D., Calvino, R., Vazquez-Rodriguez, J. M., Aldama, G., Cosin-Sales, J., Quiles, J., Gaze, D. C., and Kaski, J. C. (2004). Comparison of ischemia-modified albumin levels in patients undergoing percutaneous coronary intervention for unstable angina pectoris with versus without coronary collaterals. *Am.J.Cardiol.* 93, 88-90.

Gaze, D. C. (2009). Ischemia modified albumin: a novel biomarker for the detection of cardiac ischemia. *Drug Metab Pharmacokinet.* 24, 333-341.

Gaze, D. C. and Collinson, P. O. (2005). Cardiac troponins as biomarkers of drug- and toxin-induced cardiac toxicity and cardioprotection. *Expert.Opin.Drug Metab Toxicol.* 1, 715-725.

Gaze, D. C., Crompton, L., and Collinson, P. (2006a). Ischemia-modified albumin concentrations should be interpreted with caution in patients with low serum albumin concentrations. *Med.Princ.Pract.* 15, 322-324.

Gaze, D. C., Sinha, M., Kaski, J. C., and Collinson, P. O. (2006b). Oxidised low density lipoprotein is a poor shot term even marker in acute coronary syndrome patients who present to the emergency department. *Clin.Chem.* 2006, A128.

Goodacre, S., Cross, E., Arnold, J., Angelini, K., Capewell, S., and Nicholl, J. (2005). The health care burden of acute chest pain. *Heart* 91, 229-230.

Hamm, C. W., Ravkilde, J., Gerhardt, W., Jorgensen, P., Peheim, E., Ljungdahl, L., Goldmann, B., and Katus, H. A. (1992). The prognostic value of serum troponin T in unstable angina. *N.Engl.J Med.* 327, 146-150.

Heslop, C. L., Frohlich, J. J., and Hill, J. S. (2010). Myeloperoxidase and C-reactive protein have combined utility for long-term prediction of cardiovascular mortality after coronary angiography. *J.Am.Coll.Cardiol.* 55, 1102-1109.

Jernberg, T., Stridsberg, M., Venge, P., and Lindahl, B. (2002). N-terminal pro brain natriuretic peptide on admission for early risk stratification of patients with chest pain and no ST-segment elevation. *J Am.Coll.Cardiol.* 40, 437-445.

Keller, T., Zeller, T., Peetz, D., Tzikas, S., Roth, A., Czyz, E., Bickel, C., Baldus, S., Warnholtz, A., Frohlich, M., Sinning, C. R., Eleftheriadis, M. S., Wild, P. S., Schnabel, R. B., Lubos, E., Jachmann, N., Genth-Zotz, S., Post, F., Nicaud, V., Tiret, L., Lackner, K. J., Munzel, T. F., and Blankenberg, S. (2009). Sensitive troponin I assay in early diagnosis of acute myocardial infarction. *N.Engl.J.Med.* 361, 868-877.

Kleinfeld, A. M., Prothro, D., Brown, D. L., Davis, R. C., Richieri, G. V., and DeMaria, A. (1996). Increases in serum unbound free fatty acid levels following coronary angioplasty. *Am.J.Cardiol.* 78, 1350-1354.

Kolodgie, F. D., Burke, A. P., Skorija, K. S., Ladich, E., Kutys, R., Makuria, A. T., and Virmani, R. (2006). Lipoprotein-associated phospholipase A2 protein expression in the natural progression of human coronary atherosclerosis. *Arterioscler.Thromb.Vasc.Biol.* 26, 2523-2529.

Lonn, E., Yusuf, S., Arnold, M. J., Sheridan, P., Pogue, J., Micks, M., McQueen, M. J., Probstfield, J., Fodor, G., Held, C., and Genest, J., Jr. (2006). Homocysteine lowering with folic acid and B vitamins in vascular disease. *N.Engl.J.Med.* 354, 1567-1577.

Mann, J. F., Sheridan, P., McQueen, M. J., Held, C., Arnold, J. M., Fodor, G., Yusuf, S., and Lonn, E. M. (2008). Homocysteine lowering with folic acid and B vitamins in people with chronic kidney disease--results of the renal Hope-2 study. *Nephrol.Dial.Transplant.* 23, 645-653.

McCord, J. M. (1985). Oxygen-derived free radicals in postischemic tissue injury. *N.Engl.J.Med.* 312, 159-163.

McDonagh, T. A., McDonald, K., and Maisel, A. S. (2008). Screening for asymptomatic left ventricular dysfunction using B-type natriuretic Peptide. *Congest.Heart Fail.* 14, 5-8.

Melanson, S. E., Morrow, D. A., and Jarolim, P. (2007). Earlier detection of myocardial injury in a preliminary evaluation using a new troponin I assay with improved sensitivity. *Am.J.Clin.Pathol.* 128, 282-286.

Mingels, A., Jacobs, L., Michielsen, E., Swaanenburg, J., Wodzig, W., and Dieijen-Visser, M. (2009). Reference population and marathon runner sera assessed by highly sensitive cardiac troponin T and commercial cardiac troponin T and I assays. *Clin.Chem.* 55, 101-108.

Morrow, D. A., Rifai, N., Sabatine, M. S., Ayanian, S., Murphy, S. A., de Lemos, J. A., Braunwald, E., and Cannon, C. P. (2003). Evaluation of the AccuTnI cardiac troponin I assay for risk assessment in acute coronary syndromes. *Clin.Chem.* 49, 1396-1398.

Mueller, C., Scholer, A., Laule-Kilian, K., Martina, B., Schindler, C., Buser, P., Pfisterer, M., and Perruchoud, A. P. (2004). Use of B-type natriuretic peptide in the evaluation and management of acute dyspnea. *N.Engl.J.Med.* 350, 647-654.

Pope, J. H., Aufderheide, T. P., Ruthazer, R., Woolard, R. H., Feldman, J. A., Beshansky, J. R., Griffith, J. L., and Selker, H. P. (2000). Missed diagnoses of acute cardiac ischemia in the emergency department. *N.Engl.J.Med.* 342, 1163-1170.

Quiles, J., Roy, D., Gaze, D., Garrido, I. P., Avanzas, P., Sinha, M., and Kaski, J. C. (2003). Relation of ischemia-modified albumin (IMA) levels following elective angioplasty for stable angina pectoris to duration of balloon-induced myocardial ischemia. *Am.J.Cardiol.* 92, 322-324.

Rajavashisth, T. B., Liao, J. K., Galis, Z. S., Tripathi, S., Laufs, U., Tripathi, J., Chai, N. N., Xu, X. P., Jovinge, S., Shah, P. K., and Libby, P. (1999). Inflammatory cytokines and oxidized low density lipoproteins increase endothelial cell expression of membrane type 1-matrix metalloproteinase. *J.Biol.Chem.* 274, 11924-11929.

Reichlin, T., Hochholzer, W., Bassetti, S., Steuer, S., Stelzig, C., Hartwiger, S., Biedert, S., Schaub, N., Buerge, C., Potocki, M., Noveanu, M., Breidthardt, T., Twerenbold, R., Winkler, K., Bingisser, R., and Mueller, C. (2009). Early diagnosis of myocardial infarction with sensitive cardiac troponin assays. *N.Engl.J.Med.* 361, 858-867.

Remme, W. J. and Swedberg, K. (2001). Guidelines for the diagnosis and treatment of chronic heart failure. *Eur.Heart J.* 22, 1527-1560.

Richards, A. M., Nicholls, M. G., Espiner, E. A., Lainchbury, J. G., Troughton, R. W., Elliott, J., Frampton, C., Turner, J., Crozier, I. G., and Yandle, T. G. (2003). B-type natriuretic peptides and ejection fraction for prognosis after myocardial infarction. *Circulation* 107, 2786-2792.

Richieri, G. V. and Kleinfeld, A. M. (1995). Unbound free fatty acid levels in human serum. *J.Lipid Res.* 36, 229-240.

Richieri, G. V., Ogata, R. T., and Kleinfeld, A. M. (1992). A fluorescently labeled intestinal fatty acid binding protein. Interactions with fatty acids and its use in monitoring free fatty acids. *J.Biol.Chem.* 267, 23495-23501.

Richieri, G. V., Ogata, R. T., and Kleinfeld, A. M. (1999). The measurement of free fatty acid concentration with the fluorescent probe ADIFAB: a practical guide for the use of the ADIFAB probe. *Mol.Cell Biochem.* 192, 87-94.

Ridker, P. M. (2003). Clinical application of C-reactive protein for cardiovascular disease detection and prevention. *Circulation* 107, 363-369.

Sabatine, M. S., Morrow, D. A., de Lemos, J. A., Gibson, C. M., Murphy, S. A., Rifai, N., McCabe, C., Antman, E. M., Cannon, C. P., and Braunwald, E. (2002). Multimarker approach to risk stratification in non-ST elevation acute coronary syndromes: simultaneous assessment of troponin I, C-reactive protein, and B-type natriuretic peptide. *Circulation* 105, 1760-1763.

Sadler, P. J., Tucker, A., and Viles, J. H. (1994). Involvement of a lysine residue in the N-terminal Ni2+ and Cu2+ binding site of serum albumins. Comparison with Co2+, Cd2+ and Al3+. *Eur.J.Biochem.* 220, 193-200.

Sinha, M. K., Roy, D., Gaze, D. C., Collinson, P. O., and Kaski, J. C. (2004). Role of "Ischemia modified albumin", a new biochemical marker of myocardial ischaemia, in the early diagnosis of acute coronary syndromes. *Emerg.Med.J.* 21, 29-34.

Sinha, M. K., Vazquez, J. M., Calvino, R., Gaze, D. C., Collinson, P. O., and Kaski, J. C. (2006). Effects of balloon occlusion during percutaneous coronary intervention on circulating Ischemia Modified Albumin and transmyocardial lactate extraction. *Heart* 92, 1852-1853.

Stary, H. C. (2000). Lipid and macrophage accumulations in arteries of children and the development of atherosclerosis. *Am.J.Clin.Nutr.* 72, 1297S-1306S.

Storrow, A. B. and Gibler, W. B. (2000). Chest pain centers: diagnosis of acute coronary syndromes. *Ann.Emerg.Med.* 35, 449-461.

Thompson, A., Gao, P., Orfei, L., Watson, S., Di Angelantonio, E., Kaptoge, S., Ballantyne, C., Cannon, C. P., Criqui, M., Cushman, M., Hofman, A., Packard, C., Thompson, S. G., Collins, R., and Danesh, J. (2010). Lipoprotein-associated phospholipase A(2) and risk of coronary disease, stroke, and mortality: collaborative analysis of 32 prospective studies. *Lancet* 375, 1536-1544.

Thygesen, K., Alpert, J. S., and White, H. D. (2007). Universal definition of myocardial infarction. *Eur.Heart J.* 28, 2525-2538.

Wu, A. H., Lu, Q. A., Todd, J., Moecks, J., and Wians, F. (2009). Short- and long-term biological variation in cardiac troponin I measured with a high-sensitivity assay: implications for clinical practice. *Clin.Chem.* 55, 52-58.

Zaphiriou, A., Robb, S., Murray-Thomas, T., Mendez, G., Fox, K., McDonagh, T., Hardman, S. M., Dargie, H. J., and Cowie, M. R. (2005). The diagnostic accuracy of plasma BNP and NTproBNP in patients referred from primary care with suspected heart failure: results of the UK natriuretic peptide study. *Eur.J.Heart Fail.* 7, 537-541.

Zapico-Muniz, E., Santalo-Bel, M., Merce-Muntanola, J., Montiel, J. A., Martinez-Rubio, A., and Ordonez-Llanos, J. (2004). Ischemia-modified albumin during skeletal muscle ischemia. *Clin.Chem.* 50, 1063-1065.

7

Do We Need Another Look at Serum Uric Acid in Cardiovascular Disease? Serum Uric Acid as a Predictor of Outcomes in Acute Myocardial Infarction

Siniša Car[1] and Vladimir Trkulja[2]
[1]*Cardiologist, Department of internal medicine, Cardiology unit, General Hospital Varaždin, Varaždin,*
[2]*Professor of pharmacology, Department of pharmacology, Zagreb University School of Medicine, Zagreb, Croatia*

1 Introduction

In humans and other higher primates, uric acid (UA) is the end product of purine metabolism generated by oxidation of xanthine catalyzed by xantine oxidase (XO) (EC 1.17.3.2) (Figure 1). In other mammals, UA is further oxidized by uricase (EC 1.7.3.3) to yield highly soluble allantoin, which is then excreted from the body. From the evolutionary standpoint, the reasons for the mutations resulting in a nonfunctioning *uricase* gene (pseudogene) in higher mammals are still unclear. In contrast to allantoin, uric acid is poorly hydrosoluble (water solubility of its salts, the urates, is slightly higher) and when its serum concentrations exceed the theoretical limit of solubility (around 415 μmol/L, or 7 mg/dL), urate crystals are likely to be formed. Approximately two thirds of the daily UA turnover is eliminated by the kidney (glomerular filtration, tubular re-absorption and secretion) and one third *via* the gastrointestinal system.

Xanthine oxidase is an ubiquitous enzyme, distributed in the liver (particularly), gut (particularly), kidney, heart (capillary endothelium primarily, but has been proven in cardiomyocytes, as well), brain, as well as in plasma. Besides the conversion of hypoxanthine to xanthine and xanthine to UA, it has a number of other functions, including hydroxylation of various purines, pterins, aromatic heterocycles and aliphatic and aromatic aldehydes (for a detailed review on XO see Pacher et al., 2006). Serum levels of UA (serum uric acid, SUA) are governed by the rates of its production and elimination, and are susceptible to a variety of nutritional, genetic, pharmacological and morbidity influences (Table 1). Hyperuricemia, a state of overtly high SUA concentration, is typically defined as SUA >360 μmol/L in women and >420 μmol/L in men, whereas values 310-420 μmol/L in men and 250-360 μmol/L in women are conventionally considered as "high-normal".

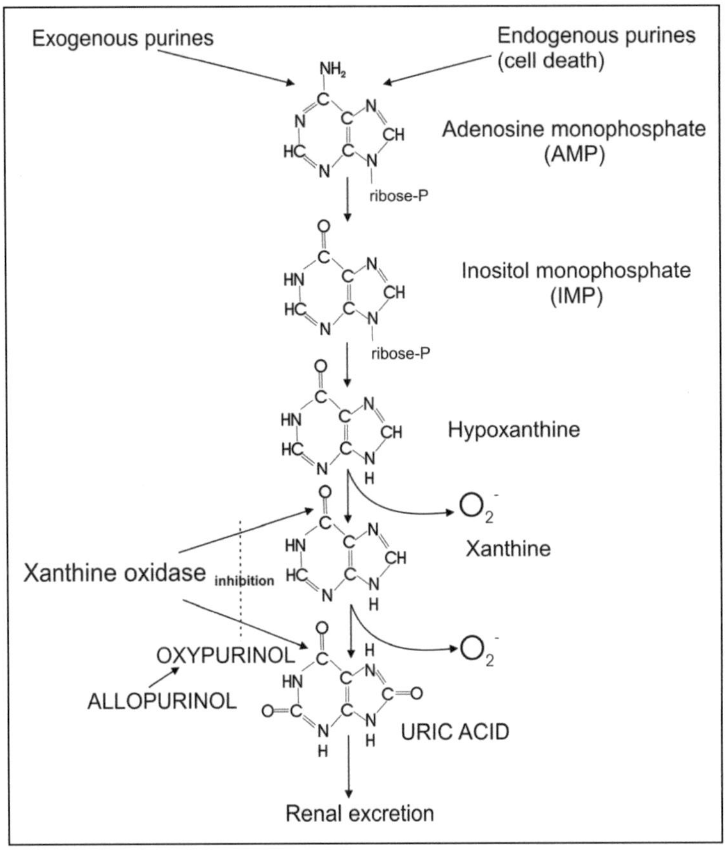

Fig. 1. Metabolism of uric acid.

*Dietary factors: increased purine intake in animal products especially internal organs (liver, kidney, brain, meat extracts), sweetbreads, anchovies, sardines, herring, mackerel, game meats, gravy, high fructose intake, alcohol
*Reduced excretion by diseased kidneys
*Malignancies, polycythemia vera, myelodysplastic syndromes, hemolytic anemias or other conditions with a rapid cell turnover
*Use of diuretics
*Mutations in proteins involved in the urate metabolism, especially xanthine oxidase, urate transporter/channel (UAT), organic anion transporters 1 and 3 (OAT1 and OAT3) and urate transporter 1 (URAT1)

Table 1. The main causes of hyperuricemia (after Lippi et al., 2008)

Ever since the late 19th century, and particularly since the 1950s, the potential role of SUA, specifically, increased SUA in cardiovascular diseases (CVD) has attracted much attention. A plethora of non-clinical, clinical and epidemiological studies have accumulated over the decades that aimed to elucidate molecular and cellular mechanisms of UA and the role of SUA as a diagnostic or a prognostic aid, or as a therapeutic target. Uric acid has a number of molecular effects potentially interesting in respect to CVD. One of the first recognized was the antioxidant potential of UA – together with ascorbic acid which recycles the UA radicals, it is the most important antioxidant in plasma that effectively scavenges the superoxide anion, hydroxyl radicals and singlet oxygen and may chelate transitional metals. Furthermore, UA blocks the reaction in which peroxynitrite (generated in reactions by which superoxide anion inactivates nitric oxide, NO) attacks and nitrosylates tyrosine residues in various proteins. Moreover, UA inhibits degradation of the extracellular superoxide dismutase (SOD3), which then is able to convert superoxide anion into hydrogen peroxide, and thus prevent NO inactivation (by the superoxide anion). Based on the knowledge about the role of oxidative stress in various aspects of CVD (e.g., endothelial function, myocardial function), it has been suggested that the loss of uricase activity in humans should be viewed as an "evolutionary benefit", protective of the cardiovascular system. Indeed, there is solid evidence that a transient rise in SUA reduces markers of oxidative stress, which then correlates well with improvements in some of the indices of cardiovascular function. For example, it has been rather well elaborated that the cardiovascular benefit of moderate wine drinking (with food) is largely due to an acute and transient wine-induced rise in SUA that counter-acts the food-induced oxidative stress. However, prolonged/excessive increase in SUA is clearly associated with cardiovascular risks or "damage" (see below), rather than with a cardiovascular benefit. Although we are still far from full understanding of molecular/cellular mechanisms of UA, the knowledge is extensive and some effects have been well documented and provide a sound mechanistic rationale. As most of the other antioxidants, under certain conditions (e.g., high concentrations, low pH, like in hypoxic tissues, low levels of other antioxidants) UA may promote oxidative stress. For example, it depletes ascorbic acid (used to re-cycle UA radicals), and thus reduces re-cycling of α-tocopherol and, consequently, β-carotene, other potent antioxidants, which, overall, may results in a reduced antioxidant activity. *In vitro*, UA (but not its precursors xanthine and hypoxanthine) exerts a number of effects on vascular smooth muscle cells: enters the cells *via* organic anionic transporters and activates transcriptional factors, like nuclear factor *kappa* B (NF-κB) and activation protein 1 (AP-1); induces the tissue renin-angiotensin-aldosterone system and angitensin II production; induces cell proliferation (via MAPK and Erk1/2 kinases); induces COX2 activity and thromboxane synthesis; induces synthesis of the monocytic chemoatractant protein 1 (MCP-1, *via* p38 MAPK) which is important in the pathogenesis of atherosclerosis; induces production of c-reactive protein (CRP) (*via* p38 MAPK). Uric acid also stimulates the mononuclear cells to production of interleukin (IL)-1β, IL-6 and tumor necrosis factor-α (TNF-α). Clearly, UA may recruit a whole armamentarium of molecular/cellular "players" that are known to be involved in the pathophysiology of vascular changes underlying CVD. Indeed, it has been repeatedly shown that infusion of UA in humans induces platelet aggregation and endothelial dysfunction with reduced NO production, an effect also seen within the kidneys. However, when discussing the potential role of UA as a "direct pathogen" in CVD, one should also keep in mind that, inherently, SUA levels are a marker of the activity of XO, an enzyme that *per se* has an important role in the oxidant-antioxidant system. While measuring SUA in humans is simple, accurate and cheap, there is no routine method to directly measure XO activity. Xanthine oxidase has been strongly implicated in CVD. The enzyme is expressed in the endothelium, but it is generally thought that XO released from the liver and the gut into the circulation and then bound to the endothelial cell is the important factor. It is in a complex relationship with NO – XO generates superoxide anion (e.g., during xanthine oxidation) that inactivates NO and tonically suppress NO synthase (NOs), whereas conversely, NO may suppress XO activity and XO is also capable of reducing nitrates and nitrites back to NO. As already mentioned, superoxide-NO reactions and reactions between the superoxide and various nitrosothiols generate peroxynitrite that can inflict oxidative and nitrosative injury to proteins, enzymes, lipids, DNA. There are observations regarding endothelial dysfunction that "shift" the focus from SUA itself to XO - while infusion of UA may induce it, uriocosuric agents, that reduce SUA, have failed to improve endothelial function; on the other hand, XO inhibitors (like allopurinol) improve the disrupted endothelial function even before changes in SUA occur. Therefore, considerations of "elevated SUA" and its role in CVD inevitably subsume its potential direct effector mechanisms, but also those effects of XO which are UA-independent and for which elevated SUA is (just) a marker.

Over the decades, at the clinical and epidemiological level, the "issue" of (S)UA and CVD has been encompassed by a controversy - should the relationship be perceived as a *causative* one, or as a mere *association*? In part, it has been fuelled by the mechanistic knowledge about the direct (possible) deleterious effects of UA and the fact that, at the same time, it might be just a marker of other events (e.g., XO activity). Additional contribution to the controversy comes from the inconsistency of observations (both "negative" and "positive" observations in many settings) and the nature of (some of) the clinical/epidemiological observations. First, SUA has been related not only to CVD or its "endpoint-events", like development of coronary artery disease (CAD) and related mortality, chronic heart failure, acute myocardial infarction or stroke, but also to a number of conditions that *per se* are CVD risk factors, e.g., hypertension, glucose intolerance, insulin resistance, dyslipidemia, obesity, metabolic syndrome, renal failure. Second, some of the studies were conducted in a way that allowed only for detection of associations, which were frequently difficult to interpret. For example, in some cases it was not possible to "isolate" an independent relationship (*association*) (independent of other risk factors) between SUA and the end point, either a direct one (of the type SUA $\Rightarrow$ endpoint) or a mediated one (of the type SUA $\Rightarrow$ other risk factor $\Rightarrow$ endpoint). Furthermore, the interpretation of associations in terms of "causes and consequences" is frequently complexed by the fact that both is possible, e.g., while there is evidence that hyperuricemia may promote renal failure, renal failure inevitably results in hyperuricemia. Generally, in biomedicine, the dilemma about causation vs. association has important practical implications - if a causative relationship is established between variables, then the "cause" clearly is a potential target for an intervention (preventive, therapeutic). It is the opinion of the authors of this text that in the specific case of SUA and CVD, this dilemma might not be as relevant. First, if there is a "marker" that can be determined easily, reproducibly and accurately and at low cost (SUA), that independently, consistently and accurately predicts future events (a reliable predictor), than, irrespective of the nature of its relationship with these "future events", it *per se* is valuable (assessment of risk). One could easily agree that despite all the existing knowledge, there is still space for improvements in risk assessment in CVD. Next, considering the nature of a potential intervention (inhibition of XO, e.g., allopurinol), it seems irrelevant whether UA itself is a cause (acting directly on the endpoint variable, or through "intervening" or "mediation" variables [other risk factors], of both) or just a marker of increased XO activity, which in fact, is the cause (or - both!) - the intervention is likely to yield a benefit. It is far beyond the scope of this text to discuss in detail all the aspects of the complex relationship between SUA and CVD. For this purpose, reader is referred to comprehensive reviews on the topic, some of which are listed at the end of this chapter (Johnson at al., 2003, Baker et al., 2005, Duan&Ling 2008, Naquibullah et al., 2007, Lippi et al., 2008, Feig et al., 2008, Doehner et al., 2008, Gagliardi et al., 2009, Bergamini et al., 2009, Kim et al., 2009 and 2010, Wechter et al., 2010). The main points could be summarized as follows:

Hypertension, metabolic syndrome, renal failure and other risk factor for CVD. There is now sufficient evidence to strongly support a claim that increased SUA is an important etiological factor in at least one form of hypertension - early-onset primary hypertension. The sequence of events includes chronic hyperuricemia in mothers that may be transferred to the fetus and result in intrauterine growth retardation and a reduced number of nephrons. The reduced number of nephrons (and renal function), together with environmental and genetic factors, contributes to permanent hyperuricemia that reduces intra-renal NO release, activates the renin-angiotensin system, promotes vascular inflammation and inhibits endothelial cell proliferation, thus leading to a vasoreactive hypertension in the first step, and eventually to a salt-sensitive hypertension (Figure 2).

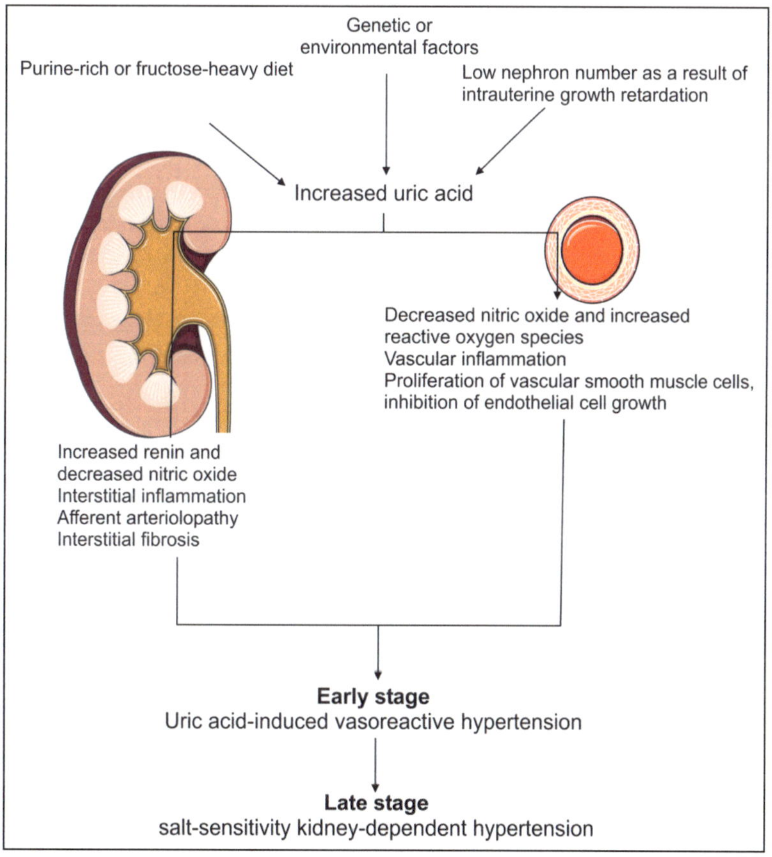

Fig. 2. Development of uric acid-induced hypertension (re-drawn and modified after Feig et al., 2008).

Otherwise, increased SUA has been repeatedly shown associated with hypertension and prehypertension. Moreover, in a number of prospective epidemiological studies in normotensive subjects, increased SUA has repeatedly consistently predicted development of hypertension independently of other risk factors. The adjusted relative risk depended on the observational period, as well as on qualification of "increased SUA". As reviewed by Feig et al. (Feig et al., 2008), in 6 studies with a total of 17 629 adult subjects, adjusted relative risks of development of hypertension (over 6-21 years) varied between 1.25 and 2.10 for "high vs. low" quartile or quintile of SUA, or for SUA levels >416 or >387 μmol/L in men (vs. lower) and >357 μmol/L in women (vs. lower) (all these cut-off points are lower than the conventional limits of hyperuricemia, see above). In the other 8 studies with a total of 25 500 adult subjects, adjusted relative risks of hypertension (over 4 to 12 years) varied between 1.10 and 1.65 for increase in SUA by one standard deviation or by 60 μmol/L. Increased SUA has been repeatedly found in patients with metabolic syndrome, obese subjects, patients with dyslipidemia or glucose intolerance. In animal models, UA may induce a correlate of human metabolic syndrome. In a sample of a general population in Japan, irrespectively of gender, SUA levels >416 μmol/L in men and >357 μmol/L in women were found to cluster with hypertension, obesity, hypercholesterolemia, hypo-HDL hypercholesterolemia and hypertriglyceridemia (Nagahama et al., 2004).

Stroke. A recent analysis of 16 prospective cohort studies that embraced 238 500 subjects and assessed predictivity of hyperuricemia (different definitions, but generally >380-416 μmol/L irrespective of gender; or >416 μmol/L in men and >360 μmol/L in women) for development of stroke, indicated that in 10/10 studies which reported on stroke incidence, adjusted relative risks (RR) were >1.0. At the same time, adjusted relative risks of stroke-related mortality were >1.0 in 10/11 studies that reported this outcome. The meta-analysis of adjusted RRs (random-effects with practically no heterogeniety) indicated RR of stroke: 1.91 (95% CI 1.06-2.75) in a mixed population; 1.42 (0.94-1.90) in men, 1.42 (1.03-1.80) in women and 1.47 (1.19-1.76) overall (Kim et al., 2009). Relative risks of stroke-related death were: 1.61 (95% CI 1.13-2.09) in a mixed population; 1.20 (1.05-1.35) in men, 1.35 (1.04-1.66) in women and 1.26 (1.12-1.39) overall (Kim et al., 2009).

Chronic heart failure (CHF). Chronic heart failure (CHF) is a typical setting in which the dilemma about UA as a "cause" or a (mere) "marker" is particularly actual (Duan & Ling, 2008, Doehner et al., 2008, Bergamini et al., 2009). Numerous animal models have clearly confirmed the role of reactive oxygen species (ROS) in pathophysiology of the heart failure – there is a clear correlation between increased markers of oxidative stress within the heart and systemically, poorer survival and a number of functional measures of cardiac functions and hemodynamic consequences. The mechanisms of direct deleterious effects of ROS within the heart include alterations of calcium metabolism and propagation of endothelial dysfunction, inflammation and cellular responses resulting in remodeling, and they sum-up with their effects on the kidneys and systemic vasculature. The sources of cardiac ROS are multiple, but there is clear evidence, including humans, of increased cardiac XO activity. It inevitably results in enhanced production of UA, besides the generation of reactive oxygen and nitrogen species. Hence, it seems practically impossible to "separate" the effects of UA *per se* from those of activated XO. Be it as it may, increased SUA in CHF patients is associated with worse functional tests and, clearly, with a worse long-term survival. An analysis in CHF patients showed doubling and tripling of the adjusted relative risk of death (over time) (i.e., "independent effect of SUA") for each 200 μmol/L increase of SUA above the cut-off point of 400 μmol/L. Moreover, the death risk was particularly increased when

SUA >565 μmol/L was combined with a score of 2 or 3 based on the heart failure survival scoring system (Anker et al., 2003). Similarly, a study in acute HF patients demonstrated an increased risk of death in patients with SUA >458 μmol/L as compared to those with SUA <416 μmol/L (adjusted RR=1.45, 95% CI 1.03-2.05) and increase in RR by around 8% (CI 1-15%) for each 60 μmol/L increase in SUA (Alimonda et al., 2009). As reviewed by Pacher et al. (2006) and Bergamini et al. (2009), several randomized trials indicated improvements in cardiac and hemodynamic parameters in CHF patients treated with allopurinol (an XO inhibitor), even with indications of improved survival, but not all trials have been "positive" and uricosuric agents seemingly were not effective.

Coronary heart disease (CAD). The link between SUA and CAD is two-fold. First, regardless of the actual mechanism (etiological factor vs. marker), increased SUA is clearly related to a number of CAD risk factors (hypertension, renal function, obesity, dyslipidemia, metabolic syndrome) and seemingly does independently predict CAD (regardless of whether a "direct" effect or "mediated" through other risk factors). A recent review and meta-analysis embraced 26 prospective cohort studies with 403 000 participants that reported on predictivity of SUA for occurrence of CAD and/or CAD-related mortality (Kim et al., 2010). The effect of SUA was expressed through a contrast of "hyperuricemia" vs "no hyperuricemia" (very different definitions in different studies; cut-offs for men ranged from 321 μmol/L to 458 μmol/L; for women they ranged from 280 μmol/L to 393 μmol/L; and for mixed population from 387 μmol/L to 416 μmol/L) or as the effect of increase in SUA by 60 μmol/L. Based on 9 studies that reported adjusted risks of CAD incidence (adjusted for known CAD risk factors), pooled RRs for CAD incidence for "hyperucemia" vs. "no hyperuricemia" were: 1.04 (95% CI 0.90-1.17) in men; 1.07 (0.82-1.32) in women; 1.32 (0.57-2.07) in mixed populations and 1.09 (1.03-1.16) overall (all random-effects estimates with very low-to-mild heterogeneity). Based on 9 studies that reported adjusted risks of CAD-related mortality (adjusted for known risk factors), pooled RRs for CAD-related mortality for "hyperucemia" vs. "no hyperuricemia" were: 1.09 (95% CI 0.98-1.19) in men; 1.67 (1.30-2.04) in women; and 1.16 (1.01-1.30) overall (all random-effects estimates with very low-to-mild heterogeneity). Based on 4 studies that reported adjusted risks of CAD-related mortality based on increase in SUA by 60 μmol/L, pooled RRs were: 1.10 (95% CI 0.96-1.24) in men; 1.17 (0.97-1.38) in women; 1.10 (1.06-1.14) in mixed population and 1.12 (1.05-1.19) overall (random-effects, low heterogeniety). Second, in animal models as well as in humans, cardiac ischemia-reperfusion injury involves increased ROS generation. The sources of ROS are, likely, multiple (as in the failing heart), but it is hypothesized that activation of XO contributes. The proposed mechanism is summarized in Figure 3: ischemia favors both intracellular accumulation of hypoxanthine and free calcium; the latter activates proteases that convert xanthine dehydrogenase to xanthine oxidase with a consequent generation of superoxide anion and UA. Several randomized trials, but not all, have shown that in patients undergoing elective coronary by-pass surgery allopurinol may reduce arrhythmias, improve cardiac index and cardiac output and reduce mortality (Wechter et al., 2010).

In contrast to the broad attention that it has received in relation to the mentioned cardiovascular disease, until the recent years SUA has practically not been investigated in the setting of the outcomes of the acute myocardial infarction (AMI) or acute coronary syndromes in general. Several studies addressing this issue have been published since 2005 and they are the main objective of this chapter. As in other SUA-CVD settings, the topic deserves some attention: an easily and reproducibly available marker with a consistent

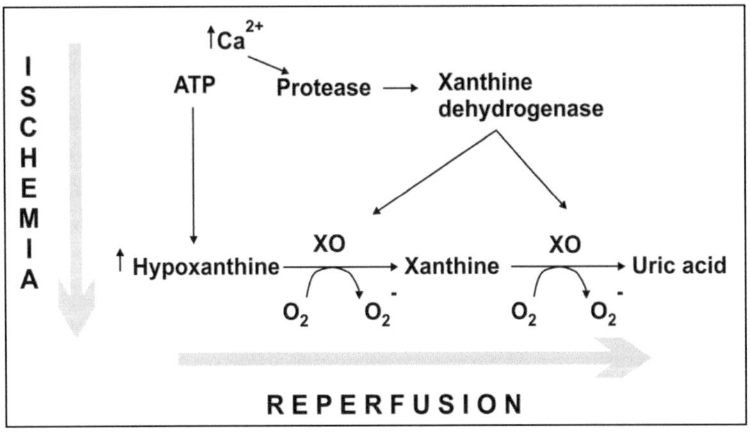

Fig. 3. Proposed effects of ischemia-reperfusion for intracardiac activation of xanthine oxidase (XO) and generation of superoxide anion (O2-) and uric acid (re-drawn and modified after Pacher et al. 2006).

predictive value may well improve risk stratification in AMI patients (and reflect on clinical decisions); considering the mechanisms relating SUA to ischemia-reperfusion (Figure 3) and other relevant intra- and extra-cardiac factors, it seems that, should a SUA-AMI outcome relationship be established, there would be a sound rationale for implementation of an intervention based on XO inhibition, regardless of whether SUA is primarily an effector or a "mere marker".

2. Do serum uric acid levels predict outcomes in acute myocardial infarction patients?

2.1 Chronology and a general description of the relevant studies

Study essentials are summarized in Table 2.

In 2005, Kojima and colleagues (Kojima et al., 2005) published the results of the Japanese Acute Coronary Syndrome Study (JACSS) - a retrospective analysis of a database on acute coronary syndrome patients generated as a result of collaboration of 35 institutions in Japan during 2002 (January - December). Patients (N=1124) were defined as consecutive AMI patients admitted to a hospital within 48 hours since the symptom onset (with SUA determined on admission). No distribution of patients by AMI type was given - whether with (STEMI) or without (NSTEMI) ST elevation. However, 943 (84%) patients underwent immediate reperfusion [predominantly by a percutaneous coronary intervention (PCI) and only sporadically by pharmacological thrombolysis] (Table 2) and could be considered as STEMI patients, whereas the remaining 181 could be considered as NSTEMI patients. Men prevailed (70%) and the mean age was 68 years. Higher on-admission SUA values were independently associated with the male sex, higher body mass index (BMI), higher serum creatinine, higher Killip's class and a history of hypertension and a previous AMI. Patients were classified based on the on-admission SUA quartiles and the analysis focused on a comparison of the outcomes between patients within the 4th quartile [(n= 276, SUA >399 μmol/L, which is higher than the cut-off value for hyperuricemia in women, and is just below the cut-off value of hyperuricemia in men (420 μmol/L)] and those within the 1st quartile [n=273, SUA <274 μmol/L, which is within the range of "low-normal SUA" in men, and just above the cut-off value of "low-normal SUA" in women (250 μmol/L)]. The primary outcome of interest was all-cause mortality (survival) during the observational period, which averaged 450 days and the maximum length was 700 days. The death-rate was higher among the 4th quartile patients (12% vs. 3%) and 4th quartile SUA values were found independently predictive of all-cause mortality: in a Cox proportional hazard regression model with adjustment for the Killip's class, age and peak creatine phosphokinase (CPK) value (selected through a stepwise procedure among a number of others, $p<0.05$), HR was 3.72 (95% CI 1.42-9.74). The analysis that considered SUA as a continuous variable indicated an adjusted death risk increase of around 22% by each increase in SUA by 50 μmol/L (HR= 1.22, 95% CI 1.11-1.35). No increase in the risk of death was found in patients within the 2nd (n=299, SUA 274-333 μmol/L) or the 3rd (n= 276, SUA 333-399 μmol/L) quartile.

In 2007, Valente and colleagues (Valente et al., 2007) reported the results of a prospective study conducted at a single PCI-performing center in Italy. The report focused on STEMI patients presenting with a cardiogenic shock and undergoing acute PCI, i.e., within 6 hours since the symptom onset (between January 2004 and June 2005) (N=45). Patients were classified as those who died during the in-hospital stay ("cases", n=20, 13 men, mean age 78 years) and those who survived (n=25, 19 men, mean age 66 years). Serum uric values taken on admission to intensive coronary care unit (ICCU) were higher in "cases" than in "survivors": (mean±SD) 434±137 μmol/L vs. 351±137 μmol/L ($p=0.040$). In a univariate test, on-admission SUA >387 μmol/L (vs. below) (which qualifies as hyperuricemia in women, but not entirely in men) was associated with higher odds of in-hospital death: OR= 6.7 (95% CI 1.4-31.8), but this association did not hold in a multivariate model (adjusted OR not reported).

The same group (Lazzeri et al., 2010) extended their study report by including all consecutive STEMI patients who underwent acute PCI (within 12 hours since the symptom onset), regardless of the clinical presentation (N=466). Patients were classified as those with on-admission (to ICCU) SUA >387 μmol/L ("high", n=100, 78.5% men, average age 72 years) and those with SUA ≤387 μmol/L ("normal", n=366, 78.6% men, average age 64 years). In-hospital mortality, the primary outcome, was higher in "high" SUA patients (9.0% vs. 2.5%). "High" on-admission SUA was found independently predictive of higher in-hospital mortality: in a logistic regression model with adjustment for age, left ventricular ejection fraction (LVEF), fibrinogen and peak troponin I levels (selected through a backward procedure among a number of others, $p<0.05$), OR was 1.82 (95% CI 1.15-2.86). With further adjustments for sex, Killip's class and diuretic use, OR=2.02 (95% CI 1.47-2.78).

In 2009, Car and Trkulja (Car&Trkulja, 2009) reported a retrospective analysis of consecutive AMI patients [N=621, 481 STEMI (77.5%), 140 NSTEMI; 64.7% men, average age 65 years) treated exclusively conservatively (between 1996 and 2001), with a low rate of fibrinolytic reperfusion (10% of STEMI patients), at a single center in Croatia, all admitted within 48 hours since the symptom onset. Outcomes of primary interest were in-hospital mortality, 30-day mortality and, for those who survived the first 30 days post-index event (considering that mortality after AMI is higher within the first 30 days than in any other subsequent 30-day period), long-term all-cause mortality (n=544; follow-up extended to up to 13 years).

In-hospital mortality was 10% and 30-day mortality was 12.4%. Higher on-admission SUA was independently predictive for both outcomes: in modified Poisson regression models (to yield relative risk, rather than odds ratio), with adjustment for age; sex; history of stroke, hypertension, AMI and HF; peak creatine phosphokinase (CPK), right bundle branch block (RBBB), serum creatinine (selected through a backward procedure, $p<0.1$) and AMI type (forced), RR for each increase in SUA by 50 µmol/L was 1.08 (95% CI 1.01-1.16) for in-hospital mortality, and it was 1.08 (95% CI 1.02-1.15) for 30-day mortality. Among those who survived the first 30-day post-index event, mortality during the subsequent period (up to 13 years) was 32.2%. Higher on-admission SUA was independently predictive of poorer long-term survival: in a Cox proportional hazard regression model, with adjustment for age, serum creatinine, heart failure at discharge, use of digitalis and SUA*age interaction (selected through a stepwise procedure among a number of others, $p<0.1$), HR for each increase in SUA by 50 µmol/L was 1.65 (95% CI 1.10-2.44).

In 2010, Rentoukas and colleagues (Rentoukas et al., 2010) reported on a small, single-center randomized controlled trial in Greece in which consecutive acute STEMI patients (June 2005 - June 2006) undergoing PCI within 3-12 hours post-symptom onset were randomized to receive allopurinol (n=21, 15 men, mean age 65 years) or placebo (n=19, 14 men, mean age 64 years) for 30 days. A loading dose of allopurinol (400 mg) was administered as soon as AMI was diagnosed, and treatment continued with 100 mg/day. During the observed 30 days, allopurinol-treated patients had lower peak CPK, peak CK-MB and lower peak troponin I levels, and a higher proportion of patients experienced a complete ST-elevation resolution (all $p<0.05$).

In 2010, Kowalczyk and colleagues (Kowalczyk et al., 2010) published a retrospective analysis of consecutive STEMI patients undergoing PCI at a single center in Poland (between 2000 and 2007). Timing of PCI relative to the symptom onset was not specified. Patients were selected as those having "impaired renal function": either having a "baseline kidney dysfunction" (BKD) defined as estimated glomerular filtration rate (eGFR) <60 mL/min71.73m^2 based on serum creatinine taken on admission or within 12 hours since admission, or having a "contrast-induced nephropathy" (CIN) defined as an increase in serum creatinine >44.2 µmol/L or >25% from the baseline value, within 48 hours since PCI. A total of 1015 such patients were included. They were classified as those with hyperuricemia (SUA >420 µmol/L determined at the same time as serum creatinine; which is in line with the definition of hyperuricemia in men, and is above the cut-off value of hyperuricemia in women) (n= 352, men 64.2%, mean age 67 years) and those without it (n= 663, men 59.6%, mean age 64 years). The observational period extended to up to 7 years post-PCI (average 3 years). Besides being older and with a higher prevalence of men, hyperuricemic patients were more frequently diabetic, had previous PCI, hypertension, eGFR <60 mL/min/1.73 m^2 and had lower LVEF at discharge. In-hospital, 30-day, 1-year and entire-period all-cause mortalities were higher in hyperuricemic vs. non-hyperuricemic patients (Table 2). The main analysis was that of all-cause mortality over the entire observed period (case-fatality rate 32.7% for hyperuricemia vs. 18.6% for no hyperuricemia). Hyperuricemia independently predicted mortality: in a Cox proportional hazard regression model with adjustment for age, cardiogenic shock on admission, diabetes, eGFR <60 mL/min/1.73 m^2, LVEF at discharge, incomplete revascularization and lack of TIMI flow grade 3 after PCI of the infarct-related artery (selected among a number of other covariates in a stepwise procedure, $p<0.05$), adjusted HR=1.17 (95% CI 1.05-1.29). In the same model but considering SUA as a continuous variable, HR (by 50 µmol/L increase in SUA)= 1.04 (95% CI 1.02-1.06).

The patients were further analyzed separately as BKD (n=503; with hyperuricemia n=225, without it n=278) and as CIN patients (n= 693, with hyperuricemia n=243, without it n=450) (these two subgroups partly overlapped - some patients with BKD later-on developed CIN). Crude mortality rates for BKD and CIN patients are summarized in Table 2. High SUA independently predicted mortality in both subgroups. BKD: adjusted HR for hyperuricemia = 1.38 (95% CI 1.23-1.53), adjusted HR by 50 µmol/L SUA increase = 1.05 (95% CI 1.03-1.07); CIN: adjusted HR for hyperuricemia = 1.21 (95% CI 1.05-1.37), adjusted HR by 50 µmol/L SUA increase = 1.06 (95% CI 1.04-1.09).

In 2011, Basar and colleagues (Basar et al., 2011) reported on their prospective observational study in 185 consecutive STEMI patients undergoing PCI within 12 hours since the symptom onset (N=185) (time-period not reported, most author affiliations in Turkey). Patients were classified as those having on-admission SUA >387 µmol/L ("high"; above the cut-off of hyperuricemia in women, but below it in men) (n= 45, 80% men, mean age 60 years) and those with on admission SUA below this level ("normal", n= 140, 80% men, mean age 58 years). Patients with "high" SUA more frequently had a history of hypertension, prior AMI, multivessel disease and had higher Killip's class at presentation. They were followed-up for 1 year. In-hospital mortality was higher in patients with "high" SUA (6.6% vs. 2.8%). The main outcomes of interest were all-cause mortality within 1-year period and proportion of patients with abnormal myocardial perfusion at 1 year post-PCI based on TIMI myocardial perfusion grade. "High" SUA independently predicted both outcomes. In a logistic regression model with adjustment for TIMI risk score, abnormal TIMI perfusion grade at discharge, LVEF at discharge, multivessel disease (selected among a number of covariates in a stepwise procedure, $p<0.1$), time to reperfusion and serum creatinine (forced covariates), OR for death was 1.29 (95% 1.14-2.08). When SUA was considered as a continuous variable (with the same adjustments), OR by 50 µmol/L increase in SUA was 1.10 (95% CI 1.02-1.14). Considering the proportion of patients with abnormal myocardial perfusion, adjusted OR (Killip class, multivessel disease, corrected TIMI time-frame count, selected based on $p<0.05$) was 2.14 (95% CI 1.17-4.19).

In 2011, Bae and colleagues (Bae et al., 2011) published a retrospective analysis of a multicenter AMI registry in South Korea. Embraced were 850 consecutive AMI patients (during 2006 and 2007), 391 (46%) of whom were depicted as STEMI patients. The remaining patients were likely NSTEMI, since typical clinical AMI presentation with an increase in cardiac enzymes was prerequisite for inclusion. Overall, 623 (73.3%) patients underwent PCI. Other reperfusion procedures were not specified. Also, time elapsed between the symptom onset and admission and timing of SUA measurement were not specified. SUA values were collected retrospectively since they had not been originally entered into the registry. Patients were classified as those who, during a 6-month period, experienced a composite outcome of death or non-fatal reinfarction or revascularization (MACE) (n=109) and those who did not (n=741). They were also classified as those with on-admission SUA >420 µmol/L (cut-off for hyperuricemia in men, and higher than that in women) (n= 172, 74.4% men, mean age 66.5 years) and those with lower SUA levels (n= 678, 67.2% men, mean age 67 years). Besides the fact that they were more frequently men and somewhat older, hyperuricemic patients more

Author/ year	Design/type	Patients	Outcomes	Univariate effects	Multivariate effects
Kojima et al. 2005	Retrospective, observational, prognostic	Consecutive AMI, type not specified; admission ≤48 hrs since onset; N= 1124 Reperfusion= 943 (84%): stent 743, balloon 146, thrombolysis 54. No reperfusion: 181 (16%)	*30-day* MACE, cardiac mortality, all-cause mortality *Long-term* All-cause mortality, follow-up maximum 700 days	**4th vs. 1st quartile SUA** *30-day MACE.* 14% vs. 5%; OR=2.83, p=0.001 *30-day cardiac death.* 11% vs. 2%; OR=6.54, p<0.001 *30-day all death.* 11% vs. 2%, OR= 5.63, p<0.001 *All-cause mortality long-term.* 12% vs. 3%, HR= 3.75, p<0.001 **SUA by 50 μmol/L** *All-cause mortality long-term.* HR= 1.28, p<0.001	**4th vs. 1st quartile SUA** *All-cause mortality long-term.* HR=3.72 (95% CI 1.42-9.74) **SUA by 50 μmol/L** *All-cause mortality long-term.* HR= 1.22 (95%CI 1.11-1.33) Ajdust: Killip's class, peak CPK and age (p<0.05)
Valente et al. 2007	Prospective, observational, prognostic	Consecutive STEMI with CS, undergoing PCI within 6 hrs since onset, N=45	In-hospital mortality	SUA >387 μmol/L (vs. below) – OR= 6.7, p=0.016	Not significant
Lazzeri et al. 2010	Extension of the above, same protocol	Consecutive STEMI under-going PCI within 12 hrs since onset, N=466	In-hospital mortality	SUA >387 μmol/L (vs. below) – 9.0% vs. 2.5%, OR=3.9, p=0.006	SUA >387 μmol/L (vs. below) OR= 1.82 (95%CI 1.15-2.86)/Adjust: age, LVEF, fibrinogen, peak Tn I (p<0.05) OR=2.02 (95%CI 1.47-2.78) / further: sex, COPD, Killip's class, use of diuretics
Car&Trkulja 2009	Retrospective, observational, prognostic	Consecutive AMI; admi-ssion ≤48 hrs since onset; N= 621, STEMI n=481 (77.5%), NSTEMI n=140 Reperfusion: 10% of STEMI (thrombolysis)	*Short-term* In-hospital and 30-day all-casue mortality *Long-term* All-cause mortality, follow-up up to 13 years; n=544 who survived first 30 days	*In-hospital mortality* SUA 50 μmol/L: RR=1.20, p<0.05 *30-day mortality* SUA 50 μmol/L: RR=1.19, p<0.05 *All-cause mortality long-term* SUA 50 μmol/L: HR=1.14, p<0.05	*In-hospital mortality* SUA 50 μmol/L: RR=1.08 (95%CI 1.01-1.16) *30-day mortality* SUA 50 μmol/L: RR=1.08 (95%CI 1.02-1.15) Ajdust: age; sex; AMI type; prior CVI, hypertension, AMI, HF; peak CPK, RBBB, serum creatinine, (p<0.1). *All-cause mortality long-term* SUA 50 μmol/L: HR=1.65 (95%CI 1.13-2.18) Adjust: creatinine, age, HF, use of digitalis, age*SUA interaction (p<0.1)
Rentoukas et al. 2010	Therepeutic, RCT, allopuri-nol vs. placebo	Consecutive STEMI under-going PCI 3-12 hrs since onset. Allop. n=21, Plac. n=19	30-day treatment and assessment: peak CPK, peak CK-MB, peak Tn I, resolution of ST elevation	Allopurinol: lower peak CPK, MB-CPK and Tn I, greater proportion of "full ST recovery" within 30 days (all p<0.05).	Not reported

Author/ year	Design/type	Patients	Outcomes	Univariate effects	Multivariate effects
Kowalczyk et al. 2010	Retrospective, observational, prognostic	Consecutive STEMI under-going PCI (time since onset not specified) with reduced renal function (N=1015), further subdivided (partly overlapping): eGFR on admission <60 mL/min/1.73m² (BKD) (n=503) and patients with PCI-induced nephropathy (CIN) (n=693)	*Short-term* In-hospital mortality 30-day all-cause mortality *1 year* All-cause mortality *>1 year* All-cause mortality	**SUA >420 μmol/L (vs. below)** *In-hospital mortality* All: 14.5% vs. 7.1%, p<0.001 BKD: 18.2 vs. 12.2%, p=0.060 CIN: 19.0% vs. 6.4%, p<0.001 *30-day mortality* All: 16.9% vs. 7.7%, p<0.001 BKD: 19.6% vs. 12.9%, p=0.04 CIN: 19.8% vs. 6.9%, p<0.001 *1-year mortality* All: 25.0% vs. 13.7%, p<0.001 BKD: 31.5% vs. 18.3%, p<0.001 CIN: 28.0% vs. 13.1%, p<0.001 *>1 year mortality* All: 32.7% vs. 18.6%, p<0.001 BKD: 41.3% vs. 25.9%, p<0.001 CIN: 35.4% vs. 16.7%, p<0.001	**SUA >420 μmol/L (vs. below)** *Overall observed period* All: HR= 1.17 (95% CI 1.05-1.29) BKD: HR= 1.38 (95% CI 1.23-1.53) CIN: HR= 1.21 (95% CI 1.05-1.37) **SUA by 50 μmol/L** *Overall observed period* All: HR= 1.04 (95% CI 1.02-1.06) BKD: HR= 1.05 (95% CI 1.03-1.07) CIN: HR= 1.06 (95% CI 1.04-1.09) Adjust: All - age, CS on admission, DM, LVEF at discharge, incomplete revascu-larization, lack of TIMI flow grade 3 after PCI of the infarct-related artery, BKD BKD – age, CS on admission. LVEF at discharge, incomplete revascularization, lack of TIMI flow grade 3 after PCI of the infarct-related artery CIN: age, CS on admission, LVEF at discharge, incomplete revascularization, BKD/ (all adjustments p<0.05)
Basar et al. 2011	Prospective, observational, prognostic	Consecutive STEMI under-going PCI within 12 hrs since onset (N=185).	In-hospital mortality 1-year impaired myocar-dial perfusion 1-year all-cause mortality	**SUA >387 μmol/L (vs. below)** *In-hospital mortality* 6.6% vs. 2.8%, p<0.01 *1-year all-cause mortality* 11.1% vs. 5.7%, OR=1.19, p<0.01 **SUA continuous** *1-year impaired perfusion* correlation *r*=0.46, p<0.001	**SUA >387 μmol/L (vs. below)** *1-year all-cause mortality* OR= 1.29 (95%CI 1.14-2.08)/Adjust: TIMI risk score, abnormal TIMI perfusion grade at discharge, LVEF at discharge, multi-vessel disease (p<0.1) + time to reperfu-sion, serum creatinine *1-year impaired perfusion* OR= 2.14 (95% CI 1.17-4.19)/Adjust: Killip multives. disease, TIMI time-frame count **SUA by 50 μmol/L** *1-year all-cause mortality* OR=1.10 (95% CI 1.02-1.14) / Adjust: same

Author/ year	Design/type	Patients	Outcomes	Univariate effects	Multivariate effects
Bae et al. 2011	Retrospective, observational, prognostic	Consecutive AMI, N=850, 391 (46%) STEMI, other not specified (likely NSTEMI - positive enzymes); 623 (73.3%) underwent PCI, other reperfusion not specified; timing admission vs. onset not specified	6-month occurrence of MACE: death or non-fatal AMI or revascularization	**SUA >420 μmol/L (vs. below)** MACE 24.4% vs. 9.9%, p<0.001 **SUA continuous** Patients with MACE (n=109) had higher SUA than those without MACE (n= 741), p<0.001	**SUA 50 μmol/L** HR: 1.24 (95% CI 1.06-1.46) / Adjust: age, BMI, systolic blood pressure, heart rate, diabetes, hyperlipidemia, previous AMI, Killip class, PCI, WBC, hemoglobin, sodium, potassium, eGFR, NT-ProBNP, hs-CRP (all univariate p<0.05).
Park et al. 2011	Retrospective, observational, prognostic	Consecutive patients undergoing PCI (N=1247), however, only 310 (24.9%) acute PCI due to STEMI (other procedures elective)	Development of acute kidney injury within 7 days post-PCI (creatinin incrase >44μmol/L or >50% vs. baseline)	**SUA >416 (M) or >387 (F) μmol/L** OR= 5.48 (95% CI 3.06-9.84)	**SUA >416 (M) or >387 (F) μmol/L** OR= 4.74 (95% CI 1.96-11.4) / Adjust: contrast amount, diabetes, hemoglobin, PCI post-AMI, eGFR <60 mL/min/1.73m^2

SUA - serum uric acid; OR - odds ratio; RR - relative risk; HR - hazard ratio (relative risk); M - male, F - female, BKD - baseline kindey dysfunction; CIN - contrast-induced nephropathy; COPD - chronic obstructive pulmonary disease; CPK - creatine phosphokinase; CPK-MB - creatine phospnokinase myocardial band; CS - cardogenic shock; CVI - cerebrovascular insult; DM - diabetes mellitus; eGFR - estimated glomerular filtration rate; HF - heart failure; hs-CRP - highly specific c-reactive protein; LVEF - left ventricular ejection fraction; MACE - major adverse cardiac events, NSTEMI - non-ST-elevation myocardial infarction; NT-ProBNP - N-termina-pro-B type natriuretic peptide; PCI - percutaneous coronary intervention; RBBB - right bundle branch block; RCT - randomized controlled trial; STEMI - ST-elevation myocardial infarction

Table 2. Summary of the studies of prognostic value of serum uric acid levels (SUA) in patients with acute myocardial infarction (AMI). Data are listed as presented in orginal publications. However, odds ratios and relative risks associated with SUA as a continuous variables were all re-calculated to 50 μmol/L increase to enable comparability of results.

frequently presented with a higher Killip class, more frequently had a history of hypertension and coronary artery disease, less frequently underwent PCI, had lower hemoglobin and serum sodium, lower eGFR, lower LVEF, and had higher potassium, high-sensitivity CRP and higher levels of pro-B-type natriuretic peptide (NT-ProBNP). Patients experiencing MACE had higher SUA levels and patients with hyperuricemia more frequently experienced MACE (24.4% vs. 9.9%, p<0.001). Higher on-admission SUA independently predicted 6-month occurrence of MACE: in a proportional hazard regression model with adjustment for age, BMI, systolic blood pressure, heart rate, diabetes, hyperlipidemia, previous AMI, Killip class, PCI, WBC, hemoglobin, sodium, potassium, eGFR, NT-ProBNP, hs-CRP (all showing univariate associations with the outcome, but not all were independently associated with the outcome), HR for MACE by 50 μmol/L increase in SUA was 1.24 (95% CI 1.06-1.46). They also noticed that SUA and NT-ProBNP additively improved the predictivity of the entire model (as judged on global chi-square increase): adding SUA or NT-ProBNP to conventional risk factors comparably increased the global chi-square, whereas adding both, yielded a model with the highest chi-square.

Park and colleagues (Part et al. 2011) recently reported a retrospective analysis of 1147 consecutive patients from a single center in South Korea (between mid 2006 and end of 2009) who underwent PCI. However, only 310 (24.9%) were STEMI patients undergoing acute PCI, whereas the rest underwent elective procedures. The report is interesting because it showed that SUA >416 μmol/L in men and >387 μmol/L (in line with "conventional" definition of hyperuricemia) independently predicted development of acute kidney injury (AKI) (increase in serum creatinine > 44 μmol/L or >50% over baseline) within 7 days from PCI. Hyperuricemia was particularly predictive of AKI when combined with eGFR before PCI <60 mL/min/1.73 m^2. Also, in univariate tests, AKI strongly predicted in-hospital mortality (19.6% vs. 0.8%, OR= 28.9 (95% CI 11.4-73.3), as did hyperuricemia - OR= 3.01 (95% CI 1.19-7.87).

From the viewpoint of predictive value of SUA for AMI outcomes, 7 out 9 of the described studies are of primary interest. The small RCT of allopurinol in STEMI patients undergoing PCI is interesting in that indicates the potential of an intervention affecting the XO-SUA system in this setting (Rentoukas et al., 2010). The study from South Korea (Park et al., 2011) reporting on consecutive PCI patients (predominantly elective, but 25% also acute) is of interest as it indicates a possible element of mechanism(s) by which increased SUA, or a condition characterized by increased SUA (specifically, hyperuricemia), might influence AMI outcomes in subjects undergoing acute PCI (potential effects on the renal function).

Most of the seven studies of primary interest were retrospective (Table 2), which, *per se*, could be viewed as a methodological drawback. However, considering the particulars of AMI and AMI treatment (an acute condition, typically handled after a standardized procedure with a detailed prospective monitoring and data recording), a retrospective data analysis is less likely to be biased in this setting than in some other situations. Clearly, however, susceptibility to some sources of bias remains (e.g., patient selection, physician's skill, accuracy in data recording, pattern of missing data etc.). The fact that data come from different parts of the world (Japan, Korea, various European and Middle-East countries) and different settings (STEMI, NSTEMI, mixed, PCI, thrombolysis or no reperfusion) should be viewed as a possibility to evaluate whether predictivity of SUA in this setting is robust and holds across genetic and cultural (e.g., nutrition, alcohol consumption, smoking habits) differences that might influence SUA levels and across different AMI types and treatment modalities.

2.2 Prediction of short-term outcomes

When considering predictivity of "on-admission" SUA levels (that is, taken at hospital admission, before any major intervention, as a part of a diagnostic work-up), one question is inevitable: what do the "on-admission" SUA levels reflect? A pre-existing condition? An acutely developed condition induced by AMI? Or, both?. Indeed, AMI *per se* causes a reduction in renal function (thus potentially reflecting on SUA levels due to a reduced excretion - studies on kinetics of creatinine elimination suggest that changes due to a sudden decline in renal function are to be expected within 5-6 hours (Hallynck et al., 1981, Hillege et al., 2003). Furthermore, as depicted in Figure 3, cardiac ischemia is likely to result in activation of XO. However, a reduction in glomerular filtration seen after AMI has been estimated at 1-3 mL/min for the period between AMI onset and day 3 post-AMI (Hillege et al., 2003), and by analogy to a failing heart (Doehner et al., 2008), increased cardiac XO activity apparently also needs certain time to occur. Therefore, it is likely that "on-admission" SUA values, when taken, for example, within first 48 hours since AMI onset are likely to largely represent the pre-existing condition. From the viewpoint of predictive power of UA, these observations are not crucial, because the question is simple: does this marker, taken at this very moment (regardless of what it represents), predict future events? They are, however, of interest when considering the possible "mechanistic" contribution of SUA to events that are to occur in a short subsequent period of time (e.g., in-hospital mortality or 30-day mortality) - clearly, the molecular/cellular mechanisms of SUA (or XO, for that matter) elaborated earlier also need to act for a certain period of time for their detrimental effects to become obvious.

In the subsequent text, word "effect" will be used to describe the relationship between SUA (as a potential predictor) and the outcomes. It does not imply causal relationship between the two, but is used simply because it is inherent to regression analysis on which all of the studies were based. Furthermore, the focus will be on adjusted estimates (ORs, RRs), i.e., those obtained in individual studies by accounting for relevant confounders. Where applicable, pooled estimates based on adjusted individual results were generated by conventional meta-analytical methodology for summary results. Since most of the studies reported on event rates >10% and used odds ratios, whereas some reported relative risks, adjusted odds ratios were corrected and transferred into relative risks as described by Zhang and Yu (Zhang&Yu, 1998) in order to allow for pooling of data.

2.2.1 Overall effect of "high" SUA (hyperuriceima)

As depicted in Table 2, in all studies that reported on short-term outcomes, i.e., in-hospital mortality and 30-day mortality, higher on-admission SUA, depicted as values above some cut-off (and regardless of this value) or treated as a continuous variable - consistently was associated with higher mortality: in STEMI patients treated with PCI, in STEMI PCI-treated patients with impaired renal function (as a pre-existing condition or contrast-induced), in a mixed population of NSTEMI and STEMI patients with poor reperfusion treatment). Hence, it appears safe to say that, regarding short-term outcomes, increased SUA (regardless of how defined) is a "robust" predictor that does not appear conditional on type of AMI and/or treatment modality. Table 3 summarizes the pooled estimate of unadjusted relative risk of in-hospital mortality for "high" SUA (based on studies in Table 2). Practically without inconsistency, the pooled estimate indicates around 2.57 times higher (unadjusted) risk of in-hospital mortality associated with "high" SUA.

Only 2 studies reported adjusted estimates of risk associated with "high SUA" in respect to in-hospital mortality, Lazzeri et al., 2010 as odds ratio, and Trkulja&Car 2009, using SUA as a continuous variables. Data from Lazzeri et al., 2010 were converted to adjusted relative risk - 1.97 (95% CI 1.45-2.66); and data from Car&Trkulja 2009 were used to calculate adjusted relative risk for "high" SUA - 1.82 (95%CI 1.13-2.93). The pooled estimate of these two adjusted RRs is 1.93 (95% CI 1.49-2.49). Hence, "high" SUA (defined here more or less consistently as SUA within the range of "hyperuricemia") apparently independently predicts in-hospital mortality.

Author	Patients	"High" SUA (μmol/L)	"High SUA" n/N	"Normal SUA" n/N	RR (95% CI)
Lazzeri 2010	STEMI, PCI	>387	9/100	9/366	3.66 (1.53-8.69)
Car&Trkulja 2009	STEMI (77.5%) poor reperfusion, NSTEMI	>420 M, >360 F	42/171	35/450	3.16 (2.09-4.75)
Kowalczyk 2010	STEMI, PCI	>420	51/352	47/663	2.04 (1.41-2.96)
Basar 2011	STEMI, PCI	>387	3/145	4/140	2.33 (0.60-8.92)
Total			105/633	95/1619	
Pooled (random) (I^2=0.5%, heterogenitey p=0.389)					2.57 (1.97-3.34)

Table 3. Meta-analysis of unadjusted relative risk of in-hospital mortality associated with "high" SUA. Valente et al., 2007 was not considered separately, because reported patients were included also in Lazzeri et al., 2010. Data for Car&Trkulja 2009 were recalculated from original data (since not reported in the original publication).

Table 4 summarizes the pooled estimate of unadjusted relative risk of "30-day mortality" for "high" SUA (based on studies in Table 2). With rather high inconsistency, the pooled estimate indicates around 2.82 times higher (unadjusted) risk of 30-day mortality associated with "high" SUA.

Author	Patients	"High" SUA (μmol/L)	"High SUA" n/N	"Normal SUA" n/N	RR (95% CI)
Kojima 2005	STEMI (84%), PCI; NSTEMI	>399	30/276	20/848	4.61 (2.68-7.92)
Car&Trkulja 2009	STEMI (77.5%) poor reperfusion, NSTEMI	>420 M, >360 F	42/171	41/450	2.70 (1.82-3.97)
Kowalczyk 2010	STEMI, PCI	>420	51/352	47/663	2.07 (1.45-2.98
Total			123/799	108/1961	
Pooled (random) (I^2=65.3%, heterogenitey p=0.056)					2.82 (1.86-4.29)

Table 4. Meta-analysis of unadjusted relative risk of 30-day all-cause mortality associated with "high" SUA. Data for Car&Trkulja 2009 were recalculated from original data (since not reported in the original publication).

No study reported an adjusted risk of 30-day mortality for "high" SUA. Car&Trkulja 2009 (Table 2) reported an adjusted RR considering SUA as a continuous variable. Original data were used to calculate RR for "high" SUA (>420 or >360 μmol/L in men and women, respectively) with the same adjustments as depicted in Table 2 – RR= 1.50 (95% CI 1.05-2.40). Hence, it appears that "high" SUA (defined more or less consistently as "hyperuricemia") independently predicts 30-day mortality after AMI.

2.2.2 Effect of high SUA in respect to gender and AMI type

All studies reporting the effects of SUA on short-term outcomes of AMI (Table 2) included patients of both sexes, but men prevailed in all studies. Two of these studies (Kojima et al., 2005, Car&Trkulja 2009) included both STEMI and NSTEMI patients, while remaining included exclusively acute PCI-treated STEMI patients (Table 2). Considering the overall effects of SUA (Table 3, Table 4), it seem reasonable to assume that the effects of SUA are consistent in both genders and both in STEMI and NSTEMI. For the purpose of this text, original data reported by Car&Trkulja 2009, apart from 8 patients who presented with cardiogenic shock (which troubles the interpretation of on-admission SUA) were analyzed for the effects of SUA on 30-day mortality by sex and type of AMI. SUA levels were considered as a continuous variable or a 3-level categorical variable: low-normal SUA values were defined as <310 μmol/l in men and <250 μmol/l in women; hyperuricemia was defined as SUA >420 μmol/l in men and >360 μmol/l in women; whereas high-normal SUA was defined as values between these limits. Figure 4 summarizes univariate effects of SUA on 30-day mortality. Mortality consistently increased across the range of SUA values, but the most prominent increase in mortality was observed at the cut-off of hyperuricemia, particularly in NSTEMI patients.

Figure 5 summarizes univariate effects of SUA on 30-day mortality in sex-by-AMI-type subgroups. Mortality consistently increased across the range of SUA values, but the most prominent increase in mortality was seen at the cut-off of hyperuricemia. The particularly prominent increase in mortality of NSTEMI is apparent in both men and women.

In multivariate analysis, a number of potential covariates were considered: pre-index event medical history, on-admission laboratory data (creatinine and eGFR [<60 mL/min/1.73 m^2], triglycerides, total and HDL and LDL cholesterol, peak CPK-MB, serum fibrinogen, white blood cells, hemoglobin, CRP), electrocardiographic particulars, pre-index event treatment and treatments delivered between the index event and 30-day post symptom onset. Multivariate model-building details are given in caption to Figure 6 which summarizes univariate and multivariate effects of SUA, as a continuous variable or as a contrast of "hyperuricemia" vs. "normal SUA", on 30-day mortality across gender, AMI type and gender-by-AMI-type subgroups. Data strongly suggest that high SUA (and specifically hyperuricemia) independently predicts 30-day mortality across all subgroups. The pronounced increase in mortality in hyperuricemic NSTEMI patients is maintained in multivariate analysis, as well. In practical terms, it may suggest that hyperuricemic NSTEMI patients might require a particularly closer monitoring. Of notion, however, the analyzed cohort was treated exclusively conservatively with very scarce use of thrombolytic reperfusion in STEMI patients.

Considering limited subgroup size/number of deaths, models in gender-by-AMI type subgroups included only selected adjustments (stepwise, $p<0.1$ to enter, $p<0.05$ to stay). Adjustments in men-STEMI: prior AMI and post-index event treatments - antiplatelets, ACE inhibitors, class I/III antiarrhythmics. Adjustments in women-STEMI: right bundle branch block and post-index event treatments - antiplatelets, ACE inhibitors, diuretics and beta blockers. Adjustments in men-NSTEMI: age. Adjustments in women-NSTEMI: prior symptomatic chronic heart failure, post-index event antiplatelet use.

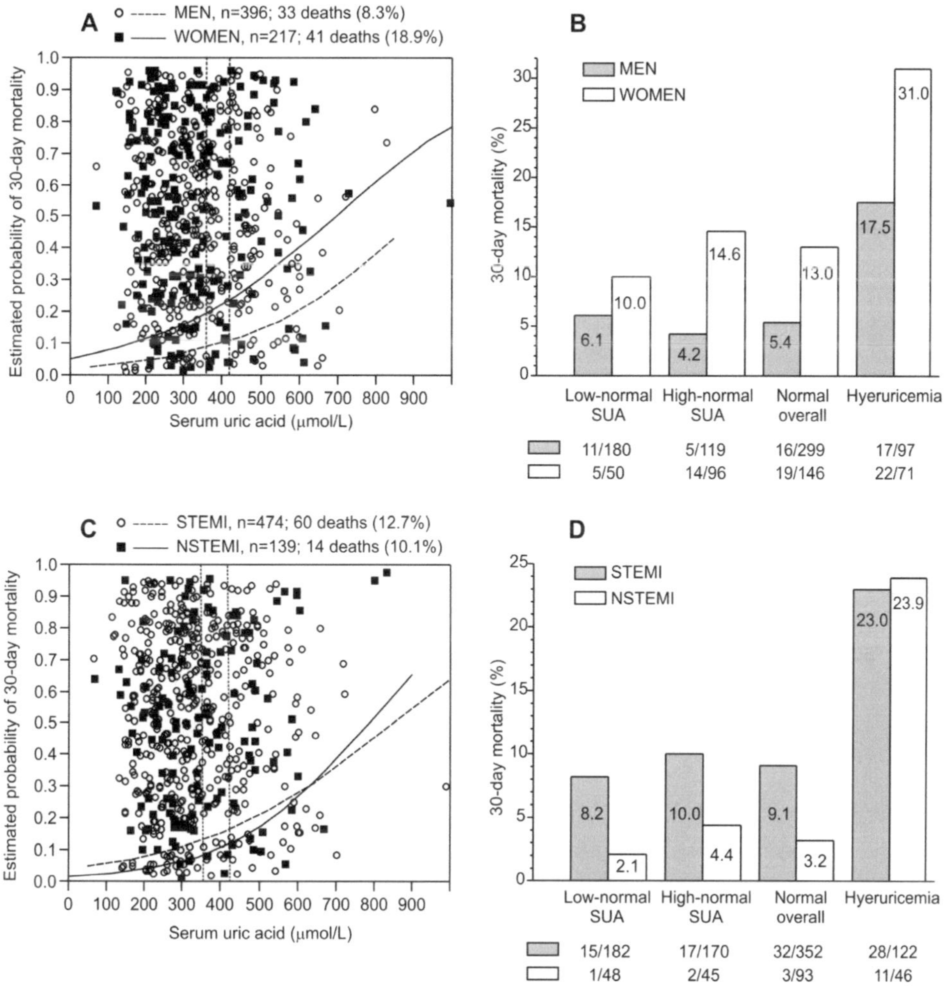

Fig. 4. Univariate effects of SUA on 30-day mortality by sex and AMI type. Estimate probability of dying across the range of SUA values (A, B) and proportion dying among low-normal, high-normal SUA and hyperuricemic patients (B, D) (based on the cohort described in Car&Trkulja 2009). Vertical lines in A and B denote the limits of hyperuricemia in men and women.

2.2.3 Effect of high SUA in respect to renal function

All studies reporting effects of SUA on short-term outcomes (Table 2) included a variable proportion of patients with reduced renal function (e.g., eGFR <60 mL/min/1.73 m^2). The study by Kowalczyk and colleagues (Kowalczyk et al., 2010) specifically included only patients with an impaired renal function (eGFR <60 mL/min/1.73 m^2 at baseline or contrast-induced renal injury). The consistency of the effects of SUA across trials suggests that, likely, effects of SUA hold in both patients with a reduced and those with a preserved renal function. No study reported specifically on patients with different levels of eGFR. For the purpose of this text, the cohort by Car&Trkulja (Car&Trkulja 2009) is re-analyzed

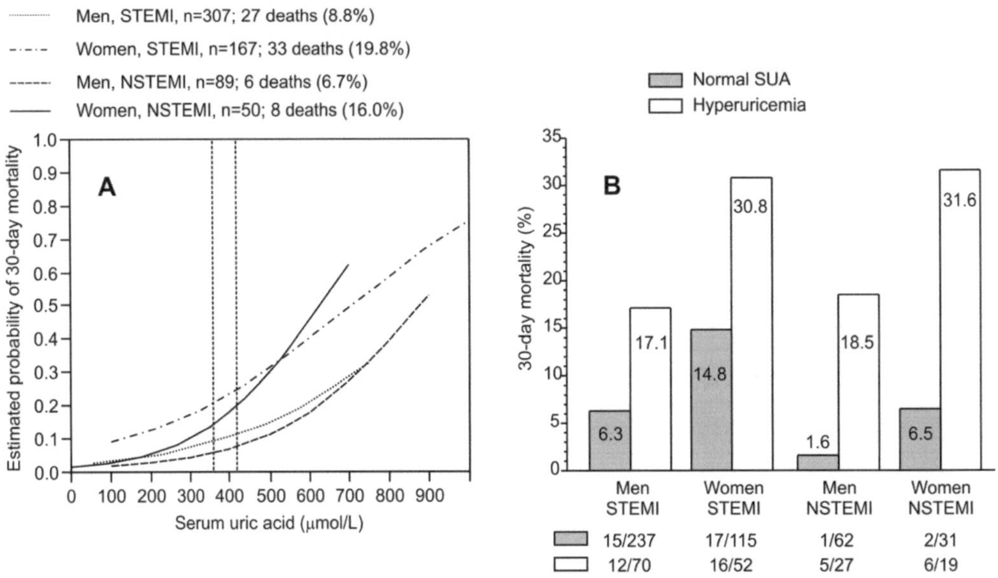

Fig. 5. Univariate effects of SUA on 30-day mortality in sex-by-AMI-type subgroups (based on the cohort described in Car&Trkulja 2009). Estimated probability of dying across the range of SUA values (A) and proportion dying among low-normal, high-normal SUA and hyperuricemic patients. Vertical lines in A denote limits of hyperuricemia in men and women.

separately for patients with eGFR <60 mL/min/1.73 m^2 and those with eGFR ≥60 mL/min/1.73 m^2. Levels of SUA values were defined as in the previous section. As shown in Figure 7, probability of 30-day mortality increased across the range of SUA values, and particularly at the level of hyperuricemia, in patients with eGFR <60 mL/min/1.73 m^2, but not in those with eGFR ≥60 mL/min/1.73 m^2. Multivariate analysis (potential adjustments as described in the previous section) demonstrated an independent association between higher SUA and particularly hyperuricemia and 30-day mortality in patients with reduced, but not in those with a preserved renal function. Univarite and multivariate SUA effects are summarized in Table 5. Reduced renal function is a well-established predictor of poor outcomes in AMI patients (specifically, eGFR <60 mL/min/1.73 m^2 has been repeatedly shown as a "break-point" of a marked increase in mortality). The present data suggest that increased SUA, i.e., hyperuricemia adds a considerable additional risk in patients with a reduced renal function. However, the current data should be viewed with a caution, since they refer exclusively to patients not treated with PCI. From a mechanistic standpoint, on the other hand, it seem plausible that detrimental effects of increased SUA are particularly obvious in patients with a reduced renal function (and not, or less so, in patients with a preserved renal function) - the potentially contributing molecular and cellular effects of SUA are more likely to manifest under the conditions of increased oxidative stress/reduce antioxidant capacity as it is seen in renal failure.

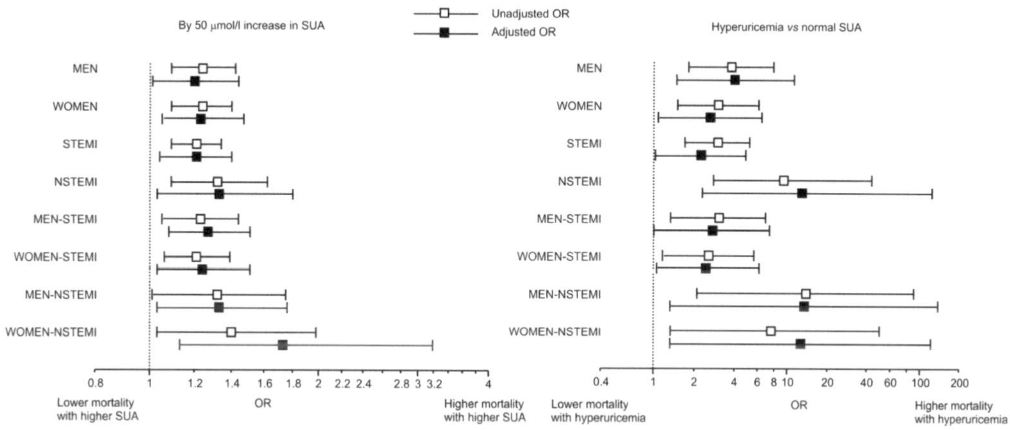

Fig. 6. Univariate and multivariate effects of SUA (as a continuous variable, by 50 µmol/L increase, left; and as a contrast of hyperuricemia vs. normouricemia, right) on 30-day mortality in subgroups by gender and type of AMI (based on the cohort described in Car&Trkulja 2009). Effects are presented as unadjusted and adjusted odds ratios (OR) (horizontal lines are 95% confidence intervals) by 50 µmol/l increase in SUA or for the contrast hyperuricemia *vs* normal SUA. Multivariate models in men, women, STEMI and NSTEMI included lag-time between symptom onset and admission and on-admission estimated glomerular filtration rate (<60 or ≥60 ml/min/1.73 m^2) as default adjustments. Other adjustments were selected in a stepwise procedure (p<0.1 to enter and p<0.05 to stay). Selected adjustments in men: prior AMI, right bundle branch block, and post-index event treatments - antiplatelets, beta blockers, diuretics, class I/III antiarrhythmics. Selected adjustments in women: age and post-index event treatments - antiplatelets, class I/III antiarrhythmics and ACE inhibitors. Selected adjustments in STEMI: sex, prior AMI, on-admission triglycerides and post-index event treatments - antiplatelets, ACE inhibitors, beta blockers, diuretics, class I/III antiarrhythmics. Selected adjustments in NSTEMI: age, on-admission total cholesterol and post-index event antiplatelet use.

	eGFR <60 (N=309)		eGFR ≥60 (N=304)	
	OR (95% CI)	P	OR (95% CI)	P
Unadjusted SUA effects				
SUA by 50 µmol/l	1.18 (1.07-1.32)	0.001	0.97 (0.74-1.27)	0.833
Hyperuricemia vs. normal SUA	2.75 (1.55-4.96)	<0.001	1.14 (0.17-4.40)	0.868
Adjusted SUA effects				
SUA by 50 µmol/l	1.24 (1.08-1.44)*	0.003	1.02 (0.74-1.36)**	0.890
Hyperuricemia vs. normal SUA	3.18 (1.49-7.03)*	0.003	1.46 (0.20-6.69**	0.659

*Adjustments, default: sex, on-admission creatinine, lag-time symptoms-admission, prior symptomatic chronic heart failure (p<0.05); selected (all p<0.05): age, post-index event treatments (till day 30 or death, whichever first) - antiplatelets, ACE inhibitors, antiarrhythmics, diuretics.
**Adjustments, default: sex, on-admission creatinine, lag-time symptoms-admission, prior symptomatic chronic heart failure; selected (all p<0.05): prior acute myocardial infarction, post-index event treatments (till day 30 or death, whichever first) - antiplatelets, beta-blockers.

Table 5. Univariate and multivariate effects of SUA on 30-day mortality in AMI patients with eGFR <60 mL/min/1.73 m^2 or ≥60 mL/min/1.73 m^2 (based on the cohort described in Car&Trkulja 2009).

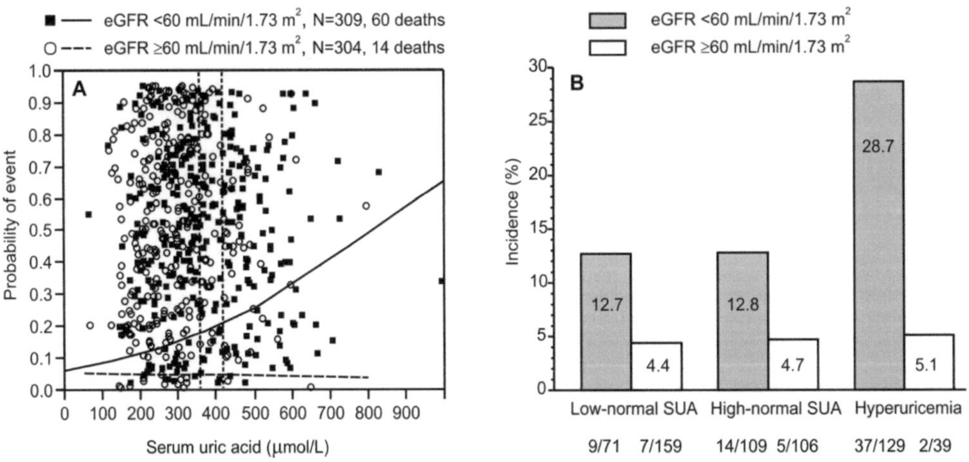

Fig. 7. Effect of SUA on 30-day mortality in AMI patients with on-admission eGFR <60 mL/min/1.73 m² or ≥60 mL/min/1.73 m² (based on the cohort described in Car&Trkulja 2009). Estimated probability of dying (A) and proportions of patients who died in the two subgroups in respect to SUA level (B). Vertical lines in A depict cut-off values of hyperuricemia in men and women.

2.3 Prediction of long-term outcomes

Prediction of medium- and long-term outcomes after AMI based on a single-point value of SUA may not be as straightforward as prediction of short-term outcomes. Namely, SUA levels may oscillate and change over time due to nutritional changes, habits (e.g., alcohol consumption, smoking) and effects of drugs, not only uricosuric or XO- inhibiting drugs, but also drugs commonly used in post-AMI patients, like thiazide diuretics or angiotensin receptor blockers. None of the studies has considered SUA as a time-varying variable. With this limitation acknowledged, all studies that reported on medium- or long-term outcomes after AMI (Table 2) consistently indicated independent unfavorable effects of SUA, either as a continuous variable or as "hyperuricemia", on mortality or other markers of poor outcomes after AMI. Kojima (Kojima et al., 2005) additionally noticed that a combination of high SUA and high(er) Killip class was particularly unfavorable in long-term. Similarly, Bae (Bae et al. 2011) showed the additive increase in risk between hyperuricemia and higher levels of NT-ProBNP. Both results actually depict the combination of a failing heart and hyperuricemia as ominous. Indirectly, these observations are in line with those suggesting that the effects of high SUA might be particularly expressed in patients with a reduced renal function - eventually, hemodynamic consequences of a failing heart would lead to a reduced renal function.

3 Conclusions and considerations for the future research

There is a sound mechanistic rationale to support a view that a condition characterized by increased SUA, regardless of whether SUA is viewed as a direct "pathogen" or a (mere) marker of some other underlying processes, might be detrimental for acute AMI patients. Clinical observations accumulated over the past 5-6 years strongly support a view that SUA should be taken into account in the process of risk stratification in AMI patients. Moreover, there are sound indications of a possibility that it could also be a useful therapeutic target. However, larger-scale prospective studies are needed to precisely isolate and quantify the

"SUA" effect, overall, and in different settings - AMI types, reperfusion procedures, renal function. Since SUA is closely associated with various other risk factors in AMI patients, the usual approach of prognostic studies based on regression analysis might not be able to meet this goal. Therefore, data mining techniques might be a valuable tool to identify clusters and/or direct and mediated relationships between different risk factor and AMI outcomes that would improve our risk-stratification methodology.

4. References

Alimonda AL, Nunez J, Nunez E, Husser O, Sanchis J, Bodi V, Minana G, Robles R, Mainar L, Marlos P, Darmofal H, Llacer A. Hyperuricemia in acute heart failure. More than a simple spectator? Eur J Int Med 2009; 20:74-79.

Anker SD, Doehner W, Rauchhaus M, Shamra R, Francis D, Knosalla C, Davos CJ, Cicoira M, Whamim W, Kemp M, Segal R, Osterziel KJ, Leyva F, Hetzer R, Ponikowski P, Coats AJS. Uric acid and survival in chronic heart failure. Validation and application in metabolic, functional and hemodynamic staging. Circulation 2003; 107:1991-1997.

Baker JF, Krishnan E, Chen L, Schumacher HR. Serum uric acid and cardiovascular disease: recent developments and where do they leave us? Am J Med 2005; 118:816-826.

Bae MH, Lee JH, Lee SH, Park SH, Yang DH, Park HS, Cho Y, Jun JE, Chae SC. Serum uric acid as an independent and incremental prognostic marker in addition to N-terminal pro-B-type natriuretic peptide in patients with acute myocardial infarction. Cric J 2011; 75:1440-1447.

Basar N, Sen N, Ozcan F, Erden G, kanat S, Sokmen E, Isleyen A, Yuzgecer H, Ozlu MF, Yildirimkaya M, Maden O, Covic A, Johnson RJ, Kanbay M. Elevated serum uric acid predicts angiographic impaired reperfusion and 1-year mortality in ST-segment elevation myocardial infarction patients undergoing percutanoeus coronary intervention. J Investig Med 2011; 59:931-937.

Bergamini C, Cicoirs M, Rossi A, Vassanelli C. Oxidative stress and hyperuricemia: pathophysiology, clinical relevance and therapeutic implications in chronic heart failure. Eur J Heart Fail 2009; 11:444-452.

Boban M, Modun D. Uric acid and antioxidant effects of wine. Croat Med J 2010; 51:16-22.

Car S, Trkulja V. Higher serum uric acid on admission is associated with higher short-term mortality and poorer long-term survival after myocardial infarction: retrospective prognostic study. Croat Med J 2009; 50:559-566.

Choi H, Atkinson K, Karlson EW, Willett W, Curhan G. Purine-rich foods, dairy and protein intake and the risk of gout in men. N Engl J Med 2004; 350:1093-1103.

Coleman LA, Roubenoff R. Gout. In: Caballero B, Allen L, Prentice A (eds). Encyclopedia of human nutrition, 2nd edition. Oxford:Elsevier, 2005, pp. 419-423.

Doehner W, Springer J, Landmesser U, Struthers AD, Anker SD. Uric acid in chronic heart failure - current pathophysiological concepts. Eur J Heart Fail 2008; 19:1269-1270.

Duan X, Ling F. Is uric acid itself a player or a bystander in the pathophysiology of chronic heart failure? Med Hypotheses 2008; 70:578-581.

Feig DI, Kang D-H, Johnson RJ. Uric acid and cardiovascular risk. N Engl J Med 2008; 359:1811-1821.

Gagliardi ACM, Miname MH, Sandos RD. Uric acid: a marker of increased cardiovascular risk. Atherosclerosis 2009; 202:11-17.

Hallynck T, Soep HH, Thomis J, Boeleart J, Daneels R, Fillastre JP, De Rosa F, Rubinstein E, Hatala M, Spousta J, Dettli L. Prediction of creatinine clearance from serum creatinine concentration based on lean body mass. Clin Pharmacol Ther 1981; 30:414-421.

Hillege HL, van Gilst WH, van Veldhuisen DJ, Navis G, Grobbee DE, de Graeff PA, de Zeeuw D. CATS randomized trial. Accelerated decline and prognostic impact of renal function after myocardial infarction and the benefits of ACE inhibition: the CATS randomized trial. Eur Heart J 2003; 24:412-420.

Johnson RJ, Kang D-H, Feig DI, Kivlighn S, Kanellis J, Watanabe S, Tuttle KT, Rodriguez-Iturabe B, Herrera-Acosta J,

Mazzali M. Is there a pathogenetic role for uric acid in hypertension and cardiovascular and renal disesas? Hypertension 2003; 41:1183-1190.

Kim SY, Guevara JP, Kim KM, Choi HK, Heitjan DF, Albert DA. Hyperuricemia and risk of stroke: a systematic review and meta-analysis. Arthritis Rheum 2009; 61:885-892.

Kim SY, Guevara JP, Kim KM, Choi HK, Heitjan DF, Albert DA. Hyperuricemia and coronary heart disease: a systematic review and meta-analysis. Arthritis Care Res 2010; 62:170-180.

Kojima S, Sakamoto T, Ishihara M, Kimura K, Miyazaki S, Yamagishi M, Tei C, Hiraoka H, Sonoda M, Tsuchihashi K, Shimoyama N, Honda T, Ogata Y, Matsui K, Ogawa H. Japanese Acute coronary syndrome study (JACSS) investigators. Prognostic usefulness of serum uric acid after acute myocardial infarction. Am J Cardiol 2005; 96:489-495.

Kowalczyk J, Francuz P, Swoboda R, Lenarczyk R, Sredniawa B, Golda A, Kurek T, Mazurek M, Podolecki T, Polnoski L, Kalarus Z. Prognostic significance of hyperuricemia in patients with different types of renal dysfunction and acute myocardial infarction treated with percutanoeus coronary intervention. Nephron Clin Pract 2010; 116:c114-c122.

Lazzeri C, Valente S, Chiostri M, Sori A, Bernardo P, Gensini GF. Uric acid in the acute phase of ST elevation myocardial infarction submitted to primary PCI: its prognostic role and relation with inflammatory markers. A signe center experience. Int J Cardiol 2010; 138:206-216.

Lippi G, Montagnana M, Franchini M, Favaloro EJ, Targher G. The paradoxal relationship between serum uric acid and cardiovascular disease. Clin Chim Acta 2008; 392:1-7.

Nagahama K, Iseki K, Inoue T, Touma T, Ikemiya Y, Takishita S. Hyperuricemia and cardiovascular risk factor clustering in a screened cohort in Okinawa, Japan. Hypertens Res 2004; 27:227-233.

Naquibullah M, Calberg MJ, Kjoller E. The pathophysiology of uric acid in relation to cardiovascular disese. Curr Cardiol Rev 2007; 3:99-103.

Pacher P, Nivorozhkin A, Szabo C. Therapeutic effects of xanthine oxidase inhibitors: renaissance half a century after the discovery of allopurionol. Pharmacol Rev 2006; 58:87-114.

Park SH, Shin WY, Lee EY, Gil HW, Lee SW, Lee SJ, Jin DK, Hong SY. The impact of hyperuricemia on in-hospital mortality and incidence of acute kidney injury in patients undergoing percutanous coronary intervention. Circ J 2011; 75:692-697.

Rentoukas E, Tsarouhas K, Tsitsimpikou C, Lazaros G, Deftereos S, Vavetsi S. The prognostic impact of allopurinol in patients with acute myocardial infarction undergoing primary percutaneous coronary intervention. Int J Cardiol 2010; 145:257-258.

Valente S, Lazzeri C, Vecchio S, Giglioli C, Margheri M, Bernardo P, Comeglio M, Chiocchini S, Gensini GF. Predictors of in-hospital mortality after percutaneous coronary intervention for cardiogenic shock. Int J Cardiol 2007; 114:176-182.

Wechter J, Phillips LJ, Toledo AH, Anaya-Prado R, Toledo-Pereyera LH. Allopurinol protection in patients undergoing coronary artery bypass graft surgery. J Invest Surg 2010; 23:285-293).

Zhang J, Yu KF. What's the relative risk? A method of correcting the odds ratio in cohort studies of common outcomes. JAMA 1998; 280:1690-1691.

8

Stress Testing and Its Role in Coronary Artery Disease

Rajkumar K. Sugumaran and Indu G. Poornima
The Gerald McGinnis Cardiovascular Institute-Allegheny General Hospital, USA

1.Introduction

Coronary Artery Disease (CAD) is the single leading cause of death of men and women in the Unites States. It accounts for about one-third of all deaths in subjects over age 35. The 2010 Heart Disease and Stroke Statistics update of the American Heart Association reported that 17.6 million persons in the United States have CAD, and that the 2006 overall death rate from cardiovascular disease was 262.5 per 100,000. CAD caused about one of every six deaths in the United States in 2006. From 1996–2006, the number of inpatient discharges from short stay hospitals with CAD, as the first listed diagnosis, increased from 6,107,000 to 6,161,000 discharges. The estimated direct and indirect cost of CAD for 2010 is $503.2 billion ($503.2 billion in equivalent Euro) (AHA, 2000). Being able to identify patients with suspected CAD early will help drive down hospital costs and ultimately decrease mortality and morbidity. Stress testing has emerged as the sole non-invasive method for risk stratifying patients with suspected CAD.

Apart from highlighting the salient advantages and disadvantages of various stress testing modalities, we will review which patients should undergo stress testing based on appropriateness criteria. Each patient needs to be managed separately based on their risk factors for significant CAD ultimately identifying those who may be at increased risk for the devastating sequeale of CAD such as acute myocardial infarction (AMI) or death.

2. Assessment of coronary artery disease risk

Identifying traditional, modifiable, and non-modifiable risk factors can help risk-stratify patients into low, intermediate, and high risk for CAD and cardiac death. Modifiable risks include hyperlipidemia (HLD), tobacco abuse, hypertension, diabetes mellitus (DM), physical inactivity, and obesity. Non-modifiable risk factors include a family history of CAD in first degree relatives under the age of 60, advanced age, and male gender (Kannel, 1976).

The frequency and predictive value of five major risk factors (hypertension, low-density lipoprotein (LDL) and high-density lipoprotein (HDL) cholesterol, glucose intolerance, and smoking) was evaluated in a study of white non-Hispanic individuals without CAD in the Framingham Heart Study and the Third National Health and Nutrition Examination Survey (NHANES III) who were 35 to 74 years of age. (Pryor, 1993).

Advanced obstructive CAD can exist with minimal or no symptoms, and can progress rapidly. The first clinical manifestation could be (MI), unstable angina, or sudden cardiac death. The rationale for early detection of CAD is that detection during the subclinical stages of the disease might allow for the reliable identification of subjects at increased risk of an adverse cardiac event. Data from more than 10,000 subjects who participated in the Multiple Risk Factor Intervention Trial (MRFIT) and the Lipid Research Clinic's Coronary Primary Prevention Trial (LRCPPT) found that the presence of asymptomatic ischemia detected during baseline treadmill exercise testing predicted an increased risk of coronary events and cardiac death at 7 to 10 year follow-up (Rautaharju, 1986; Ekelund, 1989). The relative risk of an abnormal exercise test is greatest in patients with underlying risk factors for CAD, such as smoking, hypertension, HLD, and DM.

While there is general consensus that screening is not necessary for asymptomatic patients at low risk for CAD, there may be certain groups in which screening is warranted. Although the available data are not strong enough to reach consensus on the identity of these special groups, many clinicians perform periodic exercise electrocardiogram (ECG) tests in asymptomatic individuals with multiple coronary risk factors including: HLD, systolic blood pressure greater than 140 mmHg, diastolic blood pressure greater than 90 mmHg, smoking, DM, and a history of premature AMI or sudden cardiac death in a first-degree relative under age 60. A positive test in such patients is associated with an increased risk of subsequent AMI and death (Rautaharju, 1986; Ekelund, 1989).

When starting to screen patients for CAD, there is no single ideal test. Based upon the available data, easy accessibility, and cost considerations, most would deduce that initial screening with exercise ECG testing is the most practical approach in high-risk individuals who can exercise and who do not have ECG abnormalities that can limit the detection of ischemic changes. Additionally, an exercise test provides information about the exercise capacity, which may be more predictive of outcome than ST segment changes (Roger, 1998).

The predictive value of an abnormal screening exercise test is determined by the presence or absence of risk factors for CAD. In addition, treadmill scores have been devised to estimate patient prognosis according to test results. The most popular validated treadmill score comes from Duke University and is based upon data from 2758 consecutive patients with chest pain a median age of 49 (Mark, 1987). The Duke treadmill score uses three exercise parameters:

Duke prognostic treadmill score = Exercise time (minutes based on the Bruce protocol) - (5 x maximum ST segment deviation in mm) - (4 x exercise angina [0=none, 1=nonlimiting, and 2=exercise limiting]).

Patients are classified as low, moderate, or high risk according to the score: Low-risk-score ≥+5, Moderate-risk-score from -10 to +4, and High-risk-score <-11.

Given that asymptomatic patients were excluded from these studies there are no data applying the results of the Duke treadmill score to asymptomatic patients who are screened for CAD. In addition, even among symptomatic patients, the score has limited prognostic utility in patients ≥75 years of age (Kwok, 2002). The 2002 ACC/AHA guidelines suggested that exercise radionuclide myocardial perfusion imaging or exercise echocardiography has potential use as a second test in asymptomatic patients who have an intermediate or high risk Duke treadmill score on exercise ECG testing even though the score has not been evaluated in asymptomatic patients (ACC/AHA 2002).

3. Treadmill exercise ecg testing

Also known as an exercise tolerance test, it is essential in evaluating for diagnosis and prognosis of coronary artery disease, as well as assessment of functional capacity or tolerance. Exercise ECG testing is the most commonly used noninvasive test because it is simple and inexpensive

Absolute
Acute myocardial infarction (within two days)
Unstable angina
Uncontrolled cardiac arrhythmias causing symptoms or hemodynamic compromise
Symptomatic severe aortic stenosis
Uncontrolled symptomatic heart failure
Acute pulmonary embolus or pulmonary infarction
Acute myocarditis or pericarditis
Active endocarditis
Acute aortic dissection
Acute noncardiac disorder that may affect exercise performance or be aggravated by exercise (eg, infection, renal failure, thyrotoxicosis)
Inability to obtain consent
Relative*
Left main coronary stenosis or its equivalent
Moderate stenotic valvular heart disease
Electrolyte abnormalities
Severe hypertension (systolic ≥200 mmHg and/or diastolic ≥110 mmHg)
Tachyarrhythmias or bradyarrhythmias, including atrial fibrillation with uncontrolled ventricular rate
Hypertrophic cardiomyopathy and other forms of outflow tract obstruction
Mental or physical impairment leading to inability to cooperate
High-degree atrioventricular block

Table 1. Absolute and Relative contraindications to Exercise ECG testing

The most common groups of patients that are excluded from exercise ECG testing are those patients unable to exercise sufficiently to reach 85% of maximum predicted heart rate (MPHR) and those with ECG changes at rest that can interfere with interpretation of the test. The exercise ECG cannot be interpreted in the presence of resting ST segment changes, left ventricular hypertrophy, left bundle branch block, a ventricular paced rhythm, or the Wolff Parkinson White syndrome. The patient must also be able to exercise adequately, since failure to achieve at least 85 percent of the predicted maximal heart rate is considered inadequate to rule out ischemic heart disease if the test is otherwise negative.

Achieving 85% of MPHR is the universally-accepted threshold that guarantees an adequate level of stress (ACC/AHA 2002). Some patients attain that level within the first couple of minutes on the treadmill, which is a sign of deconditioning while others may not get there until they are in the more advanced stages of the test suggesting either chronotropic

ACC/AHA guideline summary: Exercise ECG testing without an imaging modality for the diagnosis of obstructive coronary heart disease (CHD)

Class I - There is evidence and/or general agreement that exercise ECG testing for the diagnosis of CHD is indicated in patients with:
• An intermediate pretest probability of CHD based upon age, gender, and symptoms, including patients with complete right bundle branch block or less than 1 mm ST depression, in the absence of the exceptions listed in class IIb and class III.
Class IIa - The weight of evidence or opinion is in favor of the usefulness of exercise ECG testing for the diagnosis of CHD in patients with:
• Suspected variant (vasospastic) angina.
Class IIb - The usefulness of exercise ECG testing for the diagnosis of CHD is less well established in patients with:
• A high or low pretest probability of CHD.
• Digoxin therapy and less then 1 mm of ST segment depression at baseline.
• Electrocardiographic evidence of left ventricular hypertrophy and and less then 1 mm of ST segment depression at baseline.
Class III - There is evidence and/or general agreement that exercise testing for risk assessment and prognosis in patients at intermediate or high probability of CHD is not useful in the following settings:
• Patients with the following baseline ECG abnormalities: 1. Preexcitation (Wolff-Parkinson-White) syndrome. 2. Electronically paced ventricular rhythm. 3. More than 1 mm of ST segment depression at rest. 4. Complete left bundle branch block.
• An established diagnosis of CHD due to prior myocardial infarction or coronary angiography. However, testing may be warranted in such patients to assess functional capacity and prognosis.

Data from Gibbons, RJ, Abrams, J, Chatterjee, K, et al. ACC/AHA 2002 guideline update for the management of patients with chronic stable angina--summary article: a report of the American College of Cardiology/American Heart Association Task Force on Practice Guidelines (Committee on the Management of Patients With Chronic Stable Angina). Circulation 2003; 107:149.

Table 2.

incompetence or an extremely conditioned athlete. Chronotropic incompetence can be a manifestation of coronary artery disease (Sugumaran, 2010). Another prognostic factor for CAD is the amount of ST segment depression that occurs during or immediately after exercise. In general, these ECG changes have a sensitivity of 50 to 70% and a specificity of 60 to 80%.

In general, exercise ECG testing provides more information than pharmacologic stress for the following reasons: exercise documents the workload that induces ischemia, exercise capacity and hemodynamic responses are predictors of prognosis independent of ischemia as stated above and ischemia at a low workload indicates a greater likelihood of severe disease and a worse prognosis than does the same degree of ischemia at a high workload. Furthermore, the inability to exercise, without having mechanical limitations, is itself associated with increased cardiovascular risk.

The main disadvantages are that the sensitivity is lower than that of stress imaging techniques, the poor specificity with marked ST-T abnormalities on resting ECG, with digoxin use, with left bundle branch block (LBBB) pattern or pacemakers, or in female population, and it does not accurately localize the site or extent of myocardial ischemia, which is important in patients who have undergone revascularization (ACC/AHA 2002).

4. Characteristics of myocardial perfusion agents

Radionuclide myocardial perfusion imaging (MPI) involves the visualization of a radiopharmaceutical that is distributed throughout the myocardium in proportion to coronary blood flow, thereby permitting the determination of relative blood flow in various regions of the heart. Perfusion imaging is dependent upon the physical properties of the radiolabeled tracer, its delivery, and its extraction and retention by the myocyte. Both cell membrane integrity and energy utilization are necessary for intracellular extraction and retention of tracer. Thus, retained tracer activity is synonymous with myocyte viability. Revascularization of such segments can lead to improvement in left ventricular function. The ideal perfusion agent would have the following characteristics: high first pass myocardial extraction, linear relationship between uptake and flow, uptake independent of metabolic state, and a stable distribution during imaging.

4.1 Thallium-201

Thallium-201 (Tl-201) is a radioactive element that is similar to potassium analogs first used in perfusion imaging, but with superior imaging characteristics. It is cyclotron produced, and therefore requires off-site manufacturing. The principal photopeaks are gamma rays at 135 keV (2.7 percent) and 167 keV (10 percent), and mercury X-rays of 69 to 83 keV (85-90 %) (Lebowitz, 1975). The physical half-life of thallium-201 is prolonged (73 hours), limiting the overall amount that can be administered to 2 to 4 mCi. Thallium uptake is partly an active process involving the Na-K-ATPase pump. Due to the relatively small contribution of active transport, extraction and uptake of thallium is relatively unaffected by ischemia, hypoxia, or digoxin and is directly proportional to coronary blood flow (Strauss, 1975).

Following thallium's initial extraction, there is a continuous exchange between the myocyte and the extracellular compartment, resulting in a phenomenon called redistribution. Intake of thallium into the cell continues via additional extraction of thallium that still remains in the blood and recirculation of tracer that has already been washed out of the intracellular compartment. Thallium may leak out of various regions within the myocardium at different rates, based upon coronary blood flow. Thus, an area that has higher coronary flow may permit the egress of thallium at a faster rate than a region of low flow, demonstrating a "differential washout" of thallium.

Redistribution often begins as early as 20 minutes following thallium administration and may result in the partial or total resolution of perfusion defects noted shortly after stress imaging. Thus, post-stress imaging should begin within 15 minutes after the initial injection. However, the estimate of perfusion is different at three to four hours after thallium delivery than under true resting conditions, and can overestimate the extent of myocardial necrosis. This potential limitation may be overcome by a second injection of a smaller dose of thallium immediately following the redistribution images. Thallium redistribution can be affected by several factors such as changes in coronary blood flow the administration of nitrates, and consequently the recognition of reversible myocardial ischemia (Medrano, 1993).

Reverse redistribution is a finding in which the perfusion defect appears worse on the delayed redistribution perfusion images (three to four hours after thallium injection) than on the initial images. This phenomenon is thought to be related to hyperemic blood flow that causes enhanced uptake of thallium on initial post-stress images, and a more rapid clearance of thallium, producing the appearance of a perfusion abnormality (Weiss, 1986). Reverse redistribution is consistent with viable myocardium. However, its presence in a patient with a low likelihood of ischemia and without other evidence of ischemia is felt to represent an artifact.

Imaging Protocols. A single dose of 2.5-4.0 mCi of Tl-201 is injected prior to peak exercise stress or at peak pharmacologic vasodilatation, and single-photon emission computed tomography (SPECT) imaging starts 10-15 minutes later. Redistribution (rest) imaging is done 2.5-4.0 hours later. In cases where standard stress-redistribution imaging shows a fixed or minimally reversible perfusion abnormality, myocardial viability can be assessed with a rest image at 18-24 hours or following reinjection of an additional 1-2 mCi dose of Tl-201. An alternative method for viability assessment is injection of 3-4 mCi of Tl-201 at rest followed by 3- to 4-hour redistribution imaging (Henzlova, 2009).

Clinical indications	Standard exercise tests	Myocardial nuclear perfusion imaging	Stress echocardiography
Detection of coronary heart disease (sensitivity)	Good (65%)	Very good (85%)	Very good (85%)
Exclusion of coronary heart disease (specificity)	Good (85%)	Very good (90%)	Very good (90%)
Accuracy in presence of marked baseline ST-T abnormalities	Poor	Very good	Very good
Localize myocardial ischemia	Poor	Very good	Good
Assess myocardial viability	Poor	Good	Good
Preoperative evaluation	Limited	Good	Good
Prognosis for CHD or post-MI	Good	Very good	Probably very good (limited studies)
Accuracy for ischemia with regional wall motion abnormalities	---	Very good	Good
Evaluation of chest pain syndromes (resting studies)	---	Good	Probably good
Infarct quantification (resting studies)	---	Good	Modest
Cost	Relatively cheap	Expensive	Modest

Table 3. Efficacy of the different methods of stress testing in specific clinical settings

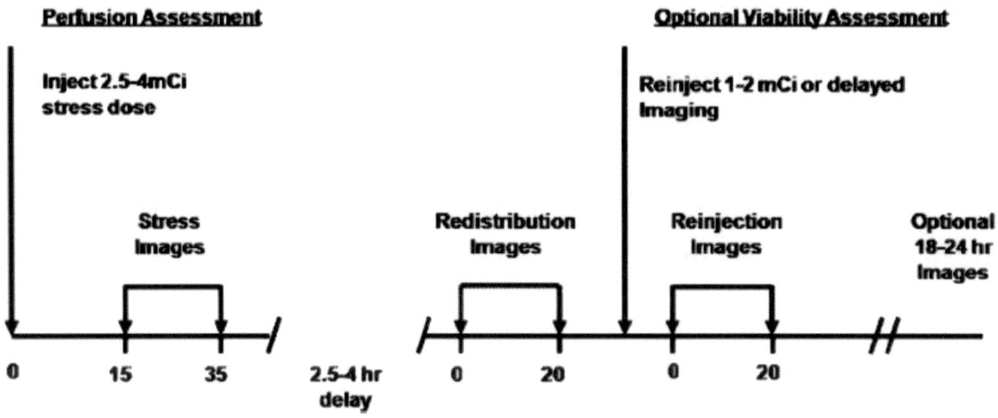

Fig. 1. Stress/redistribution/reinjection/18- to 24-hour Tl-201 imaging protocol.

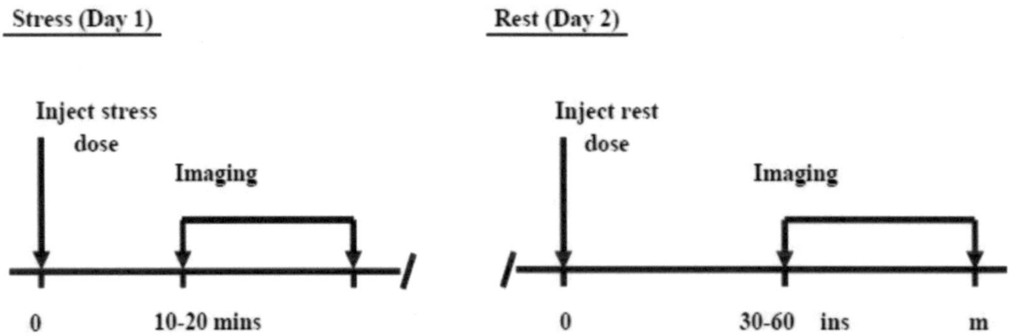

Fig. 2. Tc-99m imaging protocols: Two-day exercise stress/rest.

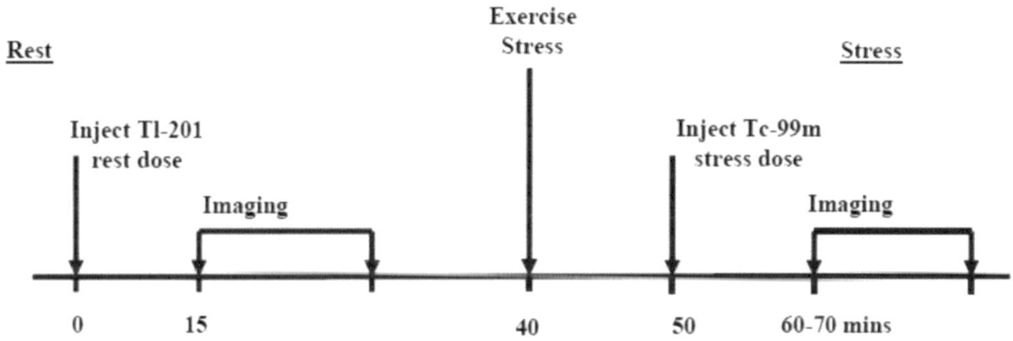

Fig. 3. Rest Tl-201/stress Tc-99m separate-acquisition dual-isotope protocol.

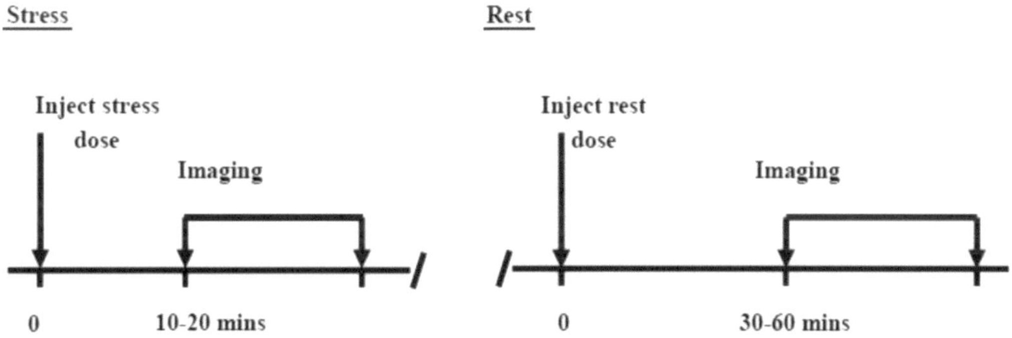

Fig. 4. Tc-99m imaging protocols: One-day exercise stress/rest.

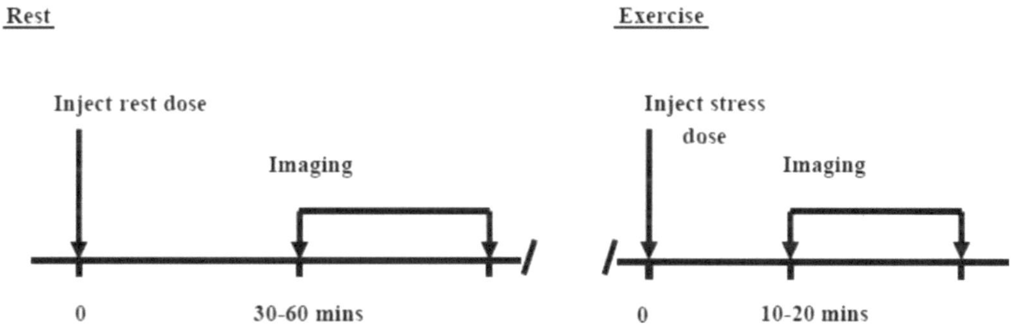

Fig. 5. Tc-99m imaging protocols: One-day rest/exercise stress.

In summary, thallium-201 has the following advantages: myocardial uptake is proportional to flow, redistribution allows a single injection for both stress and rest images The two primary disadvantages are its low photon energy resulting in more scatter and soft tissue attenuation and the longer physical half-life limiting the allowable dose which reduces image quality.

4.2 Technetium-99 labeled agents

There are several physical advantages for the use of technetium-99m (Tc-99m) perfusion tracers. The higher photon energy (140 keV) is well suited for gamma camera imaging, and may result in less photon attenuation and scatter due to soft tissue when compared with thallium-201. A half-life of six hours and favorable dosimetry permits the administration of substantially more activity, thereby resulting in a high number of emitted photons and improved image resolution. The increased photon flux also permits functional imaging with gated SPECT or first-pass techniques. Tc-99m is a generator produced product, and the workhorse of most nuclear medicine departments. As a result, it is readily available at most institutions. Three 99m Tc-labeled myocardial perfusion agents are now available in clinical practice: sestamibi, tetrofosmin, and teboroxime but only the first two are commonly used. Other tracers are in various stages of development. Each compound has unique properties that make it suitable for certain types of imaging

Clinical indications	Standard exercise tests	Myocardial nuclear perfusion imaging	Stress echocardiography
Detection of coronary heart disease (sensitivity)	Good (65%)	Very good (85%)	Very good (85%)
Exclusion of coronary heart disease (specificity)	Good (85%)	Very good (90%)	Very good (90%)
Accuracy in presence of marked baseline ST-T abnormalities	Poor	Very good	Very good
Localize myocardial ischemia	Poor	Very good	Good
Assess myocardial viability	Poor	Good	Good
Preoperative evaluation	Limited	Good	Good
Prognosis for CHD or post-MI	Good	Very good	Probably very good (limited studies)
Accuracy for ischemia with regional wall motion abnormalities	---	Very good	Good
Evaluation of chest pain syndromes (resting studies)	---	Good	Probably good
Infarct quantification (resting studies)	---	Good	Modest
Cost	Relatively cheap	Expensive	Modest

Table 4. Efficacy of the different methods of stress testing in specific clinical settings

Sestamibi Tc-99m (Cardiolite™) is in a class of compounds known as isonitriles. Sestamibi has the following general characteristics: it is a lipophilic monovalent cation with transient hepatic uptake, minimal lung uptake, and a good target-to-background ratio unlike thallium uptake. Sestamibi uptake is not dependent upon the Na-K-ATPase pump. Distribution within the myocardium is proportional to blood flow (Wackers, 1989).

Due to minimal redistribution over time, Sestamibi is well suited to the prolonged acquisition times associated with tomographic imaging. The absence of significant sestamibi redistribution necessitates two separate injections of the radiopharmaceutical, one during peak stress and a second while at rest. The lack of sestamibi redistribution permits greater flexibility in scheduling, since imaging is not mandated immediately after injection. Sestamibi can be used to quantify the area of risk in a patient suffering an acute myocardial infarction. Since sestamibi activity reflects myocardial perfusion at the time of injection, defects on these early images indicate possible areas of jeopardized myocardium.

Sestamibi can be given to patients with chest pain and nondiagnostic findings on ECG, and images taken later, even after treatment of the chest pain. Both gated SPECT and first pass imaging have been performed successfully with this agent. This evaluation may be one of the most valuable clinical attributes of sestamibi scintigraphy (DePuey, 1995).

In summary, Tc-99m sestamibi has the following advantages: myocardial uptake is proportional to flow, there is stable retention of tracer (minimal redistribution), and simultaneous perfusion and function assessment is possible

Pharmacologic test	Sensitivity, percent	Specificity, percent
Adenosine echocardiography	72	91
Adenosine SPECT MPI	90	75
Dipyridamole echocardiography	70	93
Dipyridamole SPECT MPI	89	65
Dobutamine echocardiography*	80	84
Dobutamine SPECT MPI	82	75

Table 5. Weighted mean sensitivities and specificities of pharmacologic stress tests.

Tetrofosmin (Myoview™) is a lipophilic, cationic diphosphine compound. It has good myocardial uptake with rapid clearance from the liver, lungs, and blood (Higley, 1993). As with sestamibi, there is little myocardial washout over time. Thus, high quality myocardial images can be obtained from five minutes to several hours after injection. The more rapid clearance from the liver with tetrofosmin may lead to less artifact from subdiaphragmatic activity, which is a common problem with Tc-99m sestamibi (Zaret, 1995).

Exercise tetrofosmin imaging is of prognostic value in patients with coronary heart disease, adding incremental information to that provided by clinical and exercise data. In a multicenter review of 4278 patients, the mortality rate in those with a normal exercise or adenosine tetrofosmin SPECT study was 0.6 percent per year, similar to published rates for normal thallium and sestamibi studies (Shaw, 2003).

In summary, important features of Tc-99m tetrofosmin include: myocardial uptake is proportional to flow, minimal redistribution occurs, and there may be more rapid washout from the liver than with sestamibi, permitting earlier imaging after injection.

Teboroxime (Cardiotec™) is a neutral, lipophilic perfusion agent in a class of compounds called the boronic acid adducts of technetium dioxime. Teboroxime differs from thallium and sestamibi in that its uptake appears to be relatively insensitive to myocardial injury. As a result, teboroxime may serve as a pure blood flow agent that is not dependent upon cellular viability (Heller,1996). In contrast to sestamibi, teboroxime is characterized by rapid uptake and washout, with a clearance half-time in the myocardium of only a few minutes.

Teboroxime appears to be a more accurate marker of flow than the other tracers at high flow rates, and may prove useful for quantification of coronary blood flow. The washout of teboroxime from the myocardium is rapid and flow-dependent. The short myocardial residence time of teboroxime necessitates rapid patient positioning and image acquisition, which increases the difficulty of testing. In addition, the lower count rates with such rapid imaging protocols preclude the use of gated SPECT imaging. In summary, the important features of Tc-99m teboroxime are that it is the most accurate marker of flow among single photon agents its rapid myocardial washout limits its clinical utility.

NOET is a neutral lipophilic compound with a technetium-nitrido (Tc(N)) core. Preliminary studies indicate that NOET may undergo redistribution similar to Tl-201. This property would make it attractive for myocardial perfusion studies, since it would have the clinically useful properties of Tl-201 and the more favorable imaging characteristics of Tc-99m. Small studies have demonstrated comparable accuracy to Tl-201 for the detection of coronary artery disease (Jeetley, 1995).

5. Exercise radionuclide myocardial perfusion imaging (rMPI)

SPECT imaging is performed by using a gamma camera to acquire multiple 2-D images from multiple angles. A computer performs a tomographic reconstruction algorithm to the multiple projections, yielding a 3-D dataset. Cardiac gated acquisitions are possible with SPECT, which are thereby used to obtain quantitative information about myocardial perfusion, thickness, and contractility of the myocardium during various parts of the cardiac cycle, and also to allow calculation of left ventricular ejection fraction, stroke volume, and cardiac output.

Exercise rMPI is a valuable tool for the evaluation of selected patients with known or suspected CAD. The development of 99m-Tc-labeled agents with improved imaging characteristics and ECG gated acquisition permits simultaneous assessment of myocardial perfusion and left ventricular systolic function. This in turn translates into superior diagnostic accuracy and provides important prognostic information regarding cardiac events. rMPI depicts the distribution of blood flow in the myocardium by imaging the uptake of an intravenously administered radionuclide. Abnormal uptake of a radionuclide results in a "cold spot" on the image localizing areas of relatively reduced myocardial blood flow associated with ischemia or scar. The relative regional perfusion distribution can be assessed at rest, during cardiovascular stress, or both (Strauss, 2008). The differentiation of ischemic myocardium is made by comparing images obtained at the peak of maximal exercise or during pharmacological stress with those obtained at rest. During stress, blood flow increases in normal coronary arteries. Because myocardial uptake of the radionuclide tracer is proportional to coronary blood flow, MPI radiotracer intensity is diminished in areas of hypoperfusion.

The choice among the different types of stress tests is based upon the patient's ability to exercise to a level high enough to produce meaningful results on exercise ECG testing, the possible presence of baseline electrocardiographic abnormalities that could interfere with the interpretation of exercise ECG testing, and whether or not it is important to localize ischemia or assess myocardial viability

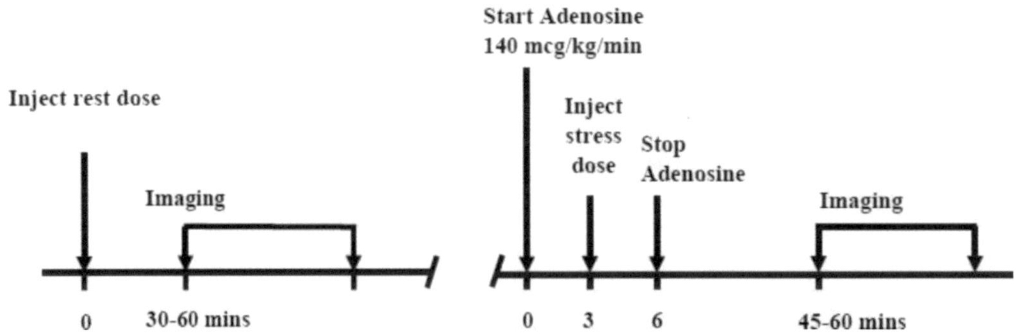

Fig. 6. Tc-99m imaging protocols: One-day rest/adenosine pharmacologic stress.

The 2002 ACC/AHA guidelines on chronic stable angina and on exercise testing published recommendations for the use of stress imaging as the initial test for diagnosis or for risk assessment in patients. Exercise rMPI is an option for diagnosis in patients with an intermediate pretest risk of CHD who are able to exercise but have baseline ECG abnormalities that can interfere with exercise ECG testing.

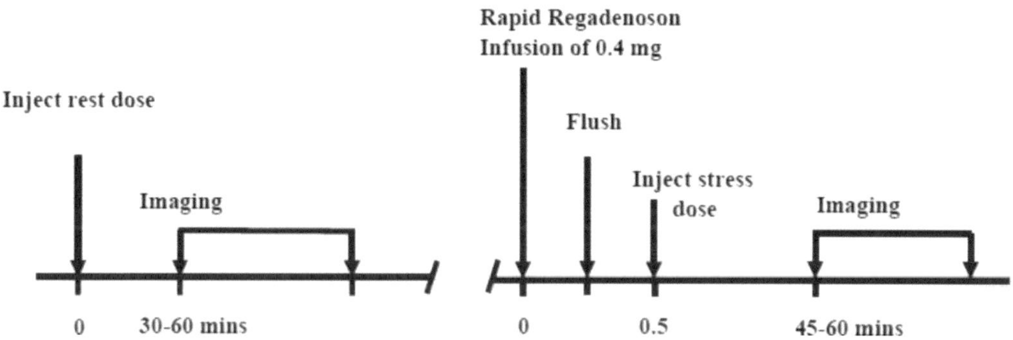

Fig. 7. Tc-99m imaging protocols: One-day rest/regadenoson pharmacologic stress.

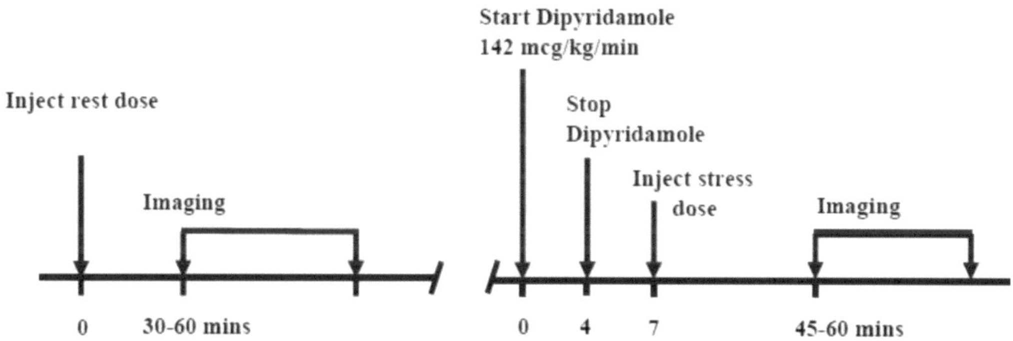

Fig. 8. Tc-99m imaging protocols: One-day rest/dipyridamole pharmacologic stress.

Patients with non-diagnostic or equivocal stress echo that were tested for ischemic symptoms would qualify for a PET scan.
Patients with non-diagnostic or equivocal nuclear testing that are being assessed for ischemic symptoms qualify for a PET scan.
Patients that can not exercise and need pharmacologic testing that have ischemic symptoms or need clearance for major surgery would qualify for a PET scan.
Patients with BMI over 40 and in some cases over 35, which are being assessed for ischemic symptoms, can go straight to a PET scan.
Patients with breast implants or large pendulous breasts, undergoing assessment for ischemic symptoms, can undergo PET imaging.
Patients with a high CAC, viewed as over 300 or 400, can often go to PET imaging. Symptoms are needed to pre-certify.
Patients with a Coronary CTA showing borderline obstructive plaque, usually in the 50-70% range, can go directly to PET imaging. Again, symptoms make it easier.
Patients with new findings of CHF and/or a cardiomyopathy can usually proceed directly to PET testing.
Patients requiring a decision regarding the need for revascularization, either from the ischemic or viability standpoint.

Table 6. Clinical Recommendations for Appropriate PET Testing

	Adenosine*	Dipyridamole*	Dobutamine
Number of Peripheral IV lines recommended	2	1	2
Radiotracer Injection	Mid infusion	3 minutes after completion of infusion	When target heart rate is reached

Table 7.

A normal exercise rMPI is associated with a low risk for future cardiac events (<1 percent annual mortality rate). In contrast, the presence of high-risk findings, such as extensive ischemia, reversible ischemia in multiple segments, transient or persistent cavity dilatation, or a left ventricular ejection fraction of <45 percent, predict an annual mortality rate above 3 percent. In the study just cited, the annual rate of cardiac death in patients with mildly abnormal, moderately abnormal, or severely abnormal perfusion defects was 2.7, 2.9, and 4.2 percent, respectively (Hachamovitch, 1998). High-risk patients should undergo coronary angiography.

Tl-201 Protocol	Stress (mCi)	Rest (mCi)	Reinjection (mCi)
Stress/Rest	2.5-4.0	-	-
Stress/Rest/Reinjection	2.5-4.0	-	1.0-2.0
Viability Only	-	3.0-4.0	-
Tc-99m Protocol	**Stress (mCi)**		**Rest (mCi)**
Two day	24-36		24-36
One day, Stress/Rest	8-12		24-36
One day, Rest/Stress	24-36		8-12
Dual isotope	24-36		2.5-4.0

Table 8. Suggested radiopharmaceutical doses for myocardial perfusion imaging protocols

	Thallium-201	Technetium-99m
Dose	2-4 mCi	20-30 mCi
Photon energy	69-83 keV	140 keV
Half-life	73 hours	6 hours
Availability	Cyclotron-produced	Generator produced; often available on site
Significant redistribution	Yes	No

Table 9. Comparison of Thallium-201 and Tecnetium-99m

6. Pharmacologic stress testing with either dipyridamole, adenosine, or regadenoson

Exercise is the preferred method of stress in SPECT rMPI. As stated earlier, patients must be able to exercise to 85% of their MPHR or 5 METs. However, there are many patients whom are unable to exercise due to physical impairments or deconditioning. When this occurs, pharmacologic stress agents are used in place of exercise. Pharmacologic stress agents are classified as either vasodilator or inotropic/chronotropic drugs. Adenosine, regadenoson, and dipyridamole produce coronary vasodilation in the presence of significant coronary stenosis; they induce heterogeneous myocardial blood flow due to differences in coronary flow reserve. The heterogeneity of myocardial blood flow during hyperemia is detectable with a perfusion tracer and SPECT or PET imaging. In patients who are unable to exercise and have contraindications to vasodilators, dobutamine is currently recommended as the stress agent in conjunction with either echocardiography or rMPI.

Adenosine (Adenoscan ™) is the most widely used pharmacologic stress agent in the United States, currently accounting for approximately 44% of pharmacologic stress MPI procedures (Malvern, 2009). It directly activates cell-surface A1 and A2 adenosine receptors in the coronary arteries, resulting in a 3.5-to 4-fold increase in myocardial blood flow (Henzlova, 2009). It is administered through a pump infusion at a weight-based dosage of 140 ug/kg/min over 6 minutes, for a total dose of 0.84 mg/kg. The radiotracer is injected at the midpoint of the infusion, depending on a 4 or 6 minute protocol. The addition of

	Thallium	Sestamibi	Tetrofosmin	Teboroxime
Class	Element	Isonitrite	Diphospine	BATO
Charge	Positive	Positive	Positive	Neutral
Lipophilic	No	No	No	Yes
Extraction	Mod-high	Moderate	Moderate	High
Retention	Moderate	High	High	Low
Redistribution	Yes	Minimal	Minimum	Yes
Start time*	<15 min	15-60 min	15-30 min	<3 min
Imaging protocol	1 day	1 or 2 days	1 or 2 days	1 day
Gated SPECT	Possible	Yes	Yes	No
First pass	No	Yes	Yes	No
Viability assessment	Yes	Yes	Yes?	No

Table 10. Characteristics of various myocardial perfusion agents

exercise (walking on the treadmill at 0% incline at 1 mi/hr) has been shown to improve the detection of ischemia as well as scan quality (Holly, 2003). Adenosine is contraindicated in patients who have second-or-third degree atrioventricular (AV) block or sinus node disease (except those with a functioning artificial pacemaker), and in patients with known or suspected bronchoconstrictive or bronchospastic lung disease, such as asthma or chronic obstructive pulmonary disease. Based on clinical trial, the most common side effects associated with adenosine were flushing (44%), chest discomfort (40%), and dyspnea (28%). These side effects are very transient lasting up to a minute and usually resolve by the end of the infusion. If necessary, to reverse these effects one may administer aminophylline 50 to 250 mg by slow intravenous injection (50-100 mg over 30-60 seconds).

Intravenous dipyridamole was the first agent approved for pharmacologic stress in MPI, in 1990, and is currently being used in roughly 26% of pharmacologic stress MPI procedures in the United States (Malvern, 2009). It induces coronary vasodilation by inhibiting the intracellular reuptake of endogenous adenosine. It is administered via pump infusion at a rate of 0.142 mg/kg/min over 4 minutes, for a total dose of 0.57 mg/kg. It is contraindicated only in patients with hypersensitivity to it, but is generally considered to be contraindicated with bronchoconstrictive or bronchospastic lung disease as well (Henzlova, 2008). The most common side effects are: chest pain (20%), headache (12%), and dizziness (12%). Similar to adenosine, aminophylline can be used to reverse the above side effects.

In April 2008, regadenoson (Lexiscan ™) was the first selective A2A adenosine receptor agonist to be approved for use in rMPI, and currently accounts for 24% of pharmacologic stress MPI procedures (Malvern, 2009). The selectivity of A2Aadenosine receptor agonists greatly reduce or even eliminate the side effects associated with the adenosine or dypyrimadole. It is administered as a rapid injection, over approximately 10 seconds. It is contraindicated in patients with sick sinus syndrome, high degree AV block, and in patients receiving oral dipyridamole therapy.

Both SPECT and positron emission tomography (PET) imaging provide useful diagnostic and prognostic information during pharmacologic stress test. However, PET is preferable in patients with prior equivocal SPECT results and, possibly, in patients with obesity or established CAD.

7. Stress echocardiography

Exercise or pharmacologic stress two-dimensional (2D) trans-thoracic echocardiography may also be used to suspect coronary artery disease by demonstrating inducible wall motion abnormalities, to assess myocardial viability prior to coronary revascularization, to risk stratify patients with known or suspected CAD, and to risk stratify patients prior to non-cardiac surgery. The high specificity of stress echocardiography compared to other modalities contributes to its utility as a cost-effective diagnostic method. The sensitivity and specificity are 76 and 88 percent respectively (Fleischmann, 1998). There are several advantages of stress echocardiography over stress rMPI, including lower cost, shorter patient time commitment, and avoidance of radiation exposure. The latter is an important issue to consider as patients often have multiple stress imaging tests during their lifetime.

Among patients who are able to exercise, exercise rMPI or exercise echocardiography can be used to identify the extent, severity, and location of ischemia in patients with an intermediate pretest probability of disease who do not have left bundle branch block or a paced ventricular rhythm but have other resting ECG abnormalities that could interfere with the interpretation of exercise ECG testing. Both may be used in patients with prior revascularization and to assess the functional significance of coronary lesions, if not already known, prior to percutaneous coronary intervention.

Exercise echocardiography or exercise rMPI is primarily recommended as the initial stress test in patients who can exercise but have baseline ECG abnormalities (i.e. LVH, ST-T changes, LBBB) that interfere with interpretation of exercise ECG testing.

In three reviews, exercise echocardiography (compared to coronary angiography) had a sensitivity of 79 to 85 percent and a specificity of 72 to 87 percent for the diagnosis of coronary artery disease (Fleischmann, 1998) (Kim, 2001) (Arruda, 2001). False negative results are more likely with sub-maximal exercise, single vessel disease, and moderate (50 to 70 percent) stenoses (Marwick, 1992).

When treadmill exercise stress is used, images are obtained immediately after exercise since imaging during exercise is not feasible. A potential limitation with this approach is that ischemia may resolve rapidly after discontinuing the exercise and a wall motion abnormality that developed during peak exercise may rapidly reverse to normal after the test is stopped. Thus, images need to be acquired as rapidly as possible (within 60 to 90 seconds after cessation of exercise). This method requires that the patient move from the treadmill into a recumbent position for imaging within a few seconds so that images can be obtained within 60 seconds after peak exercise. Due to tachypnea and tachycardia that develop at peak exercise, the heart is frequently visible for only one or two beats at end expiration. Early image acquisition is necessary since ischemia induced wall motion abnormalities may resolve rapidly as the heart rate slows, causing a decrease in the sensitivity of the test, especially for single vessel disease. Failure to achieve or exceed target heart rate also decreases sensitivity.

Some laboratories perform stress echocardiography using supine or upright bicycle ergometry. The peak heart rate and achieved double product (the product of peak heart rate and peak systolic blood pressure) are usually lower and the achieved blood pressure is higher after a bicycle protocol than a treadmill test. A typical supine bicycle protocol increases the workload by 25 W every three minutes until an endpoint is achieved. In this protocol, an exercise duration of 20 minutes is typical for a healthy adult without endurance training. The protocol can be modified during image acquisition to allow complete data collection without increasing the workload once maximum capacity is reached.

A major advantage of bicycle ergometry is that it allows continuous monitoring of wall motion during exercise. More importantly, imaging throughout the study (so that rest, intermediate, peak and recovery images are obtained) may permit detection of the onset and disappearance of transient wall motion abnormalities and improve sensitivity of detection of coronary artery disease (Park, 2007). An additional advantage of continuous imaging is that during low level stress, an improvement in a dysfunctional wall is equivalent to improvement with low dose dobutamine; therefore, a segment that improves during low level exercise has a high likelihood of viability. If segmental wall motion deteriorates beyond its resting level of dysfunction at peak stress, then the affected segment has a high likelihood of being supplied by stenosed coronary artery.

	Dipyridamole	Adenosine	Regadenoson	Dobutamine
Chemical	Pyrimidine derivative	Endogenous vasodilator of purine derivative	Purine derivative	Synthetic catecholamine
Onset and duration of action, half-life	Effect peaks at 7-15 minutes, half-life 30-45 minutes	Immediate onset, half-life less than five seconds, effects disappear rapidly after infusion	Peak 1-4 minutes after injection Half-life of ≈30 minutes	Onset 1-2 minutes, half-life 2 minutes
Mechanism of action	Blocks reuptake of endogenous adenosine causing coronary vasodilation	Stimulation of adenosine receptor A2A causing coronary vasodilation	Stimulates A2A adenosine receptor causes coronary vasodilation	Alpha-1, beta-1, and beta-2 stimulation increases myocardial O2 demand and secondary vasodilatation
Dose	140 µg/kg per min for 4 minutes (maximum 0.56 mg/kg)	140 µg/kg per min for 4-6 minutes	Regadenoson 0.4 mg/5 mL	5-40 µg/kg per min, depending upon heart rate response
Radionuclide injection	7-9 minutes after initiation of infusion	3 minutes into infusion; infusion continued for further 1-3 minutes	10-20 seconds after regadenoson	At peak stress
Hemodynamics	Slight increase in heart rate and slight decrease in blood pressure (BP)	Slight increase in heart rate and slight decrease in BP (adenosine more than dipyridamole)	Slight increase in heart rate and slight decrease in BP	Target heart rate 85 percent of maximum predicted heart rate
Side effects	Occur frequently, but minor	Same as dipyridamole but resolve rapidly; heart block more common	Dyspnea, headache and flushing	Most common chest pain, most serious nonsustained ventricular tachycardia, nonfatal myocardial infarction
Contraindications	Bronchospasm, second or third degree AV block or sick sinus syndrome (unless protected by a functioning pacemaker)	Same as dipyridamole	Second- or third-degree AV block or sinus node dysfunction Caution for bronchospasm	Recent acute coronary syndrome, hemodynamic and electrophysiologic instability

Table 11. Comparisons between different pharmacologic stress agents.

When exercise echocardiography is performed during supine or upright bicycle exercise, images are obtained during exercise so ischemic dysfunction is more likely to be captured if adequate workloads are attained. Continuous echocardiographic monitoring has another potential advantage in that it permits detection of the biphasic response of dysfunctional yet viable myocardium that is characterized by initial improvement of regional function followed by deterioration similar to the biphasic response detected during dobutamine stress echocardiography.

Dobutamine increases heart rate and myocardial contractility. The onset of action is within one to two minutes of intravenous infusion, the half-life is two minutes, and the drug is metabolized via methylation and conjugation. At a dose of 20 µg/kg per min, there is a small but significant increase in systolic blood pressure (mean 12 mmHg in one report) and at 40 µg/kg per min, the mean heart rate is 120 to 125 beats/min.

The 2007 ACC/AHA perioperative guidelines regarding stress testing in patients with left bundle branch block concluded that exercise imaging (with either echocardiography or rMPI) was suboptimal (due to low specificity) and that either vasodilator rMPI or dobutamine stress echocardiography is preferred for these patients (Fleisher, 2009).

The standard dobutamine stress test components are: graded dobutamine infusion in five three-minute stages starting at 5 μg/kg/min, followed by 10, 20, 30, and 40 μg/kg/min. An initial dose of 2.5 μg/kg/min is sometimes employed in tests evaluating viability. Low-dose stages facilitate recognition of viability and ischemia in segments with abnormal function at rest, even when viability evaluation is not the main aim of the test (Pellikka, 2007). End points are achievement of target heart rate (defined as 85 percent of age MPHR), new or worsening wall-motion abnormalities of moderate degree, significant arrhythmias, hypotension, severe hypertension, and intolerable symptoms. Atropine, in divided doses of 0.5 mg to a total of 2.0 mg, should be administered as needed to achieve target heart rate. Atropine increases the sensitivity of dobutamine echocardiography in patients receiving beta-blockers and in those with single-vessel disease (McNeill,1992).

8. Cardiac Computed Tomography Angiography (CCTA) and stress Cardiac Magnetic Resonance Imaging (CMRI)

Cardiac computed tomography angiography (CCTA) is an imaging method that uses a computed tomography (CT) scanner to look at the structures and blood vessels of the heart. In some situations a CCTA can be done instead of, or in addition to, a stress test. Both CCTA and a stress test may be used to screen patients for CAD.

Calcium scoring and CCTA have different clinical indications. Calcium scoring is primarily used for risk stratification of asymptomatic patients, while CCTA is primarily used in patients with acute or chronic chest pain. One potential use of performing a non-enhanced calcium scoring study before a CCTA is to decide whether to proceed with CCTA in patients with extensive coronary calcium. There is no established calcium score cutoff value above which CCTA will not be diagnostic, but a score of 1000 is often used. In the multicenter Assessment by Coronary Computed Tomographic Angiography of Individuals Undergoing Invasive Coronary Angiography (ACCURACY) trial, the specificity of CCTA was significantly reduced (from 86% to 53%) in patients with calcium scores greater than 400 (Budoff, 2008).

A 2008 scientific statement from the AHA indicates that the potential benefit of noninvasive coronary angiography is likely to be the greatest for symptomatic patients who are at intermediate risk for CAD after initial risk stratification, including patients with equivocal stress tests. CCTA is recommended over coronary magnetic resonance angiography (MRA) because of superior diagnostic accuracy. Neither coronary CCTA nor MRA is recommended to screen for CAD in patients who have no signs or symptoms suggestive of CAD.

The following indications were rated as appropriate for coronary CT angiography (Hendel, 2006): evaluation of chest pain syndrome in patients with intermediate pretest probability of CAD and uninterpretable ECG or inability to exercise, evaluation of chest pain syndrome in patients with uninterpretable or equivocal stress test, evaluation of acute chest pain in patients with intermediate pretest probability of CAD and no ECG changes and serial enzymes negative, evaluation of coronary arteries in patients with new-onset heart failure to assess etiology, and evaluation of suspected coronary anomalies.

A CCTA can directly estimate the amount of stenosis likely indicating an area of ischemia CCTA is not recommended in patients with either a very low pretest likelihood of coronary stenosis or a high pretest likelihood of coronary stenosis. Concerns about radiation exposure limit the use of CCTA in patients with very low likelihood of coronary disease. Patients with high likelihood of CAD are likely to require invasive coronary angiography and intervention. The usefulness of CCTA is reduced in patients with pronounced coronary calcification. In a 2008 meta-analysis (Mowatt, 2008), CCTA had a sensitivity of 99% and negative predictive value (NPV) of 100% for patient-based detection of significant CAD. The ACCURACY trial suggested that, compared with other noninvasive modalities such as stress echocardiography and stress nuclear testing, CCTA has comparable specificity but superior sensitivity and NPV.

Along with accurately depicting left and right ventricle ejection fractions, volumes, and myocardial mass, CMRI can also reveal regional wall motion abnormalities in ischemic tissue. By using T2-weighted imaging and assessment of left ventricular wall thickness, CMRI adds a level of specificity that no other stress modality can reach. Late gadolinium enhancement (LGE) or delayed enhancement CMRI is thought to reflect fibrosis and irreversibly damaged myocardium including acute and chronic MI. The possible role of LGE as a risk predictor for subsequent cardiac events was evaluated in a group of 195 patients without known prior MI, but with known or suspected CAD (Kwong, 2006). During an average follow-up of 16 months, patients with LGE on the baseline study had a higher incidence of major adverse cardiovascular endpoints (MACE) compared to those without this finding. In addition, LGE was the strongest multivariable predictor of MACE taking into account traditional clinical, angiographic, and functional variables. CMRI has been evaluated using dobutamine, dipyramidole, adenosine, or regadenoson as pharmacologic stress. The proper role of this diagnostic tool in the evaluation of patients with suspected or known coronary artery disease remains to be determined. Some of the disadvantages are: cost, availability, motion artifact, and observer bias.

CMRI or CCTA is suggested to evaluate suspected or known congenital or acquired coronary anomalies, particularly to establish the proximal course relative to the great vessels of coronary arteries with abnormal origin. CMRI is preferred in these younger patients to avoid radiation exposure and in patients with contraindications to iodinated contrast or beta blockers. In patients with no signs or symptoms suggestive of coronary artery disease, we recommended that neither CCTA nor CMRI should be used to screen for coronary disease. Noninvasive coronary angiography is reasonable for symptomatic patients who are at intermediate risk for coronary artery disease after initial risk stratification, including patients with equivocal stress test results. Diagnostic accuracy currently favors CCTA over CMRI for these patients. In patients with known or suspected congenital or acquired coronary anomalies, we suggest CCTA or CMRI. CMRI is preferred in younger patients given concerns about potential long-term effects of radiation associated with CCTA. In patients with coronary artery bypass grafts in whom it is not possible to selectively engage clinical important grafts during invasive angiography, we suggest CCTA or CMRI for evaluation of coronary artery bypass graft patency. In patients with contraindications to beta blockers or iodinated contrast or with significant renal dysfunction, CMRI is preferred to CCTA. Neither CCTA nor CMRI should be used to screen for coronary disease in patients who have no signs or symptoms suggestive of coronary artery disease.

9. Positron emission computed tomography myocardial perfusion imaging

PET is an established noninvasive method of evaluating myocardial perfusion and viability (Schelbert, 1994). This technique has the advantage of being able to assess perfusion and metabolism simultaneously. PET requires the use of positron-emitting isotopes (such as oxygen-15, carbon-11, nitrogen-13, and fluorine-18), which are incorporated into physiologically active molecules. During ischemia, myocyte metabolism is shifted to glucose from fatty acids. Thus, uptake of a glucose analog, fluorine-18 labeled deoxyglucose (FDG) by myocytes in an area of dysfunctional myocardium indicates metabolic activity and thus, viability. Regional perfusion can be simultaneously assessed with an agent that remains in the vascular space and thus demonstrates the distribution of blood flow (such as N-13 ammonia or Rb-82). As a result, PET imaging has the potential to differentiate between normal, stunned, hibernating, and necrotic myocardium. The presence of enhanced FDG uptake in regions of decreased blood flow defines hibernating myocardium by PET imaging, while a concordant reduction in both metabolism and flow is thought to represent predominantly necrotic myocardium. Regional dysfunction in presence of normal perfusion is indicative of stunning. Myocardial segments with significant reductions in both blood flow and FDG uptake have only a 20 percent chance of functional improvement following revascularization. In comparison, dysfunctional territories deemed to be hibernating by PET have approximately an 80 to 85 percent chance of functional improvement following revascularization (Lucignani, 1992).

PET MPI is indicated for the diagnosis and risk stratification of suspected CAD in patients with an intermediate or high likelihood of CAD and cannot exercise adequately or have a LBBB or paced rhythm on ECG. PET MPI is also indicated for the detection of the co-presence of CAD and for the assessment of resting myocardial perfusion in patients undergoing the assessment of myocardial viability with FDG PET.

Rubidium-82 generators are delivered to the PET center on a monthly basis. Rubidium has a half life of 75 seconds, making pharmacologic imaging necessary. The patient lies comfortably, with their head outside of the scanner, for 30 minutes. Rubidium-82 is used to obtain cardiac PET images before and after dipyridamole, the pharmacologic agent of choice at this time. Aminophylline can be given at the end of the procedure to minimize side effects, which are minimal.

PET methodology utilizes Beta (+) decay of a nucleus resulting in emission of a positron, which rapidly annihilates with an electron, giving off two 511-keV photons that travel opposite each other (180 degrees). Images are produced as the two photons are detected simultaneously in the ring shaped scanner. Spatial resolution is presently in the range of 4-6 mm, making PET superior to conventional nuclear imaging. Temporal resolution is also superior and clinical studies have consistently shown increased sensitivity and specificity with PET compared to conventional nuclear testing.

PET offers additional benefits in comparison to nuclear testing. As mentioned, the total procedure takes 30 minutes compared to 3-4 hours for nuclear testing. Technetium, the primary isotope in conventional nuclear testing, has become difficult to obtain and recently most labs are limited in their ability to test patients. PET using rubidium-82 has less radiation exposure to the patient and staff. Research in molecular and nanotechnology is within years of taking Cardiac PET imaging and its benefits to a new level.

Patients with non-diagnostic or equivocal stress echo that were tested for ischemic symptoms would qualify for a PET scan.
Patients with non-diagnostic or equivocal nuclear testing that are being assessed for ischemic symptoms qualify for a PET scan.
Patients that can not exercise and need pharmacologic testing that have ischemic symptoms or need clearance for major surgery would qualify for a PET scan.
Patients with BMI over 40 and in some cases over 35, which are being assessed for ischemic symptoms, can go straight to a PET scan.
Patients with breast implants or large pendulous breasts, undergoing assessment for ischemic symptoms, can undergo PET imaging.
Patients with a high CAC, viewed as over 300 or 400, can often go to PET imaging. Symptoms are needed to pre-certify.
Patients with a Coronary CTA showing borderline obstructive plaque, usually in the 50-70% range, can go directly to PET imaging. Again, symptoms make it easier.
Patients with new findings of CHF and/or a cardiomyopathy can usually proceed directly to PET testing.
Patients requiring a decision regarding the need for revascularization, either from the ischemic or viability standpoint.

Table 12. Clinical Recommendations for Appropriate PET Testing

Some of the disadvantages of PET include: limited availability, difficult use with exercise stress and lack of experienced/trained staff. Patients who benefit from PET MPI are those who have an equivocal SPECT MPI for diagnosis or risk stratification of known or suspected CAD, require pharmacologic stress imaging, are more prone to attenuation artifacts such as obese patients, female patients, arms down imaging, and finally those who require myocardial viability assessment

Most PET stress scans are performed using pharmacological stress with vasodilator stress being the most common. The radiotracer is injected during peak hyperemia using the same or a separate intravenous line. Exercise stress is feasible but may be cumbersome due to high radiation dose to personnel, coordination with the cyclotron and patient motion.Rubidium-82 (Rb 82) (76-second half-life) is produced by a generator and is the most widely used radiotracer for clinical PET MPI. The Sr-82 generator that produces Rb-82 is replaced every 28 days, reflecting the physical half-life of Sr-82. The use of N-13 ammonia (9.96-minute half-life) is limited to institutions that have a cyclotron on site. The longer half-life permits exercise stress.

10. Stress testing in women and diabetics

Cardiovascular diseases are the most common cause of death and disability in women in the United States (Eaker, 1999). Between the ages of 45 to 64, one in nine women develops symptoms of some form of cardiovascular disease. After age 65, the ratio climbs to one in three women, according to the National Center for Health Statistics (Mosca, 1997). Women are more likely to initially present with chest pain than a more clearly defined event such as a myocardial infarction. Women rated their chest pain as more intense, used different terms to describe the pain such as sharp or burning, had more symptoms unrelated to pain, and more frequently had pain and other sensations in the neck and throat. Women present about 10 years later than men and with a greater risk-factor burden. Women are less likely than men to have typical angina and those who present to the emergency department with new onset chest pain are approached and diagnosed less aggressively than men. The symptoms of MI in women may differ slightly from those in men. Many cases of myocardial infarction MI in women go unrecognized, particularly at younger ages or in patients with diabetes.

The symptoms of AMI in women differ from those in men, which may in part explain the greater delays in both seeking and receiving care. Women who present with episodic chest pain need to be evaluated for CAD. The likelihood of CAD is based in part upon the character of the presenting symptoms and the presence or absence of coronary risk factors.

The risk assessment must be sex specific because the risk factors themselves, as well as their relative importance, may differ between women and men. In particular, hormonal status, diabetes, smoking, and a family history of premature CAD appear to be more important in women. Women with chest pain, compared to men, have a lower rate of CAD and a higher rate of false positive results on exercise ECG testing (Diamond, 1979).

The process of establishing the diagnosis of CAD in women is similar to that in men, but several points need to be kept in mind: treadmill exercise testing has a higher false-positive rate in women, while stress imaging appears to have similar accuracy. The prevalence of significant coronary disease found at the time of angiography is lower in women than men presenting with chest pain. Women with chest pain and no evidence of atherosclerotic coronary artery disease on coronary angiography may have cardiac syndrome X or microvascular disease, or far more rarely, takotsubo cardiomyopathy or spontaneous coronary artery dissection.

Compared to individuals without diabetes, those with diabetes have a higher prevalence of CAD, a greater extent of myocardial ischemia, and are more likely to have an AMI and silent myocardial ischemia (Hammoud, 2000). The increase in cardiovascular risk is due both to diabetes and to the frequent presence of other risk factors such as hyperlipidemia and hypertension. In addition to the increase in cardiovascular events, patients with type 2 diabetes also have a high rate of asymptomatic coronary artery disease compared to the general population. Furthermore, asymptomatic patients may have coronary anatomy that does not permit optimal outcomes with percutaneous coronary intervention or coronary artery bypass graft surgery. Some diabetic patients have a blunted appreciation of ischemic pain, which may result in atypical anginal symptoms, silent ischemia, or even silent infarction. Silent ischemia in diabetes is thought to be caused at least in part by autonomic denervation of the heart.

Diabetic patients have an increased frequency of silent ST segment depression and coronary perfusion abnormalities during stress testing (Scognamiglio, 2006). Since type 2 diabetes is considered to be a CAD equivalent, the primary purpose of screening would be to identify patients whose prognosis could be improved with medical therapy or coronary revascularization. When stress testing is performed for the diagnosis of CAD in the general population, many experts recommend standard exercise ECG testing if the resting ECG is normal, since the exercise response will be an important factor in determining prognosis. If the resting ECG has abnormalities that will interfere with interpretation during exercise or if localization of ischemia is expected to be important, an exercise test with imaging can be performed. For patients who cannot exercise, pharmacologic stress testing should be performed.

The sensitivity and specificity of SPECT rMPI in the diabetic patients were 86 and 56 percent for ≥50 percent diameter stenosis and 90 and 50 percent for ≥70 percent diameter stenosis. Test performance was similar with exercise and adenosine and in the non-diabetic patients. When performing dobutamine stress echocardiography, the sensitivity and specificity were 81 and 85 percent, respectively. Currently, neither CMRI or cardiac CT is an alternative to invasive, selective coronary angiography and neither is recommended for screening asymptomatic patients, including those at high risk. Furthermore, the higher rate of extensive coronary calcification in patients with diabetes interferes with the interpretation of stenosis severity. In the patients with a normal stress rMPI, cardiac mortality was low and equivalent in diabetic and non-diabetic patients for the first two years. However, after two years, there was a sharp increase in cardiac events in the diabetic patients, with the highest risk in diabetic women.

The most cost effective approach to screening and prevention of cardiovascular events in asymptomatic patients with diabetes remains a subject of debate. The 2002 ACC/AHA guidelines for exercise testing made a more limited conclusion that the weight of evidence favors evaluation only in asymptomatic patients with diabetes who plan to begin a vigorous exercise program.

11. The future of stress testing in coronary artery disease

Noninvasive cardiac testing is used for risk stratification for patients with possible acute coronary syndromes. Several testing modalities exist, and each has unique advantages and disadvantages. Patient characteristics, costs, and local resources dictate which of the cardiac tests are chosen. Noninvasive cardiac tests are improving as new diagnostic technologies and methods are being developed. As future studies reveal the true diagnostic characteristics and capabilities of these tests, physicians can better assess patients' risk of coronary artery disease. As with all diagnostic tests, none of the cardiac tests are ideal.

The utility of a recent negative stress test is limited when it is used to determine the risk for acute coronary syndrome (ACS) in a patient presenting to the emergency department with symptoms of angina. Unfortunately, overreliance on negative stress tests is a common reason for misdiagnosis or delays in diagnosis in patients with ACS. It is critical to remember that cardiac tests are useful for risk stratification, but no test is capable of stratifying a patient's risk to zero. Evaluation of patients with acute chest pain in emergency rooms is time-consuming and expensive, and it often results in uncertain diagnoses or patients with chest pain and low risk for short-term cardiac events, outpatient stress testing is feasible, safe, and associated with decreased hospital admission rates. With an evidence-based protocol, physicians efficiently identify patients at low risk for clinically significant coronary artery disease and short-term adverse cardiac outcomes. The role of cardiac stress testing is invaluable. The future of cardiovascular medicine will be not how to treat acute coronary syndromes, but how can we predict them.

12. References

American Heart Association. *2001 Heart and Stroke Statistical Update.* Dallas, TX: AHA, 2000.

American Society of Nuclear Cardiology (ASNC) PET Myocardial Perfusion Imaging (MPI) Practice Points June 2010.

Arruda AM, Das MK, Roger VL, et al. Prognostic value of exercise echocardiography in 2,632 patients > or = 65 years of age. *J Am Coll Cardiol* 2001; 37:1036.

Budoff MJ, Dowe D, Jollis JG, Gitter M, Sutherland J, Halamert E, et al. Diagnostic performance of 64-multidetector row coronary computed tomographic angiography for evaluation of coronary artery stenosis in individuals without known coronary artery disease: results from the prospective multicenter ACCURACY (Assessment by Coronary Computed Tomographic Angiography of

Individuals Undergoing Invasive Coronary Angiography) trial. *J Am Coll Cardiol.* Nov 18 2008;52(21):1724-32.

DePuey EG, Rozanski A. Using gated technetium-99m-sestamibi SPECT to characterize fixed myocardial defects as infarct or artifact. *J Nucl Med* 1995; 36:952.

Diamond GA, Forrester JS. Analysis of probability as an aid in the clinical diagnosis of coronary-artery disease. N Engl J Med 1979; 300:1350.

Eaker ED, Chesebro JH, Sacks FM, et al. Cardiovascular disease in women. *Circulation* 1993; 88:1999.

Ekelund LG, Suchindran CM, McMahon RP, et al. Coronary heart disease morbidity and mortality in hypercholesterolemic men predicted from an exercise test: the Lipid Research Clinics Coronary Primary Prevention Trial. *J Am Coll Cardiol* 1989; 14:556.

Fleischmann KE, Hunink MG, Kuntz KM, Douglas PS. Exercise echocardiography or exercise SPECT imaging? A meta-analysis of diagnostic test performance. *JAMA* 1998; 280:913.

Fleisher LA, Beckman JA, Brown KA, et al. 2009 ACCF/AHA focused update on perioperative beta blockade incorporated into the ACC/AHA 2007 guidelines on perioperative cardiovascular evaluation and care for noncardiac surgery: a report of the American college of cardiology foundation/American heart association task force on practice guidelines. *Circulation* 2009; 120:e169.

Gibbons RJ, Abrams J, Chatterjee K, et al. ACC/AHA 2002 guideline update for the management of patients with chronic stable angina.

Gibbons RJ, et al. ACC/AHA 2002 guideline update for exercise testing: a report of the American College of Cardiology/American Heart Association Task Force on Practice Guideines (Exercise Testing) 2002.

Hammoud T, Tanguay JF, Bourassa MG. Management of coronary artery disease: therapeutic options in patients with diabetes. J Am Coll Cardiol 2000; 36:355.

Hachamovitch R, Berman DS, Shaw LJ, et al. Incremental prognostic value of myocardial perfusion single photon emission computed tomography for the prediction of cardiac death: differential stratification for risk of cardiac death: differential stratification for risk of cardiac death and myocardial infarction. *Circulation* 1998; 97:535.

Heller LI, Villegas BJ, Reinhardt CP, et al. Teboroxime is a marker of reperfusion after myocardial infarction. *J Nucl Cardiol* 1996; 3:2.

Hendel RC, Patel MR, Kramer CM, Poon M, Hendel RC, Carr JC, et al. ACCF/ACR/SCCT/SCMR/ASNC/NASCI/SCAI/SIR 2006 appropriateness criteria for cardiac computed tomography and cardiac magnetic resonance imaging: a report of the American College of Cardiology Foundation Quality Strategic Directions Committee Appropriateness Criteria Working Group, American College of Radiology, Society of Cardiovascular Computed Tomography, Society for Cardiovascular Magnetic Resonance, American Society of Nuclear Cardiology, North American Society for Cardiac Imaging, Society for Cardiovascular Angiography and Interventions, and Society of Interventional Radiology. *J Am Coll Cardiol.* Oct 3 2006;48(7):1475-97.

Henzlova MJ, Cerqueira MD, Hansen CL, et al. ASNC Imaging Guidelines for Nuclear Cardiology Procedures: Stress protocols and tracers. 2009

Higley B, Smith FW, Smith T, et al. Technetium-99m-1,2-bis[bis(2-ethoxyethyl) phosphino] ethane: human biodistribution, dosimetry and safety of a new myocardial perfusion agent. *J Nucl Med* 1993; 34:30.

Holly TA, Satran A, Bromet DS, et al. The impact of adjunctive adenosine infusion during myocardial perfusion imaging: results of the Both Exercise and Adenosine Stress Test (BEAST) trial. *J Nucl Cardiol.* 2003; 10:291-296.

Jeetley P, Sabharwal NK, Soman P, et al. Comparison between Tc-99m N-NOET and Tl-201 in the assessment of patients with known or suspected coronary artery disease. *J Nucl Med* 1995; 36:936.

Kannel WB, McGee D, Gordon T. A general cardiovascular risk profile: The Framingham study. *Am J Cardiol* 1976; 38:46-51.

Kim C, Kwok YS, Heagerty P, Redberg R. Pharmacologic stress testing for coronary disease diagnosis: A meta-analysis. *Am Heart J* 2001; 142:934.

Kwok JM, Miller TD, Hodge DO, Gibbons RJ. Prognostic value of the Duke treadmill score in the elderly. *J Am Coll Cardiol* 2002; 39:1

Kwong RY, Chan AK, Brown KA, et al. Impact of unrecognized myocardial scar detected by cardiac magnetic resonance imaging on event-free survival in patients presenting with signs or symptoms of coronary artery disease. *Circulation* 2006; 113:2733.

Lebowitz E, Greene MW, Fairchild R, et al. Thallium-201 for medical use. *I. J Nucl Med* 1975; 16:151.

Lucignani G, Paolini G, Landoni C, et al. Presurgical identification of hibernating myocardium by combined use of technetium-99m hexakis 2-methoxyisobutylisonitrile single photon emission tomography and fluorine-18 fluoro-2-deoxy-D-glucose positron emission tomography in patients with coronary artery disease. *Eur J Nucl Med* 1992; 19:874.

Malvern PA. *The Myocardial Perfusion Study Monthly Monitor.* Arlington Medical Resources Inc; 2009.

Mark DB, Hlatky MA, Harrell FE Jr, et al. Exercise treadmill score for predicting prognosis in coronary artery disease. *Ann Intern Med* 1987; 106:793.

Marwick TH, Nemec JJ, Pashkow FJ, et al. Accuracy and limitations of exercise echocardiography in a routine clinical setting. *J Am Coll Cardiol* 1992; 19:74.

McNeill AJ, Fioretti PM, el-Said SM, et al. Enhanced sensitivity for detection of coronary artery disease by addition of atropine to dobutamine stress echocardiography. *Am J Cardiol* 1992; 70:41.

Medrano R, Mahmarian J, Verani M Nitroglycerine before injection of thallium-201 enhances detection of reversible hypoperfusion via collateral blood flow: A randomized, double blind parallel, placebo-controlled trial using quantitative tomography. *J Am Coll Cardiol* 1993; 21:221A

Mosca L, Manson JE, Sutherland SE, et al. Cardiovascular disease in women: a statement for healthcare professionals from the American Heart Association. Writing Group. Circulation 1997; 96:2468.

Mowatt G, Cummins E, Waugh N, Walker S, Cook J, Jia X, et al. Systematic review of the clinical effectiveness and cost-effectiveness of 64-slice or higher computed tomography angiography as an alternative to invasive coronary angiography in the investigation of coronary artery disease. *Health Technol Assess.* May 2008;12(17):iii-iv, ix-143

Park TH, Tayan N, Takeda K, et al. Supine bicycle echocardiography improved diagnostic accuracy and physiologic assessment of coronary artery disease with the incorporation of intermediate stages of exercise. *J Am Coll Cardiol* 2007; 50:1857.

Pellikka PA, Nagueh SF, Elhendy AA, et al. American Society of Echocardiography recommendations for performance, interpretation, and application of stress echocardiography. *J Am Soc Echocardiogr* 2007; 20:1021.

Pryor DB, Shaw L, McCants CB, et al. :Value of the history and physical in identifying patients at increased risk for coronary artery disease. *Ann Intern Med* 1993; 118:81-90.

Rautaharju PM, Prineas RJ, Eifler WJ, et al. Prognostic value of exercise electrocardiogram in men at high risk of future coronary heart disease: Multiple Risk Factor Intervention Trial experience. *J Am Coll Cardiol* 1986; 8:1.

Roger VL, Jacobson SJ, Pellikka PA, et al. Prognostic value of treadmill exercise testing: a population-based study in Olmsted County, Minnesota. Circulation 1998; 98:2836.

Schelbert HR. Metabolic imaging to assess myocardial viability. *J Nucl Med* 1994; 35:8S.

Scognamiglio R, Negut C, Ramondo A, et al. Detection of coronary artery disease in asymptomatic patients with type 2 diabetes mellitus. J Am Coll Cardiol 2006; 47:65.

Shaw LJ, Hendel R, Borges-Neto S, et al. Prognostic value of normal exercise and adenosine (99m) Tc-tetrofosmin SPECT imaging: results from the multicenter registry of 4,728 patients. *J Nucl Med* 2003; 44:134.

Strauss HW, Harrison K, Langan JK, et al. Thallium-201 for myocardial imaging. Relation of thallium-201 to regional myocardial perfusion. *Circulation* 1975; 51:641.

Strauss HW, Miller DD, Wittry MD, et al. Procedure guideline for myocardial perfusion imaging 3.3 2008.

Sugumaran RK, Lollo T, Poornima IG, Chronotropic incompetence as a manifestation of coronary artery disease and its reversal with revasularization. *J Nucl Cardiol* 2010; 17:2.

Wackers FJ, Berman DS, Maddahi J, et al. Technetium-99m hexakis 2-methyoxyisobutyl isonitrile: human biodistribution, dosimetry, safety, and preliminary comparison to thallium-201 for myocardial perfusion imaging. *J Nucl Med* 1989; 30:301.

Weiss AT, Maddahi J, Lew AS, et al. Reverse redistribution of thallium-201: sign of non transmural myocardial infarction with patency of the infarct-related coronary artery. *J Am Coll Cardiol* 1986; 7:61.

Zaret BL, Rigo P, Wackers FJ, et al. Myocardial perfusion imaging with 99mTc tetrofosmin. Comparison to 201Tl imaging and coronary angiography in a phase III multicenter trial. Tetrofosmin International Trial Study Group. *Circulation* 1995; 91:313

9

Reassessing the Value of the Exercise Electrocardiogram in the Diagnosis of Stable Chest Pain

Peter Bourdillon
Imperial College, UK

1. Introduction

"Do not use exercise ECG to diagnose or exclude angina for people without known coronary artery disease" - a quote from the summary (Cooper et al, 2010) of the guidelines of the United Kingdom's National Institute for Health and Clinical Excellence (NICE) on the diagnosis of discomfort of suspected cardiac origin (NICE, 2010). Amongst other things, NICE recommends that the probability of coronary artery disease (pCAD) is determined from the person's symptoms and risk factors, and that the subsequent management depends on whether the pCAD is less than 10%, 10 to 30%, 30 to 60%, 60 to 90% or greater than 90%: if the pCAD is less than 10% or greater than 90% further testing is not required; if the pCAD is between 60 and 90%, the patient is a candidate for coronary arteriography; if the pCAD is between 10 and 60% non-invasive testing is indicated.

Ever since a meta-analysis (Gianrossi et al., 1989) of the exercise electrocardiogram (ECG), in which the sensitivity was assessed as being 68% and the specificity as 77%, the test's role in the diagnosis of coronary artery disease has been questioned. However, in 1979 Diamond & Forrester demonstrated that the greater the ST segment shift on exercise ECG, the greater the post-exercise probability of coronary artery disease (pCAD) whatever the pre-exercise pCAD. Furthermore, the Duke Treadmill Score (Mark et al., 1991) demonstrates that the greater the ST segment depression the worse the prognosis.

The purpose of this study is to show, using the data obtained from a West London population and NICE's methodology, the different impact the exercise ECG has on subsequent management, if Diamond & Forrester's method of analysing exercise ECG data is used instead of NICE's.

2. Methods

Patients with a history of chest pain referred direct from primary care to the rapid access chest pain clinic of the Hammersmith Hospital, London, between January 1999 and March 2010 were studied. Each person was asked to complete a questionnaire (Table 1) which combines questions from two previously published studies (Joswig et al., 1985; Pryor et al., 1993).

		Yes	No
1	Have you had a coronary bypass operation or a coronary angioplasty?		
2	Have you ever been told that you have had a heart attack?		
3	Have you smoked 10 or more cigarettes a day in the last 5 years?		
4	Have you ever had diabetes?		
5	Has your blood cholesterol ever been more than 6.2 or have you ever been told that your cholesterol is high?		
6	Do you get *breathless* with the pain or discomfort?		
7	Do you feel *sick* with the pain or discomfort?		
8	Is the pain or discomfort *burning* in nature?		
9	Is the pain or discomfort *prickling* in nature?		
10	Do you feel the pain or discomfort in the *middle* of the chest?		
11	Does the pain or discomfort go into *both* arms?		
12	Do you feel the pain or discomfort *deep* of the chest?		
13	Is the pain or discomfort made *worse* by moving your arms or twisting your body?		
14	Is the pain or discomfort brought on by *exertion* such as climbing stairs or walking uphill?		
15	Is the pain or discomfort brought on by *sexual intercourse*?		
16	How long does the pain or discomfort *usually* last if you stop doing whatever started it?		
	less than 30 seconds		
	between 30 seconds and 10 minutes		
	more than 10 minutes		
		Yes	No
17	Do you use glyceryl trinitrate (the spray or the small white tablet under the tongue used to treat chest pain)?		
18	How long does the pain or discomfort *usually* last if you use glyceryl trinitrate?		
	less than 30 seconds		
	between 30 seconds and 10 minutes		
	more than 10 minutes		

Table 1. The questionnaire each patient was asked to complete.

The questionnaire was translated into 5 languages commonly used in the local community, viz. Farsi, Hindi, Polish, Punjabi and Urdu. The raw data from the questionnaire were stored in a bespoke database. For a symptomatic diagnosis of Typical Angina (chest pain symptom score 3 points) the following criteria had to be met: a) 'Yes' to both question 10 and question 12 and b) 'Yes' to either question 14 or question 15 and c) 'between 30 seconds and 10 minutes' to question 16 or 'between 30 seconds and 10 minutes' to question 18 if the answer to question 17 was 'Yes'. Atypical Angina was diagnosed if any 2 of criteria a), b) and c) were met (chest pain symptom score 2 points); otherwise Non-Anginal Chest Pain was diagnosed (chest pain symptom score either 1 or 0 points).

From the questionnaire data, pCAD was calculated (Pryor et al., 1993) for routine clinical use (pCAD_DUKE). To assess the impact of NICE's guidelines, NICE's modification of pCAD_DUKE that omits the history of myocardial infarction and omits ECG data, was used to recalculate pCAD as pCAD_NICE. The doctor or nurse assessing the patient had the pCAD_DUKE available when deciding whether or not to exercise the patient.

Treadmill exercise ECGs were performed following the Bruce protocol (Bruce et al., 1949). The Mason-Likar electrode positions (Mason & Likar, 1966) were used. The maximum ST segment shift 60-80 ms after the end of the QRS was noted; it was considered less than 50 µV if the ST segment was upsloping and the end of the QRS depressed. ST segment shifts due to rhythm disturbances were ignored. From the exercise ECG the post-exercise pCAD was calculated using Bayes' Theorem of conditional probability

$$\text{post-exercise pCAD} = [100 * \text{pre-exercise pCAD} * \text{sensitivity}] / [(\text{pre-exercise pCAD} * \text{sensitivity}) + (100 - \text{pre-exercise pCAD}) * (100 - \text{specificity})]$$

and using the sensitivities and specificities in Table 2 for different levels of ST segment shift (Diamond & Forrester, 1979). Also calculated were

$$\text{the positive likelihood ratio} = \text{sensitivity}/(100 - \text{specificity}) \text{ and}$$

$$\text{the negative likelihood ratio} = (100 - \text{sensitivity})/\text{specificity}$$

ST segment shift (µV)	Sensitivity (%)	Specificity (%)	Positive Likelihood Ratio	Negative Likelihood Ratio
0 - 50	14.3	37.5	0.23	2.29
51 - 100	20.8	77.3	0.92	1.02
101 - 150	23.3	89.0	2.12	0.86
151 - 200	8.8	97.9	4.19	0.93
201 - 250	13.3	98.8	11.08	0.88
> 250	19.5	99.5	39.00	0.81

Table 2. The 6 combinations of sensitivity and specificity corresponding to the maximum ST segment shift on exercise (Diamond & Forrester, 1979). NICE's assumption of a sensitivity of 67% and a specificity of 69% for the single threshold point of 100 µV has a positive likelihood ratio of 2.16 and a negative likelihood ratio of 0.48

The post-exercise pCAD was also calculated using NICE's assumption of sensitivity 67% and specificity 69% for a ST segment shift threshold of 100 µV. NICE's sensitivity and specificity were obtained from table 14 of Mowatt et al., 2008, in which the sensitivities and specificities obtained from Kuntz et al., 1999, and from Mowatt et al., 2004, were averaged.

3. Statistics

Multivariate linear regression analysis (StatsDirect version 2.7.8; StatsDirect Ltd, Altrincham, WA14 4QA, UK) was used to perform analysis of variance (ANOVA) to determine the impact of age, sex and race on the likelihood of a patient being referred for an exercise ECG. Dummy variables were generated for sex and race. Multivariate linear regression analysis was also used to determine the impact of age, sex, race on chest pain symptom score and on exercise workload. Chi-square analysis was used to compare the numbers of exercised patients in each pCAD category with the numbers not exercised.

4. Results

All 7739 patients referred to the rapid access chest pain clinic completed the questionnaire. Following clinical assessment 5157 of the 7739 (66.6%) were exercised. 359 of 2582 (13.9%) who were not exercised had either left ventricular hypertrophy or an intraventricular conduction defect on 12 lead ECG, while 513 of 5157 (9.9%) who were exercised had either left ventricular hypertrophy or an intraventricular conduction defect ($\chi^2 = 26.9$ $P < 0.0001$).

Age	Black	South Asian	Miscellaneous	Oriental	White	**Females** Total
10 - 19	0 (1)	1.5 (2)	0 (2)		1 (2)	0.71 (7)
20 - 29	1.45 (11)	1.88 (9)	0.5 (6)	2.5 (2)	1.41 (29)	1.43 (57)
30 - 39	1.41 (36)	1.16 (12)	1.5 (16)	0.5 (4)	1.10 (58)	1.23 (126)
40 - 49	1.17 (47)	1.47 (46)	1.29 (24)	1.38 (13)	1.32 (129)	1.32 (259)
50 - 59	1.15 (51)	1.36 (66)	1.5 (18)	1.25 (8)	1.26 (178)	1.28 (321)
60 - 69	1.53 (43)	1.55 (58)	1.55 (29)	1.5 (8)	1.24 (161)	1.38 (299)
70 - 79	1.42 (33)	1.48 (35)	1.22 (9)	1.33 (6)	1.36 (176)	1.38 (259)
80 - 89	1.28 (7)	1.33 (6)	1 (2)	2 (1)	1.4 (90)	1.38 (106)
90 - 99		2 (1)			1.14 (7)	1.25 (8)
Total	1.32 (229)	1.46 (235)	1.34 (106)	1.35 (42)	1.3 (830)	1.33 (1442)

Age	Black	South Asian	Miscellaneous	Oriental	White	**Males** Total
10-19		0 (1)	1 (1)		0.66 (6)	0.62 (8)
20-29	0.25 (8)	0.9 (10)	1.66 (6)	2 (1)	1.06 (32)	1 (57)
30-39	0.9 (20)	1.34 (29)	1.06 (16)	0.5 (4)	0.87 (94)	0.96 (163)
40-49	0.92 (28)	1.12 (48)	1.27 (33)	1.2 (5)	1.04 (107)	1.08 (221)
50-59	1.12 (8)	1.53 (39)	1.48 (27)	0.8 (5)	1.19 (129)	1.28 (208)
60-69	1.30 (23)	1.47 (40)	1.41 (12)	1.33 (3)	1.37 (127)	1.39 (205)
70-79	1.07 (28)	1.53 (32)	1 (8)	1 (1)	1.35 (116)	1.32 (185)
80-89	1.57 (7)	1 (10)	2 (3)		1.41 (72)	1.40 (92)
90-99					2 (1)	2 (1)
Total	1.03 (122)	1.33 (209)	1.33 (106)	1 (19)	1.20 (684)	1.21 (1140)

Table 3. The average chest pain symptom score of females (above) and males (below) not exercised by race and decade of age. Typical angina = 3, atypical angina = 2, non-anginal chest pain = 1 or 0. The numbers in brackets are the numbers of patients.

Table 3 shows the distribution of age, sex and race of those not exercised, while table 4 shows the distribution of age, sex and race of those exercised. The distributions are similar. Black men had similar chest pain symptom scores to White men and Black men to Black women, but the South Asian, Miscellaneous and Oriental women had higher chest pain

Age	Black	South Asian	Miscellaneous	Oriental	White	**Females** Total
20 - 29	1.5 (6) 9.83	1.5 (6) 10.3	1.16 (6) 10.3		1.27 (18) 12.8	1.33 (36) 11.5
30 - 39	1.52 (17) 9.05	1.53 (28) 8.07	1.54 (11) 7.72	2 (4) 9.25	1.47 (76) 11.2	1.51 (136) 9.99
40 - 49	1.72 (84) 8.10	1.81 (103) 8.14	1.79 (64) 8.18	1.41 (17) 10.0	1.53 (236) 9.48	1.65 (504) 8.83
50 - 59	1.41 (87) 7.90	1.6 (135) 7.8	1.75 (68) 8.07	1.89 (19) 8.73	1.45 (373) 8.49	1.52 (682) 8.24
60 - 69	1.44 (90) 6.86	1.70 (98) 6.71	1.56 (41) 7.48	1.63 (19) 7.52	1.46 (363) 7.69	1.50 (611) 7.39
70 - 79	1.46 (43) 6.16	1.36 (25) 5.84	1.73 (15) 6.73	1 (1) 4	1.35 (234) 6.43	1.38 (318) 6.35
80 - 89	2 (2) 2.5	1 (1) 4			1.42 (42) 4.85	1.44 (45) 4.73
90 - 99					1 (1) 7	1 (1) 7
Total	1.51 (329) 7.50	1.65 (396) 7.54	1.69 (205) 7.94	1.66 (60) 8.68	1.45 (1343) 8.19	1.52 (2333) 7.97

Age	Black	South Asian	Miscellaneous	Oriental	White	**Males** Total
10-19					0 (1) 16	0 (1) 16
20-29	1.25 (8) 14.6	0.83 (12) 13.0	1.12 (8) 13.6		1 (26) 13.2	1.01 (54) 13.4
30-39	1.6 (30) 12.3	1.22 (84) 11.7	1.20 (43) 12.5	1.5 (6) 12.6	1.17 (173) 13.0	1.23 (336) 12.5
40-49	1.38 (68) 11.3	1.13 (143) 10.9	1.46 (84) 11.0	0.90 (11) 11.2	1.22 (396) 11.6	1.24 (702) 11.4
50-59	1.37 (43) 9.62	1.28 (146) 9.60	1.32 (92) 10.0	0.91 (12) 11.3	1.19 (472) 10.0	1.23 (765) 9.94
60-69	1.28 (53) 8.05	1.50 (111) 7.54	1.30 (43) 8.93	2 (3) 10	1.21 (419) 8.65	1.28 (629) 8.43
70-79	1.38 (42) 6.42	1.37 (51) 7.09	1.53 (13) 8.07	0.75 (4) 8.75	1.36 (188) 6.96	1.36 (298) 6.98
80-89	1.5 (4) 6.75	1 (2) 5.5	2 (2) 5.5		1.38 (31) 5.51	1.41 (39) 5.64
Total	1.38 (248) 9.66	1.27 (549) 9.69	1.35 (285) 10.5	1.08 (36) 11.1	1.22 (1706) 10.0	1.25 (2824) 9.98

Table 4. The average chest pain symptom score of females (above) and males (below) exercised and average exercise workload achieved (metabolic equivalents) by race and decade of age. Typical angina = 3, atypical angina = 2, non-anginal chest pain = 1 or 0. The numbers in brackets are the numbers of patients and the third number in a cell is the average exercise workload

symptom scores than the Black and White women. Analysis of Variance (ANOVA) showed that a higher chest pain symptom score was found in females and in those who were South Asians or in those having a Miscellaneous race (compared to being White). However, the descriptors explained only 2.4% of the variance in chest pain symptom score. ANOVA also showed that the younger the age, being male and a higher symptom score all made being exercised more likely. The descriptors explained 1.6% of the variance in the likelihood of being exercised. Table 4 also shows the workload achieved on exercise. For the 5157 patients who were exercised, younger males with low symptom scores were those who achieved the highest workload. Whites and Orientals were the races that achieved the highest workload and South Asians the lowest. The descriptors explained 36.4% of the variance.

Table 5 shows a comparison of the pre-test pCADs of the patients who were not exercised with those who were exercised. Chi-square analysis showed a significant difference in the proportions exercised and the proportions not exercised (χ^2=120.4 with 4 degrees of freedom; $P < 0.0001$). Those with a pCAD below 10% were less likely to be exercised than those with pCAD between 10 and 90%.

pre-test pCAD	not exercised	exercised	total
< 10%	853	1243 (59.3%)	2096
10 - 30%	697	1676 (70.6%)	2373
30 - 60%	470	1234 (72.4%)	1704
60 - 90%	411	834 (67.0%)	1245
> 90%	151	170 (53.0%)	321
Total	2582	5157 (66.6%)	7739

pCAD = probability of coronary artery disease

Table 5. The pre-test pCAD of the patients according to whether or not they were exercised. The "exercised" column includes the percentage (in brackets) of the patients for a given pre-test pCAD who were exercised. Patients with a pre-test pCAD of less than 10% were less likely to be exercised than those with pCAD between 10 and 90%

Table 6 shows the change in pCAD categories following exercise. In the top part of Table 6 the numbers in each cell show how the pCAD changes when 6 combinations of sensitivity and specificity are used to calculate the post-exercise pCAD. 3296 of 5157 (63.9%) changed category: 535 of the 3296 increased pCAD while 2761 reduced pCAD. Had only the 2910 patients with pre-test pCAD between 10 and 60% been exercised, 1383 (47.5%) would have had CAD ruled out and 48 (1.6%) CAD ruled in. Another 170 (5.8%) would have become candidates for coronary arteriography. Figure 1 illustrates the change in pCAD. The bottom part of Table 6 shows the change in pCAD categories following exercise when NICE's assumption of one combination of sensitivity (67%) and specificity (69%) is used to calculate the post-exercise pCAD. 2271 of 5157 (44.0%) changed category. Of those with a pre-exercise pCAD of between 10% and 60%, 793 of 2910 (27.3%) had CAD ruled out and 128 (4.4%) became candidates for coronary arteriography. Figure 2 illustrates the change in pCAD.

	Post-exercise pCAD% 6 Sensitivities and Specificities					
Pre-exercise pCAD%	< 10	10 - 30	30 - 60	60 - 90	> 90	Total
< 10	1146	73	21	3		1243
10 - 30	1287	225	119	38	7	1676
30 - 60	96	795	170	132	41	1234
60 - 90		113	393	207	121	834
> 90				77	93	170
Total	2529	1206	703	457	262	5157

	Post-exercise pCAD% Sensitivity 67% Specificity 69%					
Pre-exercise pCAD%	< 10	10 - 30	30 - 60	60 - 90	> 90	Total
< 10	1162	81				1243
10 - 30	793	760	123			1676
30 - 60		664	442	128		1234
60 - 90			371	417	46	834
> 90				65	105	170
Total	1955	1505	936	610	151	5157

pCAD = probability of coronary artery disease

Table 6. The top part of the table shows how the numbers of patients in each category changed following exercise using the 6 combinations of sensitivity and specificity as in table 2. The bottom part of the table shows how the numbers of patients in each category changed following exercise using a single combination of sensitivity (67%) and specificity (69%).

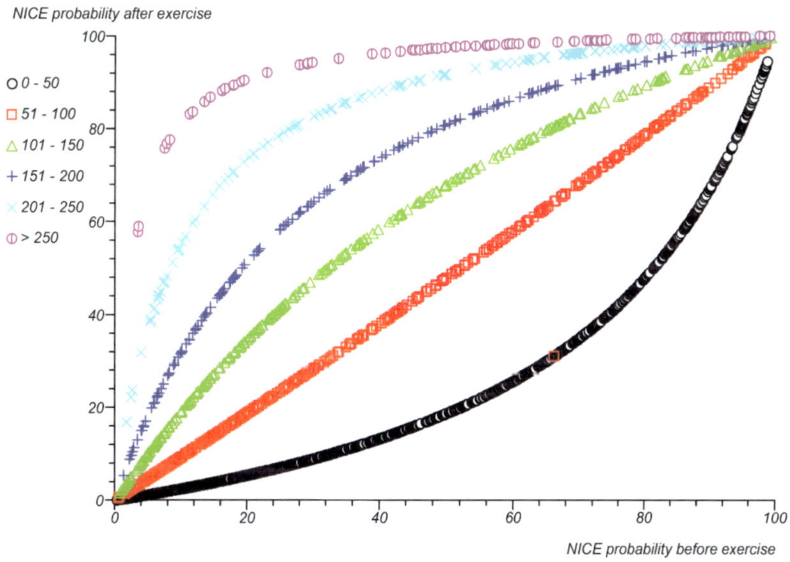

Fig. 1. The probability (%) of CAD after exercise plotted against the probability of CAD before exercise when 6 combinations (5 thresholds of ST shift) of sensitivity and specificity were used. The graph shows the discrimination that can be obtained by using several thresholds of ST shift and how CAD can be ruled out if the ST shift is less than 50 μV. The units of the thresholds in the legend are μV.

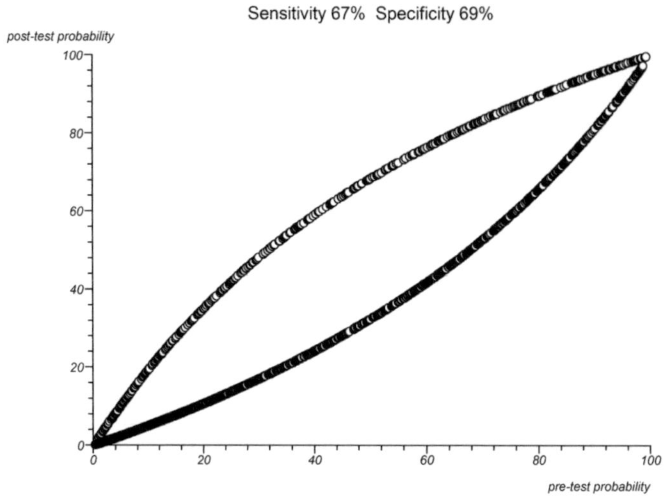

Fig. 2. The probability (%) of CAD after exercise plotted against the probability of CAD before exercise using a single threshold of 100 μV.

5. Discussion

The purpose of this study has been to try and demonstrate the superior diagnostic value of taking the amount of ST segment shift into account compared with using a single threshold point when interpreting the exercise ECG. The publication of the method used by NICE to obtain the pre-exercise probability of CAD (pCAD) made this comparison and the testing of NICE's recommendations feasible. NICE recommends firstly, that symptoms and risk factors should be used to derive pCAD and secondly, that the subsequent management depends on whether the pCAD is less than 10%, between 10 and 30%, between 30 and 60%, between 60 and 90%, or greater than 90%. Those with a pCAD of less than 10% have CAD ruled out and need no further investigation for CAD. Those with a pCAD of more than 90% have CAD ruled in. Those with a pCAD between 60 and 90% should be considered for coronary arteriography. NICE recommends that those with a pCAD between 10 and 60% need further investigation, but not exercise ECG.

In this study 5157 of 7739 consecutive patients referred to the rapid access chest pain clinic had an exercise ECG. Table 6 shows that using NICE's methodology and a sensitivity of 67% and a specificity of 69% for an ST segment shift of 100 μV, the exercise ECG rules out CAD in 793 (27.3%) of the 2910 patients with a pre-exercise pCAD between 10 and 60%, while another 128 (4.4%) become candidates for coronary arteriography. However, modifying the calculation of the post-exercise pCAD to account for increasing ST segment shift during exercise has a dramatic effect: of the 2910 patients who had a pre-test pCAD between 10 and 60% and who were exercised, 1383 (47.5%) would have had CAD ruled out and 48 (1.6%) CAD ruled in. Another 170 (5.8%) would have become candidates for coronary arteriography. The exercise ECG would therefore have defined the subsequent management of more than half the patients that had a pre-test pCAD between 10 and 60%.

The distributions by age, sex and race of patients referred for exercise ECG were similar to those of the whole cohort. Women were more likely to have angina than men. As recommended by NICE, patients referred for exercise testing were less likely to have a pCAD below 10% than those with a pCAD between 10 and 30%. The workload achieved during exercise was greater in men than in women and declined with age.

Table 2 reproduces part of table 4 of Diamond & Forrester, 1979 and adds corresponding positive and negative likelihood ratios. Diamond & Forrester reviewed 31 published papers to derive the table. From these papers they were able to derive a sensitivity and a specificity for each of the 5 thresholds. The assumption is that these are mutually exclusive events, each having their own receiver operating characteristic curve. Table 2 shows that increasing the ST segment shift above 100 μV steadily increases the likelihood of CAD, while an ST segment shift of less than 50 μV reduces the likelihood of CAD.

Table 7 shows the effect of varying the combination of sensitivity and specificity on a single ST segment shift with a threshold of 100 μV. NICE assumed for calcium scoring a sensitivity

	Post-exercise pCAD% Sensitivity 89% Specificity 43%					
Pre-exercise pCAD%	< 10	10 - 30	30 - 60	60 - 90	> 90	Total
< 10	1199	44				1243
10 - 30	1473	137	66			1676
30 - 60	21	1001	144	68		1234
60 - 90		66	511	233	24	834
> 90				90	80	170
Total	2693	1248	721	391	104	5157

	Post-exercise pCAD% Sensitivity 86% Specificity 64%					
Pre-exercise pCAD%	< 10	10 - 30	30 - 60	60 - 90	> 90	Total
< 10	1157	86				1243
10 - 30	1473	65	138			1676
30 - 60	151	871	73	139		1234
60 - 90		151	459	171	53	834
> 90				93	77	170
Total	2781	1173	670	403	130	5157

	Post-exercise pCAD% Sensitivity 68% Specificity 77%					
Pre-exercise pCAD%	< 10	10 - 30	30 - 60	60 - 90	> 90	Total
< 10	1144	99				1243
10 - 30	987	522	167			1676
30 - 60		764	280	190		1234
60 - 90			407	351	76	834
> 90				70	100	170
Total	2131	1385	854	611	176	5157

Table 7. Three parts of the table show the effect on the data of using different combinations of sensitivity and specificity. At the top is that for a sensitivity of 89% and a specificity of 43% (NICE's combination for Calcium Scoring). In the middle is that for a sensitivity of 86% and a specificity of 64% (NICE's combination for Myocardial Perfusion Scanning). Below is that for a sensitivity of 68% and a specificity of 77% (the combination from the meta-analysis of Gianrossi et al., 1989).

of 89% and a specificity of 43%; this is the combination in the top part. NICE assumed for myocardial perfusion scanning with single photon emission computed tomography a sensitivity of 86% and a specificity of 64%; this is the combination in the middle part. From their meta-analysis Gianrossi et al., 1989 obtained a sensitivity of 68% and a specificity of 77%; this is the combination in the bottom part. For ruling out CAD when the pre-exercise pCAD is between 10 and 60%, table 7 and the bottom part of table 6 indicate that NICE's combinations of sensitivity and specificity used with calcium scoring (51.3% ruled out) and with myocardial perfusion scanning (55.8% ruled out) are both superior to NICE's combination used with exercise ECG (27.3% ruled out) and to the combination used by Gianrossi et al (33.9% ruled out). However, NICE recommends using myocardial perfusion scanning only if the pre-exercise pCAD is between 30 and 60%. Consequently, only 151 of 1234 (12.2%) would have had CAD ruled out. Only the combination of 6 sensitivities and specificities resulted in any of those with a pre-test pCAD between 10 and 60% having CAD ruled in.

As NICE, 2010, assumed costs of $100 (£66), $450 (£293) and $160 (£103) for exercise ECG, for myocardial perfusion scanning and for calcium scoring respectively, the explanation for the recommendation not to use the exercise ECG may be partly due to the assumptions about the proportions of indeterminate tests. NICE assumed 24% of exercise ECGs were indeterminate, 6% of myocardial perfusion scans were indeterminate and 2% of calcium scores were indeterminate. The 24% was NICE's modification of the unsubstantiated 30% in Kuntz et al., 1999. In the present study no exercise ECG was indeterminate, although it is accepted that interpretation of ST shift in the presence of left ventricular hypertrophy or of intraventricular conduction defect is unreliable. Ten per cent of the ECGs of the patients exercised showed either left ventricular hypertrophy or an intraventricular conduction defect.

6. Study limitations

Firstly, the sensitivities and specificities of each of the 5 thresholds of ST shift used were obtained by a review of the literature (Diamond & Forrester, 1979) rather than by a formal meta-analysis. Secondly, the patients were not asked about their race. The members of the ECG team assessed a person's race. Even though there were only 5 different races from which to choose, it is likely that misclassification occurred. Thirdly, being in paper format, the answers to the questionnaire were subject to transcription errors when entered into the database. Fourthly, measurement of the maximum ST segment shift on exercise was made by the member of the ECG team supervising the test. Until June 2006 all exercise tests were checked by the author. After June 2006 a weekly tutorial session with the author enabled the ECG team to discuss ST segment shifts that were difficult to assess.

7. Conclusions

It is concluded firstly, that the exercise ECG does indeed have limited diagnostic value if a single threshold is used for the diagnosis of CAD; secondly, that the exercise ECG has considerable diagnostic value if several thresholds are used; and thirdly, that NICE's recommendation "Do not use exercise ECG to diagnose or exclude angina for people without known coronary artery disease" seems to be partly the result of an unjustified assumption about the proportion of indeterminate exercise ECGs.

8. Acknowledgements

I thank the members of the ECG Team who entered the data into the bespoke database.

Some of the data presented has previously been published as a letter (Bourdillon, 2010).

9. References

Bourdillon, P. (2010). Exercise ECG useful in finding coronary artery disease. *British Medical Journal* Vol. 340, c1971, ISSN 0959-8138

Bruce, R. Lovejoy, F Jr. Pearson, R. Yu, P. Brothers, G. & Velasquez, T. (1949). Normal respiratory and circulatory pathways of adaptation in exercise. *Journal of Clinical Investigation*, Vol. 28, No. 6, pp. 1423–1430, ISSN 0021-9738

Cooper, A. Timmis, A. & Skinner J. (2010). Assessment of recent onset chest pain or discomfort of suspected cardiac origin: summary of NICE guidance. *British Medical Journal*, Vol. 340, No. 7749, c1118, ISSN 0959-8138

Diamond, G. & Forrester, J. (1979). Analysis of probability as an aid in the clinical diagnosis of coronary-artery disease. *New England Journal of Medicine*, Vol. 300, No. 24, pp. 1350-8, ISSN 0028-4793

Gianrossi, R. Detrano, R. Mullvihill, D. Lehmann, K. Dubach, P. Colombo, A. McArthur, D. & Froelicher, V. (1989). Exercise-induced ST depression in the diagnosis of coronary artery disease. A meta-analysis. *Circulation*, Vol. 80, No. 1, pp. 87-98, ISSN 0009-7322

Joswig, B. Glover, M. Nelson, D. Handler, J. & Henderson, J. (1985). Analysis of historical variables, risk factors and the resting electrocardiogram as an aid in the clinical diagnosis of recurrent chest pain. *Computers in Biology and Medicine*, Vol. 15, No. 2, pp. 71-80, ISSN: 0010-4825

Kuntz, K. Fleischmann, K. Hunink, M. & Douglas, P. (1999). Cost-effectiveness of diagnostic strategies for patients with chest pain. *Annals of Internal Medicine*, Vol. 130, No. 9, pp. 709-718, ISSN 0003-4819

Mark, D. Shaw, L. Harrell, F Jr. Hlatky, M. Lee, K. Bengtson, F. McCants, C. Califf, R. & Pryor D. (1991). Prognostic value of a treadmill exercise score in outpatients with suspected coronary artery disease. *New England Journal of Medicine*, Vol. 325, No.12, pp. 849-853, ISSN 0028-4793

Mason, R. & Likar, I. (1966). A new system of multiple-lead exercise electrocardiography.*American Heart Journal* Vol. 71, No. 2, pp. 196–205, ISSN 0002-8703

Mowatt, G. Vale, L. Brazzelli, M. Hernandez, R. Murray, A. Scott, N. Fraser, C. McKenzie, L. Gemmell, H. Hillis, G. & Metcalfe, M. (2004). Systematic review of the effectiveness and cost-effectiveness and economic evaluation of myocardial perfusion scintigraphy for the diagnosis and management of angina and myocardial infarction. *Health Technology Assessment*, Vol. 8, No. 30, pp. 1-207, ISSN 1366-5278

Mowatt, G. Cummins, E. Waugh, N. Walker, S. Cook, J. Jia, X. Hillis, G. & Fraser, C. (2008). Systematic review of the clinical effectiveness and cost-effectiveness of 64-slice or higher computed tomography angiography as an alternative to invasive coronary angiography in the investigation of coronary artery disease. *Health Technology Assessment*, Vol. 12, No. 17, pp. 1-143, ISSN 1366-5278

National Institute for Health and Clinical Excellence. (10 June 2010). *Chest pain of recent onset: assessment and diagnosis of recent onset chest pain or discomfort of suspected cardiac origin (clinical guideline 95).* Retrieved from www.nice.org.uk/guidance/cg95

Pryor, D. Shaw, L. McCants, C Lee, K. Mark, D. Harrell, F Jr. Muhlbaier, L. & Califf, R. (1993) Value of the history and physical in identifying patients at increased risk for coronary artery disease. *Annals of Internal Medicine,* Vol. 118, No. 2, pp. 81–90, ISSN 0003-4819

Part 3

Treatment Regimens for Coronary Artery Disease

10

Effectiveness and Efficiency of Drug Eluting Stents

José Moreu[1], José María Hernández[2], Juan M Ruiz-Nodar[3], Nicolás Vázquez[4], Ángel Cequier[5], Felipe Fernández-Vázquez[6] and Carlos Crespo[7,8]

[1]*Hospital Virgen de la Salud, Toledo,*
[2]*Hospital Clínico Universitario de Málaga, Málaga,*
[3]*Hospital General de Alicante, Alicante;*
[4]*Hospital Juan Canalejo, La Coruña,*
[5]*Hospital Universitari de Bellvitge; Barcelona,*
[6]*Hospital de León, León,*
[7]*Univertisity of Barcelona Department of statistics, Barcelona,*
[8]*Oblikue Consulting S.A., Barcelona*
Spain

1. Introduction

Coronary artery disease (CAD), also known as ischemic heart disease (IHD) and coronary heart disease (CHD), is caused by the narrowing (stenosis) of one or more coronary arteries, due to atherosclerosis, restricting blood flow and reducing the supply of oxygen to the heart muscle. Transient shortages in blood flow and oxygen lead to angina pectoris and chest pain, which may radiate to the left shoulder, arms, neck, back or jaw. Stable angina symptoms do not tend to progress in intensity over time. More seriously, the rupturing of an atherosclerotic plaque (causing a thrombotic occlusion) and stenosis of the vessel can result in acute myocardial infarction (AMI) due to a critical reduction in the blood supply to the heart muscle (myocardial ischemia). High levels of morbidity and mortality associated with this infarction are a consequence of ischemia. It is vital to promptly re-establish coronary blood flow after an infarction, because sustained ischemic damages and injuries to the heart muscle may lead to sudden death or heart failure. In addition to infarction, acute symptomatic manifestations of ischemic heart disease include unstable angina, and less common conditions such as cardiogenic shock and sudden death (Thygesen, 2007).

Cardiovascular disease has a large budget impact, most of which is attributed to coronary artery disease. Therefore, effective treatment strategies are important to reduce associated costs. The total cost of coronary artery disease in the European Union (EU) is estimated to be over €49 billion and can be divided into direct health care costs (48%), productivity losses (34%) and informal care (18%) (Figure 1) (Allender, 2008). Estimated healthcare costs of ischemic heart disease in the EU approaches €24 billion, with approximately 50% of the economic burden due to in-patient care (€12.5 billion) and 25% associated with medication

(€6 billion). In 2006, mortality and morbidity associated with CAD were responsible for nearly €17 billion productivity losses across the EU, whilst informal care costs were estimated to be more than €9 billion (Allender, 2008).

In 2010, ischemic heart disease was the main cause of death worldwide, causing 12.8% of world total deaths (WHO, 2011). Regarding Spain, three out of ten deaths are due to cardiovascular disease, being the leading cause of death even though its incidence has decreased almost a point with respect to the last known data, dating back to 2008 (INE 2011). Specifically, cardiovascular disease has been responsible for 31.2% of the deaths caused in Spain during 2009, resulting in a total of 120,053 deceases. In conclusion, ischemic heart disease is one of the main causes of quality-adjusted life years lost (around 10% of disability), also producing 18% of the Spanish health expenditure, far above respiratory system diseases (13%), and poorly defined signs and symptoms (9%) (Gisbert y Brosa, 2005). Their direct health expenditure in Spain is nearly €727 million, with half of this cost being associated to hospitalizations caused by pathology, 43% to monitoring, and only 6% to pharmacological costs (MsyC, 2003).

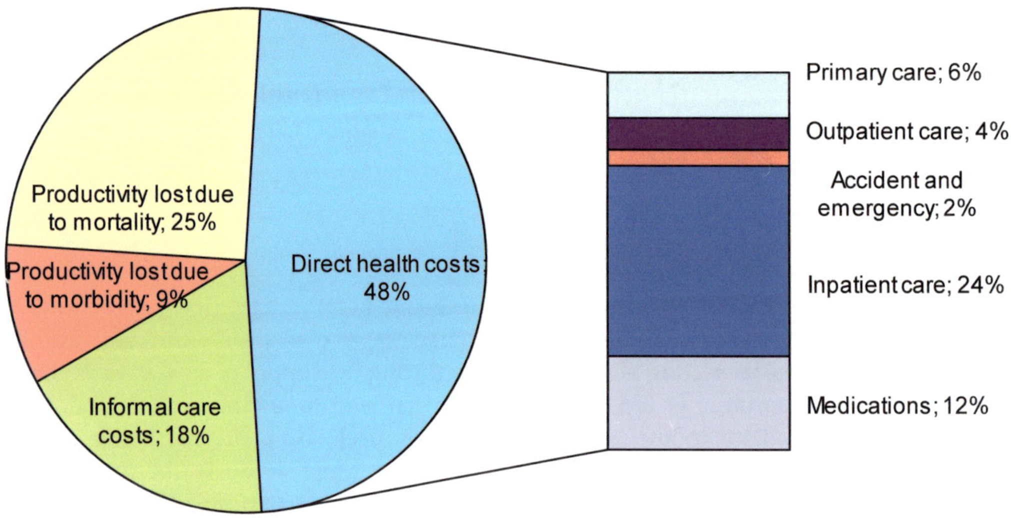

Source: Allender, 2008

Fig. 1. Costs of Coronary Disease in EU (2006).

2. Revascularization treatment of coronary artery disease: drug eluting stents

Coronary revascularization in patients with atherosclerotic heart disease has emerged as the most accepted method of treatment in the last 50 years, still offering two types of procedures: surgical and percutaneous.

The surgical technique for the implementation of vein and/or arterial grafts was developed in 1960. Since then, the procedure has not undergone many technical changes on the essentials, only an increase in the use of arterial grafts and the achievement of some procedures without extracorporeal circulation in minimally invasive surgery. However, despite the large experience learned over all these years, the results remain operator-dependent and closely related to the amount of procedures performed by each surgeon.

Percutaneous Coronary Intervention (PCI) was first carried out in 1977. It was only reserved for patients with a disease in a single coronary artery, and supported by a surgical team. A clear difference between PCI and surgery is that Evidence-Based Medicine always accompanied interventional cardiology: advances have been supported by randomized multicenter studies before being implemented in all the centers. In the 1980's, PCI spread, but it was a very operator-dependent procedure, using rudimentary catheters and with a high number of complications (acute arterial occlusion in up to 15% of the procedures and restenosis in up to 40-50%). The PCI boom began in the 90's with the development and use of intracoronary stents and the remarkable improvement in balloon catheters, which solved early acute complications freeing the PCI from the surgical services and decreasing the restenosis rates. The BENESTENT study (Serruys et al., 1994) in Europe and the STRESS study (Fischman DL et al., 1994) in America, published in August 1994, gave rise to the spread of coronary stents. PCI stopped being operator-dependent when carried out in centers with a high overall volume, and the dreamt comparison with revascularization surgery began. Until then only the results with balloon catheters in general favored bypass surgery (GABI, EAST, RITA, ERACI, CABRI, BARI studies). Numerous comparative randomized studies were carried out between surgery and PCI in all kinds of situations and with different types of lesions (AWESOME, SoS, ERACI II, ARTS). The results were rather homogenous: there were not significant differences in terms of mortality, except in diabetic patients, between both techniques and differences only appeared in favor of surgery regarding the need of repeating bypass procedures in the short to medium term (Hoffman SN et al., 2003).

Restenosis continued to be the Achilles' heel of PCI despite stents. All efforts were focused on the investigation of antiproliferative drugs linked to stents. In the year 2002, the results from the RAVEL study were published, showing a restenosis rate of 0% at 6 months after implantation of sirolimus-coated stents (Cypher®) (Morice MC et al., 2002). For several years, two kind of drug eluting stents (DES) coexisted largely; the above-mentioned sirolimus-coated stent and another stent coated with paclitaxel (TAXUS®). Many studies and registries were published on both DES in different clinical situations (SIRIUS program, TAXUS program, DIABETES I, ISAR program, COMPARE, etc...), all of them showing similar results in regard to decreased restenosis rates. The first study comparing the results of bypass surgery with PCI using sirolimus DES in patients with multivessel disease was the ARTS II study, which showed that there were not significant differences in the cardiovascular event rates between the group treated with DES and the comparative group treated with bypass surgery of the ARTS I study. However, the ARTS II study was widely criticized, because although the patients with multivessel disease included for DES treatment were more complex, the comparative surgical group was older. Two randomized multicenter studies were designed to compare the results of bypass surgery and PCI with DES in patients with multivessel disease, trying to clarify the controversies; one in diabetic patients, the FREEDOM study, and another one that included all kinds of coronary lesions, the SYNTAX study (Serruys PW et al., 2009). In the latter, 1800 patients with left main or three-vessel disease were randomized to bypass surgery or PCI with Taxus stent, provided that the surgery team and the interventionist cardiology team considered the patient a candidate for any of both interventions. At 12 months, the primary objective of non-inferiority of PCI over surgery regarding MACCE (Major Adverse Cardiac and Cerebrovascular Events) was not achieved (17.8% vs. 12.4% for CABG; P=0.002), mostly due to the increase in new bypass surgeries in the PCI group (13.5% vs. 5.9%, P<0.001). There were not significant differences in terms of mortality and Myocardial Infarctions (MI), but there was a higher number of strokes in the surgical group (2.2% vs. 0.6% with PCI; P=0.003). After a deep analysis of patients, the study showed that patients with a greater technical complexity derived from their anatomy (SYNTAX score higher than 32) may benefit more from surgery whereas patients with a low (0-22) or medium score (23-32) evolved similarly with both treatments. The analysis of the 705 patients with left main disease showed that those with isolated left main lesion or associated to one-vessel disease benefited more from PCI.

Since 2005, new DES with different drugs (with or without polymers) were incorporated , all of them involving large study projects with a similar design to that applied to the projects of the first generation DES (SIRIUS, TAXUS projects). All the drugs used belong to the "limus" family, which present the lowest Late Loss Index; specifically, tacrolimus, zotarolimus, everolimus, and biolimus. Tacrolimus DES (JANUS®) failed to prove a lower restenosis rate than conventional bare metal stents (BMS). The zotarolimus DES (Endeavour®) was the first second generation stent available. The ENDEAVOR I, II, and III studies showed an excellent balance between the benefits of stent and restenosis reduction since the very beginning, helping the stent to position properly in the European market. Subsequently and with the same drug, the Resolute® stent and the third generation of DES, the Resolute Integrity®, were introduced, following the RESOLUTE FIM study. The Xcience V® and Prime® stents, using everolimus, were developed based on the SPIRIT investigation program, that includes the SPIRIT I, II, III, IV and V studies. As with the zotarolimus stent, we currently have a third generation of everolimus-coated stents already, Xcience Prime® and Promus Element®. Finally, a fifth drug, which is being used at the moment, is the biolimus (Biomatrix® and Nobori® stents) whose results come from randomized studies as LEADERS and NOBORI.

Windecker et al., in The World Congress of Cardiology 2007, triggered an important controversy about the security of DES due to an increase in the occurrence of late subacute occlusions (Windecker S & Meier B, 2007). Kirtane et al., in an analysis of 34 observational studies between BMS and DES including 182,901 patients, showed a reduction in mortality (HR 0.78, 95% CI 0.71–0.86) and myocardial infarction rates (0.87, 95% CI 0.78–0.97) with the use of DES that remains similar after multivariate adjustment (Kirtane AJ et al., 2009). All the studies performed with second and third generation DES prove the results of this meta-analysis with similar subacute occlusion rates to BMS.

Recently, the European Society of Cardiology together with the European Society of Cardio-Thoracic Surgery, have published new guidelines on myocardial revascularization (Task Force 2010). These guidelines state that, taking into account the anatomy, the revascularization has a recommendation of Class I[1] in all cases with left main disease, two or

[1] Classes of recommendations: Class I, Evidence and/or general agreement that a given treatment or procedure is beneficial, useful, effective; Class II, Conflicting evidence and/or a divergence of opinion about the usefulness/efficacy of the given treatment or procedure; Class IIa Weight of evidence/opinion is in favor of usefulness/efficacy; Class IIb, Usefulness/efficacy is less well established by evidence/opinion; Class III, Evidence or general agreement that given treatment or procedure is not useful/effective, and in some cases may be harmful.

three-vessel disease, proximal anterior descending artery lesion and one-vessel disease with more than 10% myocardial risk. In addition, according to the clinical practice, it is only contraindicated when the optimized medical treatment leaves the patient asymptomatic. Regarding the type of revascularization (surgery or PCI), guidelines suggest an individualized assessment by the cardiology and surgery team of each centre, assuming the general indications. Patients with Syntax high risk score (>33) and two or three-vessel disease have indication Class I for surgery and Class III for PCI. Patients with medium score (23-32) and impossibility of full revascularization by PCI have Class I indication for surgery and Class III for PCI. The rest of cases have both indications.

2.1 Stent thrombosis

Thrombosis of a coronary stent is a serious complication, which appears in almost 50% of the cases as transmural acute myocardial infarction, presenting a high mortality rate (Moreno R, 2005). This complication usually takes place during the first weeks after the stent implantation, and especially in the first 24 hours. Chronologically, stent thrombosis is classified as acute (in the first 24 hours after the stent implantation), sub-acute (between 24 hours and 30 days), late (more than 30 days), and as a concept introduced more recently, very late (more than 6-12 months).

The variables associated with a higher incidence of thrombosis are the existence of a visible thrombus before stent implantation, the implantation of more than one stent, left ventricular dysfunction, a suboptimal result, a non-elective stent implantation, small vessels, a residual dissection and a slow flow.

2.1.1 Current recommendations in antiplatelet post-stent treatment

In the initial years of using stents, anticoagulants were initially administered (heparin sodium at first and oral anticoagulation later for several months) in conjunction with acetylsalicylic acid (ASA). In this way, thrombosis rate was reduced to 3-4%. However, this reduction in stent thrombosis rate was at the expense of a high incidence of hemorrhagic complications. In subsequent years, several randomized studies showed that if anticoagulation was replaced with ticlopidine (antiplatelet drug from the group of thienopyridines which works by inhibiting adenosine-deaminase) the incidence of hemorrhagic complications and stent thrombosis decreased (Hall P et al., 1996; Urban P et al., 1998; Schömig A et al., 1996; Leon MB et al., 1998; Bertrand ME et al., 1998). With the appearance of clopidogrel (thienopyridine) the secondary effects associated to ticlopidine disappeared, becoming the drug of choice together with ASA after stent implantation.

According to the Guidelines of the European Society of Cardiology, the double antiplatelet therapy in addition to ASA is recommended during 12 months after stent implantation in patients who suffer acute coronary syndrome, and during 6 months in patients with stable angina (Task Force 2010). Nevertheless, the risk of stent thrombosis with the higher assessed DES is being shown in long-term studies, despite serious doubts. On this point, the new DES is expected to offer advantages, although it will be necessary to get more evidence to eliminate uncertainty. For the second and third generation of DES, the stent thrombosis results are excellent, but the specific time of dual antiplatelet treatment with these devices is unknown and additional studies will be welcome.

3. Efficacy and effectiveness of RESOLUTE® DES: preliminary results of REDES registry

Drug Eluting Stents (DES) reduce the risk of restenosis, repeat interventions and re-hospitalization compared to BMS due to the release of potent antiprofilerative drugs from the stent surface. However, despite the success of DES in reducing repeat revascularization procedures, about 5% of patients require repeat procedures within a year. In patients with diabetes or coronary heart disease in small vessels, these rates are higher (Stone GW et al., 2004; Mauri L et al., 2010; Stolk JM et al., 2010). The incidence of myocardial infarction and death attributable to restenosis is minimal, but often causes recurrent angina.

DES have also shown to significantly reduce stent thrombosis, which can be an important clinical problem resulting in an acute myocardial infarction (60-70%), death (20-25%) or emergency bypass surgery (Ayyanatahn S et al., 2009). Nevertheless, the occurrence of late stent thrombosis, between 30 days and a year after stent implantation, is one of the most complex effects of stent placement in general, and of DES in particular.

Due to the above two points, the long-term safety of DES remains an important area of clinical research, especially in avoiding late stent thrombosis (Mauri L et al., 2007). Therefore, clinical studies with different DES are being conducted in order to demonstrate its effectiveness and long-term safety. To date, more than 100 DES randomized clinical trials in 60,000 patients have been performed, but quality varies considerably between different clinical trials, especially regarding the statistical powering and the selection of angiographic criteria instead of primary clinical endpoints. Accordingly, only a small proportion of DES can be recommended based on data from published studies as shown in Table 1 (Task Force 2010).

3.1 RESOLUTE® clinical evidence

The coronary stent Endeavor RESOLUTE® is a second generation stent indicated for improving coronary luminal diameter and reducing restenosis in patients with symptomatic ischemic heart disease in de novo arterial lesions of native coronary arteries with a reference vessel diameter of 2.25 to 4.0 mm and a lesion length ≤27mm. Its current clinical program consists of four clinical trials and two multicenter registries: RESOLUTE FIRST, RESOLUTE All Comers, RESOLUTE International, RESOLUTE US, RESOLUTE Japan, and RESOLUTE Asia.

RESOLUTE FIRST is a prospective, multicenter, non-randomized, single arm study of the use of the Endeavor RESOLUTE® stent in patients with symptomatic ischemic heart disease, whose objective was to assess the safety and efficacy in the medium and long term. 139 patients with 140 lesions were included in 12 centers of Australia and New Zealand, and 24-month data are available. The results showed that the cumulative MACE rate at 12 months was 8.5%, and 11% at 24 months. The Target Lesion Revascularization (TLR) rate at one year was 0.8%, and at 12 months there were no Target Vessel Revascularizations (TVR). At two-year follow-up, results showed a TLR, TVR, and Target Vessel failure (TVF) rates of 1.4%, 0% and 7.9% respectively. One possible stent thrombosis occurred in the first year after implantation, however no late or very late thrombosis have occurred (Meredith IT et al., 2009; Meredith IT et al., 2010).

DES	Eluted drug	Trials and references
Clinical primary endpoint reached		
BioMatrix Flex	Biolimus A9	LEADERS (Windecker el al., 2008)
Cypher	Sirolimus	SIRIUS (Moses et al., 2003)
Endeavor	Zotarolimus	Endeavor II, III and IV (Fajadet et al., 2006; Gershlic el al., 2007)
Resolute	Zotarolimus	RESOLUTE-AC (Serruys et al., 2007)
Taxus Liberté/Element	Paclitaxel	TAXUS IV and V (Stone et al., 2004; Stone et al., 2005) PRESEUS-WH (Kerelakes et al., 2010)
Xcience V	Everolimus*	SPIRIT III and IV (Stone et al., 2009; Stone et al., 2010)
Angiographic primary endpoint reached		
Nevo	Sirolimus	NEVO RES I (Ormiston et al., 2010)
Nobori	Biolimus A9	NOBORI I Phase 1 and 2 (Chevalier et al., 2007; Chevalier et al., 2009)
Yubon	Sirolimus	ISAR-Test (Mehilli et al., 2006)

Selection is based on adequately powered RCT with a primary clinical or angiographic endpoint. With the exception of LEADERS and RESOLUTE (all-comers trial), efficacy was investigated in selected de novo lesions of native coronary arteries.
*Promus Element device elutes everolimus from a different stent platform.
DES = Drug Eluting Stent

Table 1. Recommended drug-eluting stents (Task Force 2010).

The randomized clinical trial, called RESOLUTE "All Comers", collected data on more than 15 centers in Western Europe and compared the zotarolimus eluting stent Endeavor RESOLUTE® with the everolimus eluting stent Xcience V (Serruys PW et al., 2010). Between April 2008 and October 2008 data from 1,292 patients with coronary artery disease and chronic stable and acute coronary syndromes were collected: 1,140 patients with 1,661 lesions were assigned to the zotarolimus eluting stent Endeavor RESOLUTE ®and 1,152 patients with 1,705 lesions to the everolimus eluting stent Xcience V. At thirteen month follow-up the Endeavor RESOLUTE ® stent was non inferior to the Xcience V stent with respect to the primary end point of TLF, which occurred in 8.2% and 8.3% of patients respectively ($P>0.0001$ for non-inferiority). There were no significant differences between the two patient groups in the rate of death from cardiac causes, any myocardial infarction, or revascularization. The rate of stent thrombosis (definitive, probable and possible) was 2.3% in the Endeavor RESOLUTE® DES group and 1.5% in the Xcience V stent ($p = 0.17$). The lack of strict exclusion criteria in this study allows that the results are representative of actual clinical practice.

Yeung et al., in April 2011 published the 12-month follow-up data from the RESOLUTE US study (Yeung AC et al., 2011): a prospective, multicenter, observational study designed to assess the effectiveness of Endeavor RESOLUTE® DES in patients with one lesion who received a stent between 2.5 and 3.5 mm. Between August 2008 and December 2009 1,402 patients from 116 centers in U.S. were included, with an average vessel diameter of 2.59±0.47 mm and a diabetes prevalence of 34.4%. The results showed that the overall TLF rate at 12 months was 4.7% and cardiac death, myocardial infarction and TLR rates were 0.7%, 1.4% y 2.8% respectively. 0.1% of patients presented stent thrombosis.

Therefore, currently there are published data from three Endeavor RESOLUTE® studies, which have shown to reach a low rate of restenosis revascularization and clinical events such as death, myocardial infarction and stent thrombosis at one-year and two-year follow-up (Table 2). Endeavor RESOLUTE® is an effective and safe stent for the treatment of patients with coronary artery disease in de novo lesions of native coronary arteries.

	RESOLUTE FIRST (12 months)	RESOLUTE All Comers (12 months)		RESOLUTE US (12 months)
	Endeavor RESOLUTE (1 lesion)	Endeavor RESOLUTE	Xcience V	Endeavor RESOLUTE (1 or 2 lesions)
	N=130	N=1,119	N=1,126	N=1,376
MACE	8.5%	8.7%	9.7%	4.9%
Death	2.3%	1.6%	2.8%	1.3%
Cardiac death	0.8%	1.3%	1.7%	0.7%
MI	5.4%	4.2%	4,1%	1.4%
Q-wave MI	0.0%	0.7%	0.4%	0.1%
Non-Q-wave MI	5.4%	3.6%	3.6%	1.2%
TLR	0.8%	8.8%	8.2%	7.4%
TVR (non-TL)	0.0%	4.9%	4.8%	4.6%
TVR (TL)	0.8%	3.9%	3.4%	2.8%
TLF	6.2%	8.2%	8.3%	4.7%
TVF	6.9%	9.0%	9.6%	6.7%
Stent Thrombosis (according to ARC, definitive, probable)	0.0%	1.6%	0.7%	0.1%

MI: Myocardial Infarction; TLR: Target Lesion Revascularization; TVR: Target Vessel Revascularization: TVF: Target Vessel Failure*; TLF = Target Lesion Failure** ARC = Academic Research Consortium criteria.

*Defined as death from cardiac causes, any myocardial infarction (not clearly attributable to a non-target vessel), or clinically indicated target-vessel revascularization)

** Defined as death from cardiac causes, any myocardial infarction (not clearly attributable to a non-target vessel), or clinically indicated target-lesion revascularization)

Table 2. Summary of published clinical results (Endeavor RESOLUTE®).

3.2 REDES registry

Recently was completed the follow-up of a prospective, multicenter, observational, one-arm registry, called REDES, whose objective was to assess the effectiveness and the resource use associated to the Endeavor RESOLUTE® DES in patients with de novo lesions in the native coronary arteries in the Spanish clinical practice. The primary endpoint was defined as the rate of Major Adverse Cardiac Events (MACE) at 30 days, 6 months and 12 months, including cardiac death, myocardial infarction (with or without Q wave), emergency bypass artery coronary graft (CABG) and TLV (repeat CABG or PTCA). Among the secondary endpoints were collected stent thrombosis rates, procedural success, device success, lesion success, TLR, and the identification and quantification of heath resources used in the management of patients at one year after stent implantation.

The Inclusion criteria of patients were patients >18 years, signed informed consent form, drug eluting indication and the decision to use Endeavor Resolute® in all lesions. The exclusion criteria were pregnant or lactating women; patients with hypersensitivity or allergies to aspirin, heparin, clopidogrel, ticlopidine, zotarolimus, rapamycin, tacrolimus, sirolimus, cobalt, nickel, molybdenum or contrast media; patients who have contraindications for antiplatelet therapy and/or anticoagulants; patients with lesions not allowing the full inflation of angioplasty balloon; patients with other DES different from Endeavor Resolute® in other previous lesions; patients with a current medical condition associated with a life expectancy of less than 12 months; and patients who are participating in another study or have completed another study in the last 30 days before registry inclusion. Also, no restriction was placed on the total number of treated lesions, treated vessels or number of stent implanted.

This study allows to know the clinical data and resource use in actual clinical practice with the Endeavor Resolute® stent. The lack of data on resource use and costs associated with treatment of coronary artery disease with DES, as well as their possible alternatives, make more relevant the studies which collect the actual resource use in routine clinical practice and allow to know the associated costs. These studies are the first step to know if stents are an effective and efficient treatment, and help make decisions within the National Health System. During the last years the inclusion of this information in protocols and data collection forms has been increasing in different studies.

3.2.1 Clinical results

Between January 2009 and February 2010 450 patients with 744 lesions from six Spanish hospitals were included. After reviewing the selection criteria, two patients were excluded, leaving 448 evaluable patients with 742 lesions. The exclusions were due to a myocardial infarction within 24 hours before the primary angioplasty procedure that led into a cardiogenic shock and death before obtaining the signed informed consent, and one patient whose clinical history showed a previous DES with another drug.

The mean age of patients was 64.5 years and 78.3% were male, 34.1% had diabetes, 63.4% hypertension, 59.8% hyperlipidemia, and 28.6% smoked at the time of surgery. In addition to clinical risk, 31.9% of patients had a previous myocardial infarction, 20.1% a previous PCI and 4.5% a previous CABG. Most patients had lesions in 1 (55.6%) or 2 (29.9%) vessels, and left anterior descending artery was the most frequently treated. Also, it should be noted that 14.2% of lesions had moderate to severe calcification, 18.9% presented a tortuosity greater than 45 °, and 11.9% bifurcation (Table 3).

Characteristic	All valuable patients (n=448)
Age, yrs	64.5 ± 10.9
Male	78.3%
Prior MI	31.9%
Q-wave MI	21.9%
Non-Q-wave MI	10.0%
Prior PCI	20.1%
Prior CABG	4.5%
Diabetes Mellitus	34.1%
IDDM	8.9%
Hyperlipidemia	59.8%
Hypertension	63.4%
History of smoking	
Current	28.6%
Ex-smoker	28.3%
Family history of cardiovascular disease	13.4%
Worst status	
Silent ischemia	6.9%
Stable angina	28.3%
Unstable angina	31.0%
MI	33.9%
Target lesion coronary artery (% total lesions)	
Left anterior descending	46.0%
Left circunflex	18.1%
Right	27.0%
Left main	1.3%
Other	7.6%
Number of treated vessels	
1	55.6%
2	29.9%
3	8.9%
4	4.5%
5	1.1%
TIMI flow grade 3	83.2%
Thrombus	6.7%
RVD, mm	2.89±0.46
Lesion length, mm	18.08±10.36
Minimum lumen diameter, mm	0.73±0.87
%diameter stenosis	83.22±12.58
Type B2/C lesion	48.6%

CABG= coronary artery bypass grafting; IDDM= insulin-dependent diabetes mellitus; MI= myocardial infarction; MLD= minimum lumen diameter; PCI= percutaneous coronary intervention; RVD=reference vessel diameter; TIMI=thrombolysis in myocardial infarction

Table 3. Baseline clinical, lesion and procedural characteristics.

The mean vessel diameter was 2.89 ± 0.46mm and the average lesion length 18.08 ± 10.36mm. The Endeavor Resolute® stent was implanted in 95.5% of lesions treated, with a lesion success of 99.7%, a device success of 95.3%, and a procedure success of 94.7%.

Preliminary results showed that the MACE rate was 1.3%, 3.6% and 4.8% at 30 days, 6 months and 12 months respectively; and the rate of definite, probable and possible stent thrombosis according to the Academic Research Consortium criteria, was 0.7% and 1.4% at 30 days and one year follow-up (Table 4). The 21 MACE, which occurred in 20 patients were 6 cardiac deaths, 4 myocardial infarctions, 11 not programmed revascularizations in the same vessel or lesion treated during the intervention. 5 patients died from probable or possible stent thrombosis, one from a possible heart failure or ventricular arrhythmia not related to the stent, and the remaining non-cardiac death was due to a metastatic renal tumor that was detected a month after the inclusion of the patient in the study. Half of the stent thrombosis occurred within 4 days after surgery and most of restenosis revascularizations were performed by PTCA and only one was performed by CAGB. During the one-year follow-up 13 scheduled PTCA were performed in different vessels than those previously treated.

	30 days	6 months	12 months
	N = 445	N = 443	N = 441
MACE	1.3%	3.6%	4.8%
Death	0.5%	1.6%	1.6%
Cardiac death	0.5%	1.3%	1.3%
MI	0.5%	0.7%	0.9%
Q-wave MI	0.2%	0.2%	0.2%
Non-Q-wave MI	0.2%	0.5%	0.7%
TLR	0.5%	1.6%	2.5%
Stent Thrombosis (according to ARC, definitive, probable)	0.7%	0.7%	0.7%
Definitive	0.5%	0.5%	0.5%
Probable	0.2%	0.2%	0.2%
Possible	0.0%	0.7%	0.7%

MACE = Major Cardiac Adverse Event; MI = Myocardial infarction; TLR = Target Lesion Revascularization; ARC = Academic Research Consortium criteria

Table 4. Clinical outcomes at 30 days, 6 months and 12 months.

If we compare these results with those obtained in the previously published study RESOLUTE All Comers, the MACE and stent thrombosis rates are better. The revascularization rate was lower considering that the proportion of diabetic patients of the REDES study was higher (34.1% vs. 23.5%), but the percentage of lesions in small vessels was lower (39.9% vs. 67.8%). The lack of strict exclusion criteria in this study such as patients with MI, multivessel disease, small vessels, long lesions, bifurcation, or tortuosity make this study representative of routine clinical practice and show actual results of the Endeavor Resolute® stent effectiveness even in patients who had suffered an MI within 72 hours prior to surgery. Therefore, the REDES study results are comparable to and even better than those obtained in previously published studies showing that the Endeavor Resolute® stent is safe and effective, and considering that a large percentage of patients had a high level of complexity.

3.2.2 Resource utilization and costs

The importance of identifying the use of health resources and costs associated with a procedure has increased considerably in recent years; however, there are still few studies that include this part in their objectives. Therefore, the REDES registry, in addition to providing the clinical results of Endeavor RESOLUTE® stent, also included the objective of identifying and quantifying the resource use from patient hospitalization until one year after the surgery in order to know the average cost of the intervention with Endeavor Resolute stent in Spain and at one-year follow-up.

To calculate the costs of the analysis, both the resource data of the REDES study and the e-Salud database were used. The e-Salud database is a private database of health care costs in Spain that can be accessed to obtain the unavailable costs with their maximum and minimum limits.

Table 5 shows the results in more detail. The average cost of the procedure was €7,076.96, but the costs of pre-hospitalization, testing and analysis, and medication before the procedure must be added to have a more realistic view of the patient's cost. These costs were €2,011.93, €1,003.36 and €112.96 respectively. Patients were hospitalized for 2.45 days before the procedure, which involves an additional cost to be taken into account. Only the direct healthcare costs were calculated for the analysis.

Procedure	% patients	Time (hours)	Cost/Hour	Assumption	Total Costs €2011
Hemodynamist	100%	1.27	33.24		42.07
Nursing	100%	1.73	15.10		26.16
Catheterization lab.	100%	1.73	388.21	Yes	671.60
Observation unit	100%	2.93	55.71		163.41
		Days	**Cost/Day**		
Post procedure no ICU	100%	1.90	820.15		1,557.92
Post procedure ICU	100%	0.72	1,479.1		1,066.40
		Number	**Unit Costs**		
Standard balloons	100%	1.04	561.95		584.53
Cutting balloons	100%	0.03	561.95		17.56
Endeavor Resolute®	100%	1.95	1,495.33		2,910.55
BMS	100%	0.05	841.42		39.44
DES	100%	0.03	1,495.33		43.39
Complications					**117.36**
TOTAL					**7,076.98**

Table 5. Procedure costs

Analysis and tests	% patients	Average use	Unit Costs	Total Costs
Pre-procedure no ICU (days)	100%	2.45	820.15	2,011.93
Cardiac stress tests	15.18%	1.03	149.13	23.30
ECG	100.00%	3.07	20.73	63.57
CK analysis	74.11%	2.52	3.51	6.54
CK-MB analysis	68.08%	2.76	12.62	23.73
Troponin analysis	81.92%	2.92	15.57	37.28
Creatine analysis	88.17%	2.03	3.84	6.87
Eco Doppler	31.25%	1.06	104.21	34.66
IVUS	6.03%	1.04	77.98	4.87
Angiographies	97.54%	1.06	622.10	645.70
Contrast medium	100.00%	253.59	0.62	156.85
TOTAL				**1,003.36**

Table 6. Pre-hospitalization, Analysis and tests costs (pre-procedure).

The average one-year follow-up cost per patient was €1,502.29, including drug treatment and diagnostic tests, emergency room visits and hospitalizations for different causes. Hospitalizations are a key point in calculating annual costs and cost-effectiveness analysis. In spite of the stents effectiveness in the treatment of coronary artery stenosis, these patients have many comorbidities and frequently visit the hospital. Although the drug treatment has the smallest weight on the total cost, it is also interesting to look at the evolution of drug treatment in the patients. At first, nearly 100% of the patients had antiplatelet therapy, and at one-year follow-up only 25% had al least one antiplatelet drug.

In conclusion, the total annual cost of a patient with coronary artery stenosis who is treated with Endeavor RESOLUTE® stent is €11,707.5 in Spain, where the cost of the procedure represents over 60%. The cost is similar to or slightly lower than that referred by other previously published studies on DES (Moreu et al., 2009). The higher initial cost of DES may be largely offset in the long term by reducing the number of hospitalizations and revascularizations, especially compared to other treatment alternatives, as it can be observed in several published cost-effectiveness analysis discussed below.

4. Economic evaluation studies on Drug Eluting Stents

Despite DES are more efficient reducing restenosis incidence, they have higher costs than conventional stents. This has opened a discussion around the use of DES. The arguments against have often focused on concerns that higher acquisition costs lead to a significant and unacceptable increase of healthcare costs. The arguments in favor are focused on the potential of DES to compensate their higher acquisition cost with the reduction of the number of repeat revascularizations and the costs associated with them (Macaya, 2004; Valdés, 2004).

Therefore, from this discussion several studies have come up comparing costs and cost-effectiveness of different alternatives (Table 9). The TAXUS I-IV series of clinical trials

30 day follow-up				
	% patients	Average use	Unit costs	Total costs
Emergency room	7.21%	1.00	126.21	9.10
Blood transfusion	0.45%	2.50	132.62	1.49
No. hospitalizations	2.70%	1.00		
ICU		3.92	1479.10	156.57
no ICU		4.58	723.83	89.66
Hemodynamist		1.33	33.24	1.20
Nursing		1.50	15.10	0.61
TOTAL (per patient) 258.63				
6 month follow-up				
	% patients	Average use	Unit costs	Total costs
Emergency room	10.25%	1.24	126.21	16.10
Blood transfusion	0.23%	1.00	132.62	0.30
No. hospitalizations	8.66%	1.13		
ICU		0.61	1479.10	87.69
no ICU		5.32	723.83	376.88
Hemodynamist		1.41	33.24	4.59
Nursing		1.55	15.10	2.29
TOTAL (per patient) 487.85				
12 month follow-up				
	% patients	Average use	Unit costs	Total costs
Emergency room	12.44%	1.20	126.21	18.90
Blood transfusion	0.46%	3.00	132.62	1.83
No. hospitalizations	6.98%	1.06		
ICU		0.29	1479.10	31.92
no ICU		5.81	723.83	312.38
Hemodynamist		1.06	33.24	2.61
Nursing		1.11	15.10	1.25
TOTAL (per patient) 368.88				

Table 7. Emergency room and hospitalization costs.

	Pre-procedure	Discharge	30 days	6 months	12 months
Aspirin	96.65%	99.11%	68.69%	65.60%	25.35%
Clopidogrel	83.48%	99.55%	68.47%	64.92%	15.67%
Ticlopidine	0.22%	0.00%	0.00%	0.00%	0.00%

Table 8. Antiplatelet treatment.

evaluated the efficiency of the Taxus DES for percutaneous coronary intervention. Thus, the TAXUS-IV study, the first randomized trial of this series that incorporated a big pre-specified cohort of patients managed in accordance with routine clinical practice without the need of angiographic follow-up, demonstrated that the use of paclitaxel-eluting stents increases hospitalization costs in $2,028 at first, although it was partially offset at one year by a reduction in the follow-up cost of $1,456 on the DES arm (Bakhai A et al., 2006). In this way, the average cost at one year was $14,583 for DES versus $14,011 for BMS (p-value<0.001). Then, the cost-effectiveness ratio for paclitaxel-eluting stents was $4,678 for avoided revascularization and $47,798 for Quality Adjusted Life Year (QALY) gained (Bakhai A et al., 2006).

Study	Type of evaluation and synthesis	Interventions	Study population	Country	Period of study
AETMIS, 2004	Cost-utility analysis	DES (sirolimus and paclitaxel coated) versus BMS	Régie de l'Assurance Maladie du Québec (RAMQ) database, unselected patients. Repeat revascularisation risk with DES taken from meta-analysis of published trials	Canada	6-13 months
Bagust et al., 2006	Cost-utility analysis	DES (sirolimus and paclitaxel coated) versus BMS	Cardiothoracic Centre (CTC) Liverpool population, unselected patients. Subgroup characteristics determined from a meta-analysis of published trials and CTC database	UK	1 year
Bakhai A et al., 2006	Cost-effectiveness analysis and Cost-utility analysis	DES (paclitaxel coated) versus BMS	Patients undergoing percutaneous coronary revascularization: results from the TAXUS-IV Trial	USA	1 year
Bischof M et al., 2009	Cost-utility analysis	DES (sirolimus and paclitaxel coated) versus BMS	unselected patients with symptomatic ischaemic coronary artery disease	USA	1+ year
Brophy JM et al., 2005	Cost-effectiveness analysis	DES (sirolimus) versus BMS	Hypothetical cohort of patients undergoing PCI	Canada	9 months
Brunner et al., 2007	Cost-effectiveness analysis and Cost-utility analysis	DES (sirolimus and paclitaxel coated) versus BMS	826 patients included in the BASKET study- 'real-world setting'	Switzerland	18 months
Cohen, 2004	Cost-effectiveness analysis and Cost-utility analysis	DES (sirolimus) versus BMS	1,058 patients with plannned PCI of a single complex coronary artery stenosis (single native coronary artery). The lesion was de novo, 15-30 mm in length with a reference vessel diameter of 2.5-3.5 mm. SIRIUS trial	USA	1 year

Eisenstein EL et al., 2009	Cost-utility analysis	DES (zotarolimus) versus BMS	1,197 patients included in the ENDEAVOR II study	USA	4 years
Ekman M, 2006	Cost-effectiveness analysis	DES (paclitaxel coated) versus BMS	Unselected patients	Sweden	1 year & 2 years
Greenberg, 2004	Cost-effectiveness analysis	DES (sirolimus) versus BMS	Unselected patients	USA	2 years
Goeree R et al., 2009	Cost-effectiveness analysis and Cost-utility analysis	DES (sirolimus and paclitaxel coated) versus BMS	All stent procedures in the province of Ontario between December 1, 2003, and March 31, 2005, with a minimum subject follow-up of 1 year.	Canada	2 years
Gulizia et al., 2004	Cost-effectiveness analysis	DES (sirolimus) versus BMS	Data obtained from literature and adapted to Sicilian population, using data form a survey conducted in seven local catheterisation laboratories	Italy	1 year
Kaiser et al., 2005	Cost-effectiveness analysis	DES (sirolimus and paclitaxel coated) versus BMS	836 patients included in the BASKET study- 'real-world setting'	Switzerland	6 months
Lord SJ et al., 2005	Cost-effectiveness analysis and Cost-utility analysis	DES (sirolimus and paclitaxel coated) versus BMS	Unselected patients	Australia	1 year
Mittman et al., 2005	Cost-effectiveness analysis	DES (sirolimus and paclitaxel coated) versus BMS	Patients treated in the trials (SIRIUS, TAXUS) and Babapulle meta-analysis	Canada	1 year
Moreu et al., 2009	Cost-effectiveness analysis	DES (zotarolimus) versus BMS	Unselected patients, based on Endeavour trials	Spain	5 years
Shrive et al., 2005	Cost-utility analysis	DES (sirolimus) versus BMS	Unselected patients, based on Canadian database of 7,334 patients undergoing PCI between 1998 and 2000	Canada	Patients' lifetime
Tarricone et al., 2004	Cost-effectiveness analysis	DES (sirolimus) versus BMS	Patients suffering from stable or unstable angina, with de novo lesion(s). Case mix derived from unselected population of 1,809 patients	Italy	1 year
Van Hout et al., 2005	Cost-effectiveness analysis	DES (sirolimus) versus BMS	238 patients with stable or unstable angina with planned PCI for single de novo coronary lesions. SIRIUS trial	The Netherlands	1 year

Table 9. DES Economic Evaluations

Although the TAXUS-IV study was carried out in U.S., it can be extrapolated to the Spanish level, because in demographic terms its inclusion criteria make this study representative of the conditions in Spain (Stone et al., 2004; Stone, 2004). In Spain, the average age of patients with a percutaneous coronary intervention is 63 years old, as opposed to 62.5 years old from TAXUS-IV study. The male proportion in the Spanish population with coronary disease is 74%, whereas in the TAXUS-IV study it was 72%. The proportion of diabetic people in the Spanish population who suffer from heart disease is nearly 25%, as opposed to 24.2% in the TAXUS-IV study.

Since the TAXUS clinical trials were not performed in Spain, the data from the mentioned TAXUS-IV study were used to estimate the economic impact of the implantation of this stent in a Spanish hospital (Russel et al., 2006). The relevant cost data related to hospitalized patients that were considered for this estimation were collected from the Spanish costs database. The cost of a percutaneous coronary intervention was calculated based on the cost of Taxus versus BMS and multiplying by 1.54, assuming a standard mean of 1.54 stents per intervention. For the number of revascularization patients treated, a mean of 370 patients was assumed given the big difference in the number of patients treated in the Spanish hospitals. Some hospitals treat less than 200 patients per year, whereas other hospitals treat more than 1,000 (López-Palop et al., 2004).

The analysis showed an expected cost at 12 months of €6,934 per patient for Taxus group and €6,756 for BMS group, i.e. 2.6% more than the Taxus group. Although the the cost for the Taxus group is higher due to higher costs of materials, 84% of this difference was compensated later with a lower probability of repeat revascularization. The cost for each repeat revascularization avoided with Taxus was estimated at €1,568. At 24 months, the cost difference decreased to 1.8% and the low probability of repeat revascularization compensated 91% of the increment in the initial cost of the procedure.

It is important to emphasize that this cost difference requires a specific analysis in the case of high risk revascularization patients. These patients include those who have small vessels, suffer long lesions and, specially, diabetic patients, who, as said, represent the 25% of the population with coronary disease. In their case, at 12 months the BMS cost is already 3% higher than the Taxus cost, and the percentage increases to 4.5% at 24 months.

The budget impact analysis was carried out considering two different settings. In the first setting, 90% of all patients of percutaneous coronary intervention receive Taxus instead of conventional stents, and 20% of patients who receive coronary surgery become Taxus patients. In this setting, the budget impact is 0.5% higher than in the base setting, although due to the reduction of surgery and reintervention, the capacity to treat patients in the surgery room increases in 8.5% with the same fixed costs and the same infrastructure.

The second setting considers the treatment of 90% of the high-risk patients, while those not included in this group are treated with conventional stents. In this case, the savings compared to the base setting is nearly 1% and the increment of the surgery room capacity was 5% (Russell et al., 2006).

The Cypher sirolimus-eluting stent was assessed after the SIRIUS clinical trial, which was carried out in 2004 in U.S. (Cohen et al., 2004). The patient characteristics were very similar to TAXUS-IV study, being the average age 62 years, 72.6% the average of male patients and

25% the proportion of diabetic patients. The economic analysis could be extrapolated to the Spanish market too, although this study has not been carried out yet in Spain.

The cost difference in initial treatment was $ 2,856 higher in the case of the Cypher stent. However, follow-up and reintervention costs were significantly lower in this case, becoming $ 2,571 lower than with conventional stents. The total costs at one year for Cypher were $ 309 higher than conventional stents (Cohen et al., 2004).

The cost-effectiveness study concluded that the cost-utility per QALY was $ 27,540, within the acceptable thresholds from the hospital perspective. In addition, in some cases of the study where the lesion was longer than 25 mm, 3 stents were used instead of two long lengths. This would have reduced the number of stents by intervention from 1.4 to 1.3, therefore, the costs per patient would have decreased about $ 136. This study, compared with the previous one showed no significant differences in the costs for treating high-risk patients (Cohen et al., 2004). The analysis indicated that DES was economically dominant in patients with long lesions in small vessels.

The Taxus stent has also been studied in Sweden by a decision model based on the revascularization rate, the resource use with its Swedish unit costs and the utilities based on the literature (Ekman M, 2006). From the public financing perspective, the average cost per patient treated at one year was €7,913 and €7,328 for Taxus stents and conventional stents respectively (Ekman M, 2006). The cost per repeat revascularization avoided was € 5,126 at one year and € 3,900 at 2 years. The results were more favorable in high risk patients: €47,791 per QALY and €838 per repeat revascularization avoided at 12 months. The budget impact was assessed too with 2 hypothetical scenarios and a baseline scenario. In the first scenario, 80% of high-risk patients were treated with DES instead of conventional stents, and the budget impact analysis increased 0.8%. In the second scenario, in addition to 80% of high-risk patients treated with DES instead of conventional stents, 20% of surgery patients with multivessel disease were treated with DES, and the budget impact analysis decreased 0.8%(Ekman M, 2006).

On the other hand, from the RAVEL study, Randomized Study with the sirolimus-eluting Bx Velocity balloon expandable stent in the Treatment of Patients with de novo native coronary artery lesions, it was demonstrated that the sirolimus DES generated an increase in the cost of the procedure of €1,284 per patient, although the net cost per year only resulted in an increase of €54 per patient (Van Hout et al., 2005).

After the TAXUS-IV, SIRIUS and RAVEL studies, it was necessary to carry out a study that compared Taxus and Cypher with each other and included an evaluation against conventional stents. This study was conducted in Switzerland in the state of Basel, and was named BASKET (Basel Kosten Effektivitäts Trial).

The BASKET study (Kaiser et al. 2005; Pfisterer et al., 2009) included more than 850 patients randomized into 3 similarly sized groups: those who received an uncoated stent, those who received Taxus and those who received Cypher. Thus, the study was planned and carried out in order to compare the increased cost-effectiveness of the three alternatives in patients with percutaneous coronary intervention.

At six months it was observed that the use of DES reduced the adverse cardiac events rate in a 44%, especially in terms of revascularization, myocardial infarction or acute coronary syndrome. There were not significant differences in efficacy between the two DES (Kaiser et al., 2005). This behavior continued for three years (Pfisterer et al., 2009), time in which the BASKET study was reevaluated. After these years it was also observed that these differences were more pronounced in patients who received long stents, while those who received shorter stents had fewer differences in effectiveness between DES and uncoated stents.

Regarding the compared cost of the three options, at six months the initial higher cost of Taxus and Cypher could not be compensated, with a cost €1,702 higher than in the case of the conventional stents. After six months, due to the reduction of adverse events, this cost was finally €902 higher (Kaiser et al., 2005). The cost-effectiveness in preventing adverse cardiac events was €18,311 higher for DES, although this was reduced significantly in the subgroups of high risk patients such as diabetics, people over 65 years old, patients with more than a treated segment, and so on. The cost-utility ratio between DES versus standard stents was €73,283 per QALY using EQ-5D index, and €54,546 by visual analogue scale (Kaiser et al., 2005).

Also, at 18 months, a higher total cost was observed in patients with DES compared to BMS (€11,808 [SD 400] per patient with DES and €10,450 [SD 592] per patient with BMS, mean difference of €1,358 [SD717], $p < 0.0001$), due to the high cost of the stent shown in the study (Brunner-La Rocca et al., 2007). Therefore, the calculation of cost-effectiveness ratio was €64,732 per major adverse cardiac events avoided, and €40,467 per QALY gained. The stent cost, the number of events, and QALYs were the main causes for not reaching an acceptable cost-effectiveness ratio.

In patients at low risk, the probability that DES reached an Incremental Cost-Effectiveness of €10,000 or less to prevent major adverse cardiac events was 0.016, but was 0.874 in patients at high risk. In this way, it denotes the major differences between Incremental Cost-Effectiveness of patients at low risk and high risk. When the cost-utility ratio is assessed, a similar pattern can be observed, being low-risk patients 41% less effective and more expensive with a probability of being cost-effective of 0.11 (threshold below €40,000 per QALY) whereas in the case of high-risk patients 76% of patients were more effective and cheaper than BSM, being the probability of cost-effectiveness of 0.975.

In the study of Shrive FM et al. (2005), it was estimated a cost per QALY of 58,721 Canadian dollars using the sirolimus DES compared to conventional stents. In diabetic patients and patients older than 70 years old the use of DES is more cost-effective. In this way, other short-term Canadian study (9 months) found that the cost per repeat revascularization avoided was 23,067 Canadian dollars and that the most cost-effective strategy was the use of DES in high-risk populations (7,800 Canadian dollars) (Brophy et al., 2005). Delimiting the vision to a hospital perspective, the cost-effectiveness ratio for avoided revascularization showed values in a range from 12,527 to 29,048 Canadian dollars (AETMIS, 2004).

Many other economic evaluation studies have focused on the comparison of DES vs. BMS combining various types of DES. Thus in Australia, from a National Health System perspective, the incremental cost per repeat revascularization avoided was 3,750 Australian dollars with sirolimus and 6,100 Australian dollars with paclitaxel at 12 months (Lord SJ et al., 2005). On the other hand, the cost per QALY was 46,829 Australian dollars and 76,467 Australian dollars with sirolimus and paclitaxel respectively. The authors concluded that limiting DES to patients at high risk may improve the cost-effectiveness (Lord SJ et al. 2005).

In UK, where a treatment is considered cost-effective below €42,000 or with a neutral cost at 12-month follow-up from a public financing perspective, DES were not cost-effective in comparison to BMS except for a selected group of patients (Bagust et al., 2006). In the same way, a Swiss study of Kaiser et al. showed a higher cost per patient for DES compared to BMS with an average of €10,544 against €9,639 from a health system financing perspective. Thus, the average cost difference between the 2 types of stents was €1,702 per patient, showing a cost per cardiac event avoided of €18,311 and a cost per QALY of €50,000 (Kaiser et al., 2005). Again, the subgroup analysis showed that DES were more cost-effective in high-risk patients (older than 65 with multivessel disease).

The latest studies, which assessed both Taxus and Cypher, indicated that in patients not selected previously DES are not cost-effective and they are becoming more cost-effective in high-risk patients (Bischof M et al., 2009 , Goeree R et al., 2009). In this way, the Bischof study, based on 17 randomized trials, showed that the cost of BMS was $25,460, the cost of sirolimus was $28,250 and $29,299 for paclitaxel (Bischof M et al., 2009). It all means that the probability of being cost-effective in the United States (threshold of $100,000 per QALY) was 8.3% and 2.8% for sirolimus and paclitaxel, respectively (Bischof M et al., 2009). For the Ontario study the differences in the revascularization rate were observed mainly in patients with two or more risk factors. Therefore, the cost per repeat revascularization and the cost per QALY were above the threshold (Goeree R et al., 2009).

The latest alternative of DES on the market was Endeavor, a zotarolimus coronary stent. Endeavor has demonstrated its effectiveness and safety with the Endeavor-I study and its benefits in the Endeavor-II study (Fajadet et al., 2007). The latter showed that Endeavor reduces the probability of suffering an adverse cardiac event from 14.4% to 7.3% and the restenosis rate was 35% for BMS and 13.2% for Endeavor.

With clinical data from the Endeavor II study (Randomized Controlled Trial to Evaluate the Safety and Efficacy of the Medtronic AVE ABT-578 Eluting Driver Coronary Stent in De Novo Native Coronary Artery Lesions), Endeavor clinical and economic benefits were assessed in U.S compared to BMS (Eisenstein EL et al., 2009). The clinical data, the resource use and the follow-up of 1,197 patients were used (598 Endeavor vs. 599 BMS), applying the quality of life of secondary sources over 4 years of follow-up.

The use of Endeavor versus BMS at 4 years reduced the target vessel revascularization rate (10.4 vs. 21.5, P <0.001), but the analysis showed no significant differences regarding mortality or non-fatal myocardial infarction. Applying a discount of 3% no difference in QALYs was observed (1.093 vs. 1.090; p = 0.69), or the total health costs ($ 21,483 vs. $ 21,680, P = 0.78) (Eisenstein EL et al., 2009).

Using the data from the ENDEAVOR-II, Moreu et al. performed a Markov model with monthly cycles to compare the efficacy data of Endeavor with other therapeutic alternatives and draw an economic of the Spanish market. Data on resource use associated with the different options and the unit costs were obtained from local data and were validated by experts. These costs were expressed in 2007 Euros with a time horizon of 5 years (Moreu et al., 2009).

This analysis showed that the cost per restenosis avoided by Endeavor was €6,851 at 1 year and €10,831 at 5 years, and costs for adverse cardiac event avoided were €7,003 and € 11,322 respectively. In this way, the lower incidence of complications with Endeavor compared to BMS resulted in an improvement of quality-adjusted survival of patients, which was progressive and strongly associated with the simulation period of the analysis, being almost 0 at 1 year. Thus, an increment of QALYs is perceived over time, since the values of cost per QALY gained is €132,877, €34,229 and €10,505 to 1, 2 and 5 years respectively (Moreu et al. 2009),

This study also included a comparison with other alternatives such as surgery, and showed that Endeavor is a less expensive option, with savings decreasing over the period of analysis.

Therefore, this study coincided with the cost-effectiveness analysis of the BASKET study, in which the higher costs of DES compared to conventional stents were mainly due to the higher initial cost of the procedure. The results at 2 years showed that these short-term higher costs are partially offset by further reductions in the incidence of complications and revascularization need. In addition, cost-effectiveness ratios also decrease with time (Moreu et al. 2009; Kaiser et al., 2005).

5. Discussion

The risk of repeat revascularizations using BMS is between 5% and 14% in the published registries, which is much lower than that observed in clinical trials (over 30%). Therefore, the absolute reduction of repeat revascularization with DES compared to BMS, or the marginal improvement of DES, is very limited in actual life. This leads to a higher cost combination for DES compared to BMS and low improvements in the quality of live by a low latitude, which make it more difficult to obtain favorable cost-effectiveness ratios to DES in all the countries.

In the recent years, there has been a growing interest in economic evaluation of health technologies, with a progressive increment of the number of articles in medical journals. Nevertheless, this increment does not translate into an increment in the quality of the studies, and the lack of methodological strength has been the general trend. This is because economic evaluation is relatively a new field (its use in the healthcare system began, with few exceptions, in the nineties when the health cost soared and new technologies with higher prices progressively appeared) which uses methods and concepts alien to medical knowledge and causes confusion in the terms use and the followed objectives.

The economic evaluation try to determine which technology is more efficient or, which is the same, what technology produces better health outcomes depending on the resources invested, once the costs, risks and benefits are identified, measured and compared.

The economic implications of the use of DES have lead to the proliferation of economic evaluation studies throughout the world. In short, in relation to the use of DES, it is widely acknowledged that its cost is the true limiting factor; for example, in our area the price of DES is 60-80% higher than conventional stents. Although many studies concluded that DES may be cost effective in large subgroups of patients, under real conditions, the DES cost-effectiveness do not come out favorably compared to BMS (Neyt M et al. 2009; Hill RA et al. 2007; Kuukasjärvi P et al., 2007).

In the current global economic crisis, the presentation of studies with data from the actual clinical practice which demonstrate a reduction in the final costs with the DES use in the national health system is crucial to decision making and efficiency. Therefore, the stents are still one of the crosshairs of Health Technology Assessment bodies. Since 2006, 8 HTA have been published with a moderate to high quality, which showed different conclusions based on the published clinical evidence, especially in terms of mortality. Five of them reviewed the published economic evidence and concluded that DES are more effective in high-risk patients, despite the great disparity between studies and the great variance in the results and cost-effectiveness ratios.

In conclusion, in the last years a great effort has been made to improve the safety and efficacy of new coronary stents. However, studies with larger patient populations and a long-term follow-up are necessary to evaluate the effectiveness of the new stents and then show that DES are a cost-effective treatment, because they will remain an important part of treatment of PCI in the near future.

6. Acknowledgement

REDES study was funded by Medtronic Ibérica. S.A.

7. References

Agence d'évaluation des technologies et des modes d'intervention en santé (AETMIS). Analyse économique des stents coronariens à élution médicamenteuse : une perspective québécoise. Rapport préparé par James Brophy et Lonny Erickson. (AETMIS 04-04). Montréal : AETMIS, 2004, xi-40 p.

Allender S, Scarborough P, Peto V, Rayner M, Leal J, Luengo-Fernandez A, et al. European cardiovascular disease statistics European Heart Network. 2008.

Ayyanatahn S, Hersh D, Coplan NL, Garratt K. The problem of stent thrombosis associated with drug-eluting stents and the optimal duration of dual antiplatelet therapy. Prev Cardiol 2009; 12:59-64.

Bagust A, Grayson AD, Palmer ND, Perry RA, Walley T. Cost effectiveness of drug eluting coronary artery stenting in a UK setting: cost-utility study. Heart. 2006;92:68-74.

Bakhai A, Stone G, Mahoney E, Lavelle T, Shi C, Berezin R, Lahue B, Clark M, Lacey M, Russell M, Ellis S, Hermiller J, Cox D, Cohen DJ, for the TAXUS-IV Investigators. Cost-effectiveness of paclitaxel-eluting stents for patients undergoing percutaneous coronary revascularization: results from the TAXUS-IV Trial. J Am Coll Cardiol. 2006;48: 253–261.

Bertrand ME, Legrand V, Boland J, et al. Randomized multicenter comparison of conventional anticoagulation versus antiplatelet therapy in unplanned and elective coronary stenting. The Full Anticoagulation versus Aspirin and Ticlopidine (FANTASTIC) study. Circulation 1998; 98:1597-1603.

Bischof M, Briel M, Bucher HC, Nordmann A. Cost-effectiveness of drug-eluting stents in a US medicare setting: a cost-utility analysis with 3-year clinical follow-up data. Value in Health 2009 12(5):649-656.

Brophy JM, Erickson LJ. Cost-effectiveness of drug-eluting coronary stents in Quebec, Canada. Int J Technol Assess Health Care. 2005;21:326-33.

Brunner-La Rocca HP, Kaiser C, Bernheim A, Zellweger MJ, Jeger R et al. Cost-eff ectiveness of drug-eluting stents in patients at high or low risk of major cardiac events in the Basel Stent KostenEff ektivitäts Trial (BASKET): an 18-month analysis. Lancet 2007; 370: 1552–59.

Chevalier B, Serruys PW, Silber S, et al. Ramdomized comparison of Nobori, biolimus A9-eluting coronary stent with a TAxus ® paclitaxel-eluting coronary stent in patients with stenosis in native coronary arteries: the NObori 1 trial. EruoIntervention 2007; 2:426-434.

Chevalier B, Silber S, Park SJ. Randomized comparison of the Nobori Biolimus A9-eluting coronary stent with the Taxus Liberte paclitaxel-eluting coronary stent in patients with stenosis in native coronary arteries: the NOBORI 1 trial-Phase 2. Circ Cardiovasc Interv 2009; 2:88-195.

Cohen DJ, Bakhai A, Shi C, Githiora L, Lavelle T, Berezin RH, Leon MB, Moses JW, Carrozza JP Jr, Zidar JP, Kuntz RE; SIRIUS Investigators. Cost-effectiveness of sirolimus-eluting stents for treatment of complex coronary stenoses: results from the Sirolimus-Eluting Balloon Expandable Stent in the Treatment of Patients With De Novo Native Coronary Artery Lesions (SIRIUS) trial. Circulation. 2004 Aug 3;110(5):508-14.

Eisenstein EL, Wijns W, Fajadet J, Mauri L, Edwards R, Cowper PA, Kong DF, Anstrom KJ . Long-term clinical and economic analysis of the Endeavor drug-eluting stent versus the Driver bare-metal stent: 4-year results from the ENDEAVOR II Trial (randomized controlled trial to evaluate the safety and efficacy of the Medtronic AVE ABT-578 eluting driver coronary stent in de novo native coronary artery lesions) . JACC Cardiovasc Interv. 2009 Dec;2(12):1178-87.

Ekman M, Sjögren I, James S. Cost-effectiveness of the Taxus paclitaxel-eluting stent in the Swedish healthcare system. Scand Cardiovasc J. 2006;40:17-24.

Fajadet J, Wijns W, Laarman GJ, Kuck KH, Ormiston J, Münzel T, Popma JJ, Fitzgerald PJ, Bonan R, Kuntz RE; ENDEAVOR II Investigators. Randomized, double-blind, multicenter study of the Endeavor zotarolimus-eluting phosphorylcholine-encapsulated stent for treatment of native coronary artery lesions. Clinical and angiographic results of the ENDEAVOR II Trial. Minerva Cardioangiol. 2007 Feb;55(1):1-18.

Fajadet J, Wijns W, Laarman GJ, et al. Randomized, double-blid, multicenter study of the Endeavor zotarolimus-eluting phophorylcholine-encapsulated stent for treatment of native coronary artery lesions: clinical and angiographic results of ENDEAVOR II trial. Circulation 2006; 114:798-806.

Fischman DL, Leon MB, Baim DS, Schatz RA, Savage MP, Penn I, Detre K, Veltri L, Ricci D, Nobuyoshi M, et al. : A randomized comparison of coronary-stent placement and balloon angioplasty in the treatment of coronary artery disease. Stent Restenosis Study Investigators. N Engl J Med 1994;331(8): 496-501.

Gerlishlick A, Kandzari DE, Leon MB, et al. Zotarolimus-eluting stents in patients with native coronary artery disease: clinical and angiographic outcomes in 1,317 patients. Am J Cardiol 2007; 100: 45M.55M.

Gisbert R, Brosa M. Evolución del coste de la enfermedad en España: 1980-2000. XXV Jornadas de Economía de la Salud. Barcelona, julio de 2005.

Greenberg D, Bakhai A, Neil N, Berezin R, Ho K, Cutlip D, Kuntz R, Cohen DJ. Modeling the impact of patient and lesion characteristics on the cost-effectiveness of drug-eluting stents. J Am Coll Cardiol. 2003; 41(suppl):538A. Abstract.

Goeree R, Bowen JM, Blackhouse G, Lazzam C, Cohen E, Chiu M, Hopkins R, Tarride JE, Tu JV. Economic evaluation of drug-eluting stents compared to bare metal stents using a large prospective study in Ontario. Int J Technol Assess Health Care. 2009 Apr;25(2):196-207.

Gulizia M, Martelli E, Tamburino C, Tolaro S, Frasheri A, Giambanco F, Grassi R, Fiscella A, Milazzo D. [Potential impact of drug-eluting stents in Sicily: results from a multicenter survey and cost-benefit analysis of drug-eluting stents versus bare metal stents]. Ital Heart J Suppl. 2004 Aug;5(8):630-8.

Hall P, Nakamura S, Maiello L, et al. A randomized comparison of combined ticlopidine and aspirn therapy versus aspirin therapy alone after successful intravascular ultrasound-guided stent implantation. Circulation 1996; 93:215-222.

Hill R, Bagust A, Bakhai A, et al. Coronary artery stents: a rapid systematic review and economic evaluation. Health Technology Assessment 2004;8(35):1-242. Available from: http://www.nice.org.uk/pdf/StentsAssessmentreport.pdf

Hill RA, Boland A, Dickson R, Dündar Y, Haycox A, McLeod C, Mujica Mota R, Walley T, Bagust A. Drug-eluting stents: a systematic review and economic evaluation. Health Technol Assess. 2007 Nov;11(46):iii, xi-221.

Hoffman SN, TenBrook JA, Wolf MP, Pauker SG, Salem DN, Wong JB: A meta-analysis of randomized controlled trials comparing coronary artery bypass graft with percutaneous transluminal coronary angioplasty: one- to eight-year outcomes. J Am Coll Cardiol. 2003 Apr 16;41(8):1293-304.

Instituto Nacional de Estadística [Statistical Institute]. Mortality by cause. 2011 [cited Juny 2011] Available: http: www.ine.es

Kaiser C, Brunner-La Rocca HP, Buser PT, Bonetti PO, Osswald S, Linka A, Bernheim A, Zutter A, Zellweger M, Grize L, Pfisterer ME; BASKET Investigators. Incremental cost-effectiveness of drug-eluting stents compared with a third-generation bare-metal stent in a real-world setting: randomised Basel Stent Kosten Effektivitäts Trial (BASKET). Lancet. 2005 Sep 10-16;366(9489):921-9.

Kereiakes DJ, Cannon LA, Feldman RL, et al. Clinical and angiographic outcomes after treatment of a novo coronary stenoses with a novel platinum chromium thin-strut stent : primary results of the PERSEUS trial. J Am Coll Cardiol 2010; 56:264-271.

Kirtane AJ, Gupta A, Iyengar S, Moses JW, Leon MB, Applegate R, Brodie B, Hannan E, Harjai K, Jensen LO, Park SJ, Perry R, Racz M, Saia F, Tu JV, Waksman R, Lansky AJ, Mehran R, Stone GW. Safety and efficacy of drug-eluting and bare metal stents:

comprehensive meta-analysis of randomized trials and observational studies. Circulation 2009;119:3198–3206.

Kuukasjärvi P, Räsänen P, Malmivaara A, Aronen P, Sintonen H. Economic evaluation of drug-eluting stents: a systematic literature review and model-based cost-utility analysis. Int J Technol Assess Health Care. 2007 Fall;23(4):473-9.

Leon MB, Baim DS, Popma JJ, et al. A clinical trial comparing three antithrombotic-drug regimens after coronary artery stenting. Stent Anticoagulation Restenosis Study Investigators. N Engl J Med 1998; 339:1665-1671.

Lord SJ, Howard K, Allen F, Marinovich L, Burgess DC, King R, et al. A systematic review and economic analysis of drug-eluting coronary stents available in Australia. Med J Aust. 2005;183:464-71.

López-Palop R, Moreu J, Fernández-Vázquez F, Hernández Antolín R. Registro Español de Hemodinámica y Cardiología Intervencionista. XIII Informe Oficial de la Sección de Hemodinámica y Cardiología Intervencionista de la Sociedad Española de Cardiología (1990-2003) Rev Esp Cardiol. 2004;57:1076-89.

Macaya C [Is systematic use of drug-eluting stents justified? Arguments against]. Rev Esp Cardiol. 2004;57: 109-15.

Mauri L, Hsieh WH, Massaro JM, Ho KK, D'Agostino R, Cutlip DE. Stent thrombosis in randomized clinical trials of drug-eluting stents. N Engl J Med 2007;356:1020-9.

Mauri L, Massaro JM, Jiang S et al. Long-term clinical outcomes with zotarolimus-eluting versus bare-metal stents. J Am Coll Cardiol Intv 2010; 3:1240-9.

Mehilli J Kstrati A, Wessely R. Ramdomized trial oof a nonpolymer-based rapamycin-eluting stent versus a polymer-based paclitaxel-eluting stent for the reduction of a late lumen loss. Circulation 2006; 113: 273-279.

Meredith IT, Worthley SG, Whitbourn R, Walters D, McClean D, Horrigan M, Popma JJ, Cutlip DE, DePaoli A, Negoita M, Fitzgerald PJ. Clinical and Angiographic results with the next-generation Resolute stent system. A prospective, multicenter, first in human trial. JACC: Cardiovascular interventions 2009;2(10):977-985.

Meredith IT, Worthley SG, Whitbourn R, Walters D, McClean D, Orminston J, Horrigan M, Wilkins GT, Hendriks R, Matsis P, Muller D, Cutlip DE. Long-term clinical aoutcomes with the next-generation Resolute stent system: a report of the two-year follow-up from the RESOLUTE clinical trial. Eurointervention 2010;5(6):692-697.

Ministerio de Sanidad y Consumo. Plan Nacional de Cardiopatía Isquémica 2004-2007. 2003 [cited Juny 2011] Available: http://www.anisalud.com/ficheros/PNCI.pdf

Mittmann N, Brown A, Seung SJ, Coyle D, Cohen E, Brophy J, et al. Economic evaluation of drug eluting stents. Technology report no. 53. Ottawa: Canadian Coordinating Office for Health Technology Assessment; 2005.

Moreno R Drug-eluting stents and other anti-restenosis devices. Rev Esp Cardiol 2005; 58:842-862.

Moreu J, Cequier A, Brosa M, Rodríguez JM, Crespo C, Hernández JM, Vázquez N, Fernández F, Ruiz-Nodar JM, Brasseur P. Evaluación económica e impacto presupuestario del stent recubierto Endeavor en España. Gac Sanit. 2009 Nov-Dic;23(6):540-7.

Morice MC, Serruys PW, Sousa JE, Fajadet J, Ban Hayashi E, Perin M, Colombo A, Schuler G, Barragan P, Guagliumi G, Molnàr F, Falotico R; RAVEL Study Group. Randomized Study with the Sirolimus-Coated Bx Velocity Balloon-Expandable Stent in the Treatment of Patients with de Novo Native Coronary Artery Lesions. A randomized comparison of a sirolimus-eluting stent with a standard stent for coronary revascularization. N Engl J Med. 2002;346(23): 1773-80.

Moses JW, Leon MB, Popma JJ, et al. Sirolimus-eluting stent versus standard stents in patients with stenosis in a native coronary artery. N Engl J Med 2003:349:1315-1323.

Neyt M, Van Brabandt H, Devriese S, De Laet C. Cost-effectiveness analyses of drug eluting stents versus bare metal stents: a systematic review of the literature. Health Policy. 2009 Jul;91(2):107-20.

Ormiston J et al. Six months results of the NEVO RES-ELUTION I (NEVO RES I Trial), a randomized multi-center comparison of the NEVO sirolimus-eluting coronary stent with the TAXUS Liberté paclitaxel-eluting stent in de novo coronary artery lesions. Circ. Cardiovasc Interv 2010.

Pfisterer M, Brunner-La Rocca HP, Rickenbacher P, Hunziker P, Mueller C, Nietlispach F, Leibundgut G, Bader F, Kaiser C; BASKET. Long-term benefit-risk balance of drug-eluting vs. bare-metal stents in daily practice: does stent diameter matter? Three-year follow-up of BASKET. Eur Heart J. 2009 Jan;30(1):16-24.

Rusell S, Antoñanzas F, Mainar V. Impacto económico del stent coronario Taxus: implicaciones para el sistema sanitario español. Rev Esp Cardiol. 2006;59(9):889-96.

Serruys PW, de Jaegere P, Kiemeneij F, Macaya C, Rutsch W, Heyndrickx G, Emanuelsson H, Marco J, Legrand V, Materne P, et al.: A comparison of balloon-expandable-stent implantation with balloon angioplasty in patients with coronary artery disease. Benestent Study Group.. N Engl J Med. 1994 Aug 25;331(8):489-95.

Serruys PW, Morice MC, Kappetein AP, Colombo A, Holmes DR, Mack MJ, Ståhle E, Feldman TE, van den Brand M, Bass EJ, Van Dyck N, Leadley K, Dawkins KD, Mohr FW; SYNTAX Investigators. Percutaneous coronary intervention versus coronary-artery bypass grafting for severe coronary artery disease. N Engl J Med 2009 Mar 5;360(10):961-72.

Serruys PW, Silber S, Garg S, van Geuns RJ, Richardt G, Buszman PE, Kelbaek H, van Boven AJ, Hofma SH, Linke A, Klauss V, Wijns W, Macaya C, Garot P, Di Mario C, et al. Compariosn of Zotarolimus-Eluting and Everolimus-Eluting coronary stents. N Engl J Med 2010;363:136-146.

Schömig A, Neumann FJ, Kastrati A, et al. A randomized comparison of antiplatelet and anticoagulant therapy after the placement of coronary stents. N Engl J Med 1996; 334:1084-1089.

Shrive FM, Manns BJ, Galbraith PD, Knudtson ML, Ghali WA. Economic evaluation of sirolimus-eluting stents. CMAJ. 2005;172:345-51.

Smith SC Jr, Feldman TE, HIrshfeld JW Jr, et al. ACC/AHA/SCAI 2005 Guideline Update for Percutaneous Coronary Intervention-Sumary Article: A Report of the American College of Cardiology/American Heart Association Task Force on Practice Guidelines (ACC/AHA/SCAI Writing Committee to Update the 2001 Guidelines for Percutaneous Coronary Intervention) J Am Coll Cardiol. 2006;47(1):216-35.

Stone GW, Ellins SG, Cox DA. Et al. A polymer-based, paclitaxel-eluting stent in patients with coronary artery disease. N. Engl J Med 2004; 350:221-231

Stone G, Ellis S, Cox D, Hermiller J, O'Shaughnessy C, Mann J, et al. One-Year Clinical Results With the Slow-Release, Polymer-based, Paclitaxel-eluting TAXUS Stent: The TAXUS-IV trial. Circulation. 2004;109: 1942-7.

Stone GW. 2-year clinical results of the TAXUS-IV Trial. Transcahtehter Cardiovascular Therapeutics Congress; Washington DC, 29th September 2004. Available from: www://bostonscientific.com/templatedate/imports/collateral/coronary/bsc_TaxusIV_24month.pdf.

Stone GW, Ellis SG, Cannon L et al. Comparison of a polymer-based paclitaxel-eluting stent with a bare metal stent in. Patients with complex coronary artery disease: a randomized controlled trial. JAMA 2005; 294:1215-1223.

Stone GW, Medei M, Newman W, et al. Randomized comparison of everolimus-eluting and paclitaxel-eluting stents; two year clinical follow-up from the clinical evaluation of the Xcience V everolimus eluting coronary stent system in the treatment of patients with de novo native coronary artery lesions (SPIRIT) III trial. Circulation 2009; 119:680-686.

Stone GW, Rizvi A, Newman W, et al. Everolimus-eluting versus paclitaxel-eluting stents in coronary artery disease. N Engl J Med 2010; 362: 1663-1674.

Stolker JM, Kennedy KF, Lindsey JB, et al. Predicting restenosis of drug-eluting stent placed in real-world clinical practice: derivation and validation of a risk model from the EVENT registry. Circ Cardiovasc Interv 2010;3:327-34.

Tarricone R, Marchetti M, Lamotte M, Annemans L, de Jong P. What reimbursement for coronary revascularization with drug-eluting stents? Eur J Health Econ. 2004 Dec;5(4):309-16.

Thygesen K, Alpert JS, White HD. Universal definition of myocardial infarction. Eur Heart J. 2007 Oct;28(20):2525-38.

The Task Force on Myocardial Revascularization of the European Society of Cardiology (ESC) and the European Association for Cardio-Thoracic Surgery (EACTS): Guidelines on myocardial revascularization European Heart Journal 2010;31: 2501–55.

Urban P, Macaya C, Rupprecht HJ, et al. Randomized evaluation of anticoagulation versus antiplatelet therapy after coronary stent implantation in high risk patients: the Multicenter Aspirin and Ticlopidine Trial after Intracoronary Stenting (MATTIS). Circulation 1998; 98:2126-2132.

Valdés M. ¿Está justificado el uso de stents con fármacos? Argumentos a favor. Rev Esp Cardiol. 2004;57: 99-108.

Van Hout BA, Serruys PW, Lemos PA, van den Brand MJ, van Es GA, Lindeboom WK, et al. One year cost effectiveness of sirolimus eluting stents compared with bare metal stents in the treatment of single native de novo coronary lesions: an analysis from the RAVEL trial. Heart. 2005; 91: 507–12.

Windecker S., Meier B: Late Coronary Stent Thrombosis. Circulation 2007: 116: 1952-1965.

Windecker S., Serruys PW, Wandel S, et al. Biolimus-eluting stent with biodegradable polymer versus sirolimus-eluting stent with durable polymer for coronary revascularization (LEADERS: a randomized non-inferiority trial. Lancet 2008:372: 1163-1173.

World Health Organization (WHO). The Top 10 causes of death. Fact sheet N°310. June 2011

Yeung AC, Leon MB, Jain A, Tolleson TR, Spriggs DJ, McLaurin BT, Popma JJ, Fitzgerlad PJ, Cutlip DE, Massaro JM, Mauri L, et al. Clinical evaluation of the Resolute Zotarolimus-Eluting Coronary Stent System in treatment of the novo lesions in native coronary arteries. J Am Coll Cardiol 2011;57.

11

Coronary Revascularization in Diabetics: The Background for an Optimal Choice

Giuseppe Tarantini and Davide Lanzellotti
Department of Cardiac, Thoracic and Vascular Sciences, University of Padua Medical School
Italy

1. Introduction

Coronary artery disease (CAD) is more extensive and severe in diabetic than non-diabetic patients both in randomized trials and registries (see table 1 and 2). Compared with non-diabetic, diabetic patients have smaller vessel size and poorer coronary collateral vessels development. Diabetes mellitus (DM) is a major risk factor for poor outcome after percutaneous coronary intervention (PCI) and is specifically associated with higher rates of restenosis. A potential mechanism underlying this phenomenon, suggested by angiographic and ultrasonic studies, is a higher degree of late luminal loss and neointimal hyperplasia in diabetic compared to non-diabetic patients . The increased rate of restenosis in diabetic patients may have an impact on their prognosis. In a study of 603 diabetic patients undergoing balloon angioplasty between 1987 and 1995, the occlusive form of restenosis has been associated with poor survival and was an independent predictor of mortality (Van Belle 2001). Finally, DM constitutes an independent predictor of early stent thrombosis, both in the bare-metal- and drug-eluting-stent era. Current guidelines favor coronary artery bypass graft (CABG) surgery over PCI in most diabetic patients with multivessel disease (MVD). However, substantial variability exists in the current medical practice suggesting a lack of clinical consensus.

2. Clinical case: how to treat?

A 74-year-old, diabetic man without a history of cardiovascular disease was admitted because of rest angina and non ST elevation acute coronary syndrome, without significant ST segment changes at electrocardiogram and with mild hypokinesia of the mid lateral left ventricular wall at 2D echocardiography. Cardiac troponin I peaked at 10ng/L. He underwent coronary angiography (18-hour after admission) that revealed a three vessel disease. The ramus intermedium had a TIMI 2 flow (Figure 1). Left ventriculography revealed mid inferior and lateral hypokinesia with an estimated ejection fraction of 60%. Should the patient be referred for CABG surgery or treated by PCI?

3. Answers from evidence-based medicine: clinical trials

3.1 Plain angioplasty vs CABG

With the advent of coronary angioplasty, several randomized, controlled trials have compared angioplasty to traditional surgery. The first was proposed Andreas Gruentzig six

REGISTRY	TOTAL n°Pt	DM %	ALL		NO DM		DM	
			MVD%	3VD%	MVD%	3VD%	MVD%	3VD%
NHLBI PTCA Registry (1985-86) (Kip 1996)	2431	13,5	49,6	19,1	48,8	17,7	54,4	27,7
NHLBI DYNAMIC REGISTRY Phase 1- 2 (1997-99) (Laskey 2002)	4629	23	57,8	25,2	55,3	23,1	66,0	32,3
BARI Registry (Detre 1999)	2010	16,9	100	31,9	100	29,7	100	43
Northern New England CVD study (1992-96) (Niles 2001)	2766	100	100	45	0	0	100	45
(Natali 2000)	2253	11,9	40,7	18,9	38	16,7	61	35

Table 1. Prevalence of multiple vessel disease in diabetic vs non-diabetic patients in clinical registries.DM: Diabetes Mellitus, MVD: Multi-Vessel Disease; 3VD: 3-Vessels Disease

TRIAL	TOTAL n°Pt	DM %	ALL		NO DM		DM	
			MVD%	3VD%	MVD%	3VD%	MVD%	3VD%
ARTS (Serruys 1999)	1205	17,3	96,1	29	95,9	27,8	97,4	32,9
ARTS-II (Serruys 2005)	607	26,2	99,7	53,6	99,8	54,7	99,4	50,3
BARI (The BARI investigators 1996)	1829	19,3	100	41	100	40	100	46
MASS-II (Hueb 2004)	611	31,1	100	58,6	100	57,9	100	60,1
SYNTAX (Serruys 2009)	1800	25,1	100	79,5	100	78,5	100	82,6
BARI 2D (Frye 2009)	1773	100	68	32	0	0	68	32
CARDIA (Kapur 2010)	510	100	94,4	59,7	0	0	94,4	59,7

Table 2. Prevalence of multiple vessel disease in diabetic vs non-diabetic patients in randomized clinical trials. DM: Diabetes Mellitus, MVD: Multi-Vessel Disease; 3VD: 3-Vessels Disease.

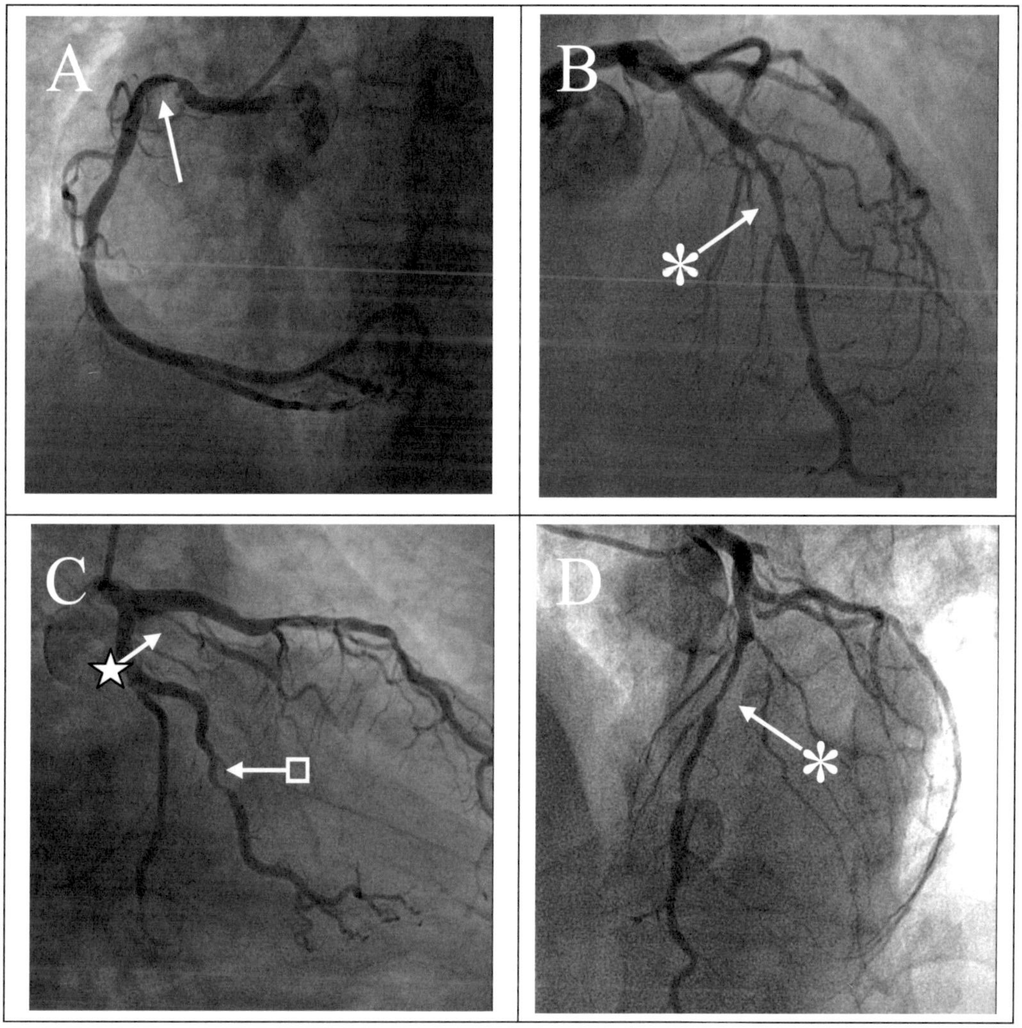

Fig. 1. A stenosis at the first tract of the right coronary artery **(A, arrow)**; a stenosis in the mid descending coronary artery **(B,D, arrows with asterisk)**; a stenosis in the obtuse marginal ramus and a subocclusion of the ramus intermedium **(C, arrows with square and with star, respectively)** All the stenosis were categorized as critical by the operator by visual assessment.

years after the execution of the first procedure, when angioplasty had reached a degree of maturity. National Heart, Lung, and Blood Institute (NHLBI) funding for the first comparison of bypass surgery and angioplasty was finally obtained, and the Emory Angioplasty versus Surgery Trial (EAST) began in 1987 (King 1994). A second multicenter randomized trial, the Bypass Angioplasty Revascularization Investigation (BARI) (the BARI investigators 1996), was also approved by the NHLBI and began 1 year later. The outcomes of these two trials were consistent with other trials (Pocock 1995) confirming the overall equivalence of angioplasty and bypass surgery for patients suitable for angioplasty. However the 5-year outcome of the BARI trial demonstrated a clear advantage for surgery in the subset of patients with DM (the BARI investigators 1997). Cardiac mortality at 5 years was 5.8% in the CABG group and 20.6% in the percutaneous transluminal coronary angioplasty group (*P*=0.0003). A review of the long-term results of the EAST trial showed a similar trend (King III 2000). A meta-analysis of the trials of MVD patients with 5-year follow-up, reported a risk difference for death of 2.3% (*P*=0.025), or, in other words, 2.3 fewer deaths in the surgery group than in the interventional group at 5 years (Hoffman 2003). At 8 years, the risk difference was 3.4 fewer deaths in the surgery group per 100 patients treated. This difference in survival did not become established until after the 3-year of follow-up. In 3 of the trials considered in this meta-analysis the diabetic population was identified. Those trials were the EAST, Coronary Angioplasty versus Bypass Revascularization Investigation (CABRI trial participants, 1995), and BARI studies. The long-term survival in the BARI trial was mainly driven by events occurring during the follow-up period. After myocardial infarction, the patients who had undergone previous bypass surgery had a dramatically lower mortality rate than those treated with angioplasty (relative risk, 0.09; 95% CI, 0.03 to 0.29). This protective effect after myocardial infarction was much more dramatic than the effect in patients who did not have infarction. The differences in completeness of revascularization, re-occlusion of dilated arteries, or progression of disease may all have contributed to the superiority of surgery. To note, the marked benefit seen in diabetic patients was limited to that large majority receiving internal mammary artery grafting to the anterior descending coronary artery. Because internal mammary artery grafts are patent in approximately 90% of the patients in late follow-up, they may serve as a protective conduit to the most important coronary artery. On the contrary, this protection would not be afforded in the angioplasty group, even if restenosis did not occur, because of potential progression of disease or plaque rupture in that proximal or mid anterior descending vessel.

Thus, neither the BARI DM findings nor the resulting Clinical Alert (McGuire 2003), that pointed out the superiority of bypass surgery, had measurable impact on the overall clinical practice patterns because they resulted obsolete before the results were available. Moreover, the results of the BARI trial were not duplicated in the BARI registry (constituted of those patients eligible, but not randomized), where diabetic patients treated by CABG or balloon angioplasty had similar survival rate and cardiac mortality (Detre 1999). These discrepancies might be explained by differences in measured and unmeasured clinical and angiographic characteristics of the patients enrolled in the registry, who underwent revascularization not by randomization but on the basis of the clinical judgment. Therefore, the primacy of surgery in the treatment of diabetic patients with MVD began to be discussed.

3.2 Bare-metal stent vs CABG

Coronary stents represented the most important improvement in the acute outcomes of patients undergoing PCI. This is clearly shown by the comparison between the diabetic patients in the 1985–1986 NHLBI PTCA registry and the contemporary patients in the 1997–2002 NHLBI Dynamic Registry (Srinivas 2002). Stenting was used in 87.5% of the latter registry and in none of the former, and resulted in greater angiographic success (94.8% versus 78.1%), less abrupt closure (0.9% versus 2.2%) and reduction of the hard end points of death (1.9% versus 4.3%), myocardial infarction (1.0% versus 7.4%), and in-hospital CABG surgery (0.8% versus 6.2%). In stent-PCI era, there were no revascularization trials specific to diabetic patients with MVD; however, 4 trials evaluated revascularization strategies using stent compared with CABG in such patients. They were the Arterial Revascularization Therapy Study (ARTS)(Serruys 1999), the Stent or Surgery trial (SOS) (SOS investigators, 2002), the Argentina Randomized Trial of Angioplasty versus Surgery (ERACI II) (Rodriguez 2001, 2003), and the Medicine, Angioplasty, or Surgery Study (MASS II) (Hueb 2004). Each of these was a strategy trial comparing CABG with stent-PCI. The ARTS trial was composed of 1205 patients with MVD randomized to CABG or stenting and followed up for 3 years. Overall survival without stroke or myocardial infarction was 87.2% for PCI and 88.4% for CABG. Repeat revascularization was substantially less than previous balloon angioplasty trials for patients randomized to stenting (21.2% at 1 year and 26.7% at 3 years). In this trial, however, DM was a strong independent predictor of events at 3 years. Among the 208 patients with DM, the ARTS I trial showed that mortality rate was not significantly different between stent-PCI and CABG, and the composite of major adverse events at 1 year was significantly higher in patients randomized to stent-PCI compared to CABG (81.3% versus 52.7%), mainly due to the higher incidence of repeat revascularization, while the incidence of death, myocardial infarction and cerebrovascular events was not different. When the ARTS trial was compared with the BARI trial for 1-year mortality, there was an apparent improvement among diabetic patients treated by stent. The 1-year mortality for diabetic patients in BARI randomized to surgery was 6.4%, compared with ARTS, 3.1%. Likewise, in the BARI PTCA group, the 1-year mortality in diabetic patients was 11.2%, compared with ARTS, 6.3%. A pooled analysis of the 4 stent trials failed to detect a difference at 5-year follow-up between stenting and surgery in diabetic patients with multivessel disease in term of death, myocardial infarction and cerebrovascular events, but an higher rate of repeat revascularization (6.3% CABG versus 25% stent) was observed. Such improvement in outcomes may reflect selection differences between BARI and ARTS or may reflect improving medical management of diabetic patients during the stent era. It should be emphasized that these randomized trials, however, might have introduced several selection bias. Because of the restrictive nature of enrollment, only the 5–12% of the total population was considered eligible for revascularization. Moreover, among the selected individuals, only 20–25% were diabetic; therefore, the results of these trials may not have captured the complex scenario of the impact of the clinical assessment in choosing PCI versus CABG in diabetic patients with MVD. To this regard in the MASS II trial, Pereira et al observed a reduced survival rate in the group randomized to a strategy of revascularization that differed from the choice of the physician (i.e., their physicians would not have chosen PCI or CABG for those patients) (Pereira 2006). They also found that the presence of three-vessel disease was the main predictor of the discordance between the choice of PCI or CABG made by randomization and that selected by physicians. Similarly, comparing the outcome of the BARI eligible diabetic patients with MVD treated by stent-PCI and included in the NHLBI Dynamic Registry with that of the diabetic patients randomized to plain angioplasty in the BARI trial, it is noteworthy that fewer lesions were attempted in the registry group (1.53 versus 2.56), and a dramatic decrease in abrupt closure and in in-hospital bypass graft surgery (1.9% versus 11.2% in BARI) was observed. Moreover the 1-year survival for NHLBI Dynamic Registry patients with characteristics similar to those of the BARI patients was 92.1%, compared to 93.6% and 88.1% of the BARI surgery and BARI PTCA patients respectively. These were not concurrent patient groups and may reflect either the significant differences between randomized and registry patients or the improved medical management of patients in the stent era.

More recently, a study conducted by Hannan and coworkers evaluated patients who underwent revascularization procedures in the New York's cardiac registries, to evaluate the rates of death and subsequent revascularization within three years after the procedure in various groups of patients with multivessel coronary artery disease (Hannan 2005). When the subgroup of patients with DM was analyzed, the adjusted hazard ratios for mortality were still lower after CABG than after stenting in all anatomical subgroups, particularly in the patients who had three-vessel disease and those with involvement of the proximal LAD artery. Restenosis, of course, remained the limiting Achille's heel of the PCI in diabetics. Thus, even in the stent era, although some improvements in PCI outcome were observed, CABG remained the gold standard for diabetics with significant and extensive multi-vessel CAD.

3.3 Drug-eluting stent vs CABG

The introduction of Drug-eluting stents (DES) significantly decreased the need for target-lesion revascularization, successfully addressing the problem of restenosis observed with the bare-metal stents. Two randomized studies, the Diabetes and Sirolimus-Eluting Stent (DIABETES) Trial (Sabaté 2005) and the SCORPIUS (German Multicenter Randomized Single Blind Study of the CYPHER Sirolimus-Eluting Stent in the Treatment of Diabetic Patients with De Novo Native Coronary Artery Lesions) (Baumgart 2007) study, compared clinical outcomes between bare-metal stents and DES in diabetic patients. The DES markedly reduced the rates of repeat revascularization in both studies. A collaborative network meta-analysis compared the risk of revascularization between the two first-generation DES - sirolimus- and paclitaxel-eluting stent - and bare-metal stents in diabetic patients (Stettler 2008). The risk of target-lesion revascularization was reduced by 71% and 62%, respectively, in favour of paclitaxel-eluting stent and sirolimus-eluting stent compared with bare-metal stents in diabetic patients, similarly to the results observed in non-diabetic patients. The absolute reduction in repeat revascularization was more pronounced in diabetic than non-diabetic patients, due to the higher baseline risk of restenosis, so the use of DES should be strongly recommended when PCI is the revascularization choice in diabetic patients. The diabetics in TAXUS IV (Dangas 2004), SIRIUS (the Sirolimus-Eluting Stent in de Novo Native Coronary Lesions trial)(Moses 2003), DECODE (Chan 2008), and DIABETES trials had single digit target lesion revascularization rates (7.8%) with DES versus 24.7% with bare-metal stents (Hillegass 2008). Although a recent meta-analysis of four trials suggested an increased risk of death with sirolimus-eluting stent compared to bare-metal stents in diabetic patients (Spaulding 2007), this finding was not confirmed in a larger analysis of 14 trials (Kastrati 2007). The safety and efficacy of the two first-generation DES in patients with and without DM was also addressed by others (Stettler 2007, 2008). Of note, in trials with less than 6 months duration of clopidogrel therapy, the risk of death associated with sirolimus eluting stents was more than twice the risk associated with bare-metal stents, whereas trials with clopidogrel of 6 months or longer showed no increase in risk with sirolimus eluting stents compared with bare-metal stents. This observation suggests that the above-mentioned increase in the risk of death associated with the use of sirolimus eluting stents in diabetic patients was most likely due to the restricted duration of clopidogrel therapy below 6 months in early trials.

In summary, DES demonstrate to be effective in reducing the need for target lesion revascularization and to have a similar safety profile, with comparable rates of death, cardiac death, and myocardial infarction to bare-metal stents in diabetic patients. But can DES be advocated for the treatment of diabetics with MVD instead of CABG?

Several registries have compared clinical outcome of patients with MVD treated by DES-PCI or CABG. The ARTS II (Serruys 2005) was a non-randomized registry to determine the safety and efficacy of sirolimus-eluting stents in 607 patients with multivessel disease. In order to make the results of this registry as comparable as possible to the randomized ARTS I trial, comparing bare-metal stents with CABG, the same inclusion and exclusion criteria, the same protocol definitions, and the same primary endpoint were chosen. Nevertheless, as compared with ARTS I, patients included into ARTS II had more three-vessel disease, a higher incidence of DM, and were treated with more and longer stents. At 1 year of follow-up, the incidence of repeat revascularization was 8.5% in ARTS II and therefore significantly lower than in the historical bare-metal stents arm of ARTS I (21.3%, RR = 0.44, 95% CI 0.31–0.61), but still higher than in the historical CABG arm of ARTS I (4.2%, RR = 2.03, 95% CI 1.23–3.34). Conversely, the combined endpoint of death, myocardial infarction, or stroke was lower in ARTS II (3.0%) than the CABG-ARTS I group (8.0%, RR = 0.37, 95% CI 0.30–0.51). In a stratified analysis, diabetic patients had a higher rate of major adverse cardiac and cerebrovascular events (MACCE) (15.7% versus 8.5%, RR = 1.85, 95% CI 1.16–2.97, $P = 0.09$) and repeat interventions (13.4% versus 6.8%, RR = 1.97, 95% CI 1.16–3.34, $P < 0.01$) compared with non-diabetic patients. There were no significant differences between ARTS II and the CABG arm of ARTS I in MACCE at 1 year. More recently, the 3-year follow-up data of ARTS II have been reported and compared to the historical groups of ARTS I. Similarly to the 1-year data, MACCE were similar in ARTS II (19.4%) and the CABG arm of ARTS I (16.2%, $P = 0.21$) but they were more frequent in the bare-metal stents arm of ARTS I (34%, $P < 0.001$). Freedom from revascularization remained higher within the CABG arm of ARTS I (93.4%) followed by the DES arm ARTS II (85.5%, $P < 0.001$) and topped in the by the bare-metal stents arm of ARTS I (73.7%, $P < 0.001$). Similarly, the ERACI III study enrolled 225 patients with multivessel disease who were treated with DES and respected the same inclusion and exclusion criteria as the randomized ERACI II trial comparing bare-metal stents with CABG (Rodriguez 2007). The need for repeat revascularization was lowest among patients undergoing CABG in ERACI II (15.4%), followed by DES-treated patients of ERACI III (21.3%) and topped by bare-metal stents -treated patients in ERACI II (38.5%, $P = 0.05$). The results of ARTS II and ERACI III have to be cautiously interpreted in the light of the non-randomized nature of the study. Consistent with that, the registry data of Hannan and colleagues, who assessed the clinical outcome of patients with MVD treated by CABG ($n = 7437$) or DES ($n = 9963$) in the New York State (Hannan 2008) showed that the rates of death (HR = 0.97, 95% CI 0.77–1.20, $P = 0.75$) and death or myocardial infarction (HR = 0.84, 95% CI 0.69–1.01, $P = 0.07$) were similar for diabetic patients irrespective of revascularization strategy. This was in contradiction with the previous report from the same investigators comparing bare-metal stents to CABG, where the latter group was associated with improved survival among diabetic patients with three-vessel disease, showing a potential benefit of DES-PCI over bare-metal stent-PCI.

The UK-based CARDIA (Coronary Artery Revascularization in DM) trial directly compared CABG with PCI (predominant DES use: 71%) in diabetic patients with multivessel disease in a randomized, non-inferiority study. Due to recruitment difficulties, only 510 of 600 planned patients (85%) were randomized (Kapur 2008). The primary endpoint, a composite of death, non-fatal MI, and stroke, assessed at 1 year showed similar outcome for PCI (11.6%) and

CABG (10.2%, $P = 0.63$) with no significant differences in rates of death (PCI: 3.2%, CABG: 3.3%, $P = 0.83$) and myocardial infarction (PCI: 8.4%, CABG: 5.7%, $P = 0.25$), although non-fatal strokes tended to be less common with PCI (0.4%) than CABG (2.5%, $P = 0.09$). Repeat revascularization procedures were more frequent with PCI (9.9%) than CABG (2.0%, $P < 0.001$) at 1-year follow-up. These findings were in line with the subgroup of diabetic patients ($n = 512$ patients) included in the Synergy between Percutaneous Coronary Intervention with Taxus and Cardiac Surgery (SYNTAX) trial (Serruys 2009), a large-scale randomized study (n = 1800 patients) comparing CABG with DES in the treatment of patients with MVD. The composite endpoint of death, MI, and stroke at 1 year was similar for CABG (10.3%) and PCI (10.1%), whereas repeat revascularization was more common with the latter [13.7% subsequent revascularization procedures with an initial strategy of multivessel DES versus 5.9% with CABG (p < 0.001)]. To note, the excess in repeat revascularization was smaller than any prior large randomized trial, in a much more complicated coronary anatomic setting. Moreover, there was a significant interaction between SYNTAX score and treatment group (P = 0.01); patients with low or intermediate scores in the CABG group and in the PCI group had similar rates of major adverse cardiac or cerebrovascular events, whereas among patients with high scores, the event rate was significantly increased in the PCI group. Thus, although PCI did not meet the test of noninferiority against CABG, the creation by the authors of a semiquantitative method (SYNTAX score) to characterize the three vessel disease might help to guide, in daily practice, the "clinical sense" to differentiate between patients and (non randomized) types of revascularization on a case-by-case basis. The prognostic role of the clinical judgment in the selection of the most appropriate strategy of coronary revascularization, already discussed in the plain angioplasty era (BARI registry) and in the bare-metal stent era (MASS II study), was confirmed by others also for DES-PCI (Tarantini 2009). Thus, in this regard, the use of SINTAX score might reduce the gap between the art and the science of the most appropriate coronary revascularization choice, and thus promises to have an important role in clinical practice.

The PCI guidelines have emphasized the long term benefit conferred by CABG in diabetic patients with MVD, but clinician's judgment on the revascularization strategy remains an important factor that is unadjustable by using standard clinical variables. This concept has been captured in the BARI 2D study (aggressive medical therapy versus revascularization)(Frye 2009), and among the diabetic patients with MVD randomized in the revascularization arm, the choice of PCI or CABG was on clinical basis and the anatomical complete revascularization was not required. The predictors for surgical choice was the presence of three vessel disease, proximal left anterior descending artery, total occlusion, complex multiple lesions (Kim 2009). The recent published appropriateness criteria for coronary revascularization (Patel 2009), developed to mimic common situations encountered in everyday practice that includes information on symptom status, extent of medical therapy, risk level as assessed by noninvasive testing, and coronary anatomy, gives to the choice of revascularization by PCI an high level of appropriateness in case of patients with DM and double vessels disease, but an "uncertainty" for diabetic patients with three vessels disease. This means that coronary revascularization may be acceptable and may be a reasonable approach for the indication but with uncertainty implying that more research and/or patient information is needed to further classify the indication .

4. Invasive physiological assessment: the role of fractional flow reserve

In patients with MVD, it is often difficult to determine which lesions are responsible for reversible ischemia. Noninvasive stress tests are often not able to accurately detect and localize ischemia. Therefore, the coronary angiogram is the standard for decision making about revascularization in such patients. In randomized trials evaluating coronary revascularization either by PCI or CABG, as well as in daily practice in most catheterization laboratories, lesions with a diameter stenosis of ≥50% on the angiogram are generally considered for revascularization. Coronary angiography, however, may result in both underestimation and overestimation of a lesion's severity and is often inaccurate in predicting which lesions cause ischemia even for lesions graded 70% to 80%. The fractional flow reserve (FFR) is an accurate and selective index of the physiological significance of a coronary stenosis that can be easily measured during coronary angiography. An FFR value of ≤0.80 identifies ischemia-causing coronary stenoses with an accuracy of >90%. In the randomized FAME (Fractional Flow Reserve Versus Angiography for Multivessel Evaluation) study (Tonino 2009), FFR-guided percutaneous coronary intervention (PCI) with drug-eluting stents was compared with angiography-guided PCI in patients with MVD. The 1-year results of this study showed that FFR guidance of PCI significantly decreased the combined end point of death, myocardial infarction, and repeat revascularization. It is noteworthy that only 46% of the patients with MVD enrolled resulted to have a functional MVD (≥2 coronary arteries with an FFR ≤0.80). This result is consistent with the results of prior studies (Sant'Anna 2007). If we compare the FAME with the SYNTAX study in which PCI was guided by angiography alone, not surprisingly, the clinical outcome was similar to that in the angiography group in the FAME study. In contrast, the clinical outcome in the FFR group in the FAME study was similar to that in the group of patients in SYNTAX who underwent coronary-artery bypass grafting (table 3).

Characteristic	**Angiography--Guided PCI (N = 546)**	**CABG (N = 549)**	**Angiography--Guided PCI (N = 496)**	**FFR--Guided PCI (N = 509)**
Mean age (yr)	65.1	64.5	64.2	64.6
Diabetes (%)	Unknown	Unknown	25.2	24.2
Unstable angina (%)	27.8	27.3	35.8	29.4
Mean EuroSCORE value	3.7	3.7	3.7	3.8
Mean SYNTAX score	14.5	14.5		
Low	17.3	17.3		
Intermediate	27.4	27.5		
High	39.8	41.0		
MACCE (%)				
All patients	19.1	11.2	15.8	11.0
Patients with low SYNTAX score	17.2	14.7		
intermediate SYNTAX score	18.6	10.1		
high SYNTAX score	7.9	6.4		
Death or MI (%)	7.9	6.4	7.9	5.1
Mean hospital stay (days)	3.5	9.3	3.7	3.4

Table 3. Characteristics of Patients and Outcomes in the SYNTAX and FAME Trials.

5. Progression of coronary disease in diabetics: the role of secondary prevention

A pooled analysis of individual patient level data from 4 second-generation stent trials pointed to the impact of progression of disease. Although not specific for diabetic patients, 5-year follow-up documented that late cardiac events were 2-fold related to the progression of the disease instead of restenosis at the originally treated site (Cutlip 2004). Events caused by the treated lesion occurred in 20.3% of the patients, most of them in the first year as result of restenosis. There were very few target lesion–specific events after the first year. Conversely, events related to untreated segments of the coronary tree continued and affected 37.9% of the patients by 5 years. At the end of 5 years, only 8.9% of patients had events limited to restenosis of the target lesion originally treated, whereas 37.9% had events that included nonrestenotic segments. The need to focus on more aggressive long-term prevention was also highlighted by a study from Denmark. A multipronged approach to prevention of vascular disease progression has gained traction in recent years. A small multifactorial intervention study in patients with type 2 DM illustrates this point (Gaede 2003). Patients were randomized to a conventional treatment according to national guidelines of Denmark or to receive intensive behavioral modification and pharmacological therapy targeting hyperglycemia, hypertension, dyslipidemia, and microalbuminuria in addition to aspirin therapy. Hemoglobin A1c values were improved in patients with the intensive therapy, and the end points of cardiovascular death, nonfatal infarction, stroke, revascularization, and amputation were reduced more than 50% (HR, 0.47; 95% CI, 0.24 to 0.73). This data was confirmed also in the more recent Action in DM and Vascular Disease: Preterax and Diamicron Modified Release Controlled Evaluation (ADVANCE) study (Patel 2008) .The profound importance of slowing disease progression, as noted above, is also highlighted by the fact that attempts at secondary prevention efforts in past randomized trials were substandard when judged by contemporary best practice. The average Low Density Lipoprotein (LDL) levels in patients on entry to the BARI trial were virtually identical to those at the end of 5 years: 143 mg% at the beginning and 141 mg% at the end. Although there is no evidence in the BARI trial that there was a specific difference in outcomes between groups who had their lipoprotein profiles improved and those who did not, the above finding is certainly proof that secondary prevention did not approximate the more rigorous clinical standards of contemporary practice. Today, pharmacological antiatherosclerotic intervention in diabetics is directed toward the hyperinsulinemia, hyperglycemia, hypertension, hyperlipidemia, and hypercoagulability that accompany DM. In addition, the Heart Outcomes Prevention Evaluation (HOPE) (Yusuf 2004) revealed that ACE inhibitors can specifically improve vascular outcomes independently of their effect on blood pressure in the diabetic subgroup. Although the United Kingdom DM study, UKDG, indicated that aggressive glycemic control per se did not reduce large-vessel vascular events in that population (UK Prospective Diabetes Study Group 1998), there are other lines of evidence to indicate that aggressive risk factor control directed toward lipids can have positive effects on long-term outcomes. Importantly, in the Scandinavian Simvastatin Survival Study (4S) (The Scandinavian Simvastatin Survival Study Group 1994), diabetics who were placed on statins had atherosclerotic event rates comparable to those of the treated non-diabetic group: a 30% to 40% reduction compared with placebo . Moreover, a subanalysis on diabetic population of the The Lescol Intervention Prevention Study (LIPS) study (Serruys 2002) that was a multinational randomized controlled trial, showed a 51% reduction in the in major adverse cardiac events from the routine use of fluvastatin, compared with controls, in patients undergoing percutaneous coronary intervention (PCI, defined as angioplasty with or without stents). This evidence supports the hypothesis that aggressive risk factor control will favorably influence the long-term outcomes in the diabetic population and assist in eliminating the gap between PCI and CABG patients. In addition, other treatments, including long-term dual antiplatelet therapy with aspirin and clopidogrel, show promise in minimizing atherothrombotic events in the diabetic population. Although they have not been specifically studied in the context of DM and MVD, they also hold the potential to minimize long-term events after successful revascularization.

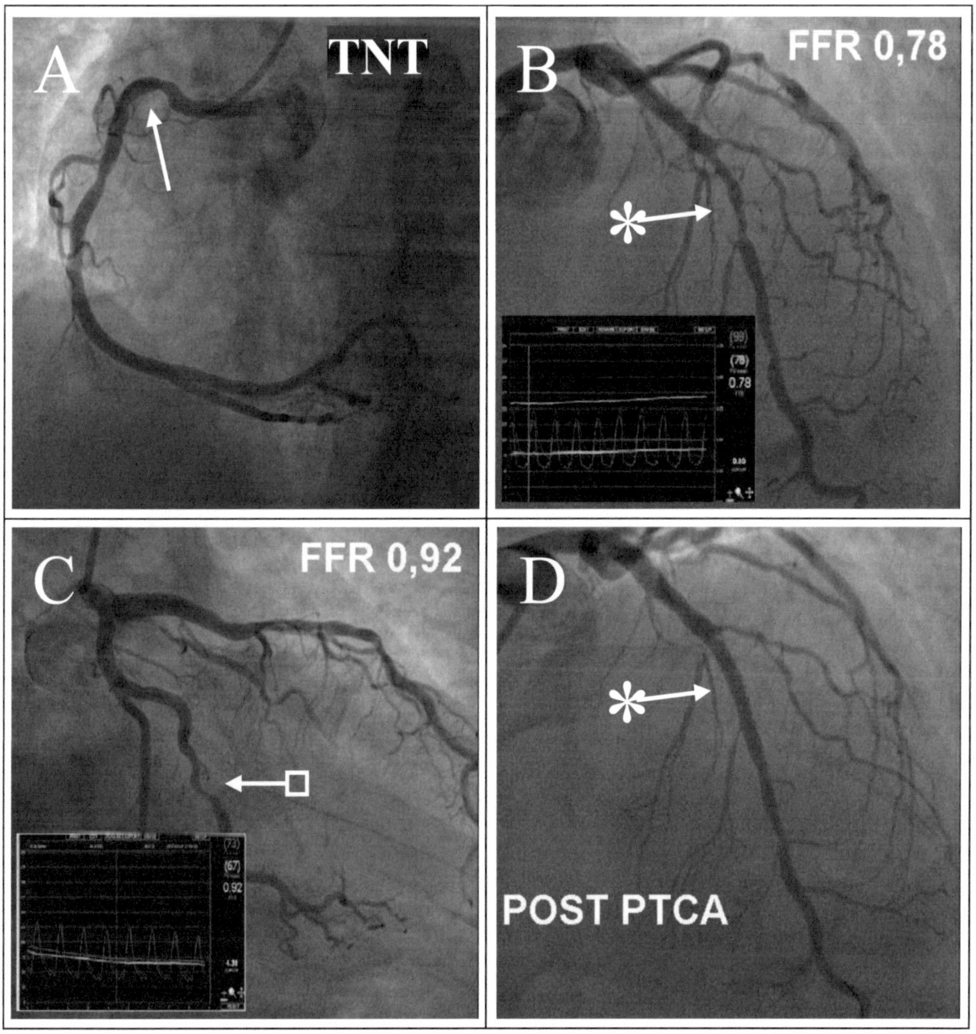

Fig. 2. The right coronary artery stenosis appeared only moderate after intracoronary nitroglicerin bolus **(A, arrow)**. The FFR was below the ischemic threshold of 0.80 **(B, arrow with asterisk)** and was stented with good angiographic result **(D, arrow with asterisk)**. The FFR of the obtuse marginal ramus stenosis was 0,92, so the lesion wasn't treated **(C, arrow with square)**.

6. Clinical case: how did we treat?

The TIMI risk score of the patients was 3 and the syntax score 13. We treated first the culprit lesion on the ramus intermedium. The lesion on the right coronary was only moderate after intracoronary nitroglicerin bolus. Then, we made a FFR estimation of the left descending artery and the obtuse marginal ramus lesions after intracoronary and intravenous infusion of adenosine (see figure 2).

Thereafter, we treated by DES-PCI only the left descending artery lesion, that resulted significant by FFR. The patient was discharged with dual antiplatelet therapy and high dosage of statin with a target of LDL < 70 mg%. At 3-year of follow-up the patients remained asymptomatic and with negative stress test.

7. Conclusions

Compared with non-diabetic, diabetic patients have more extensive atherosclerosis and a worse clinical outcome following revascularization procedures. Notwithstanding, the therapeutic benefit of revascularization is particularly pronounced in this high-risk subgroup of patients. The best strategy of coronary revascularization in diabetic patients depends on the clinical setting and anatomical factors (see figure 3).

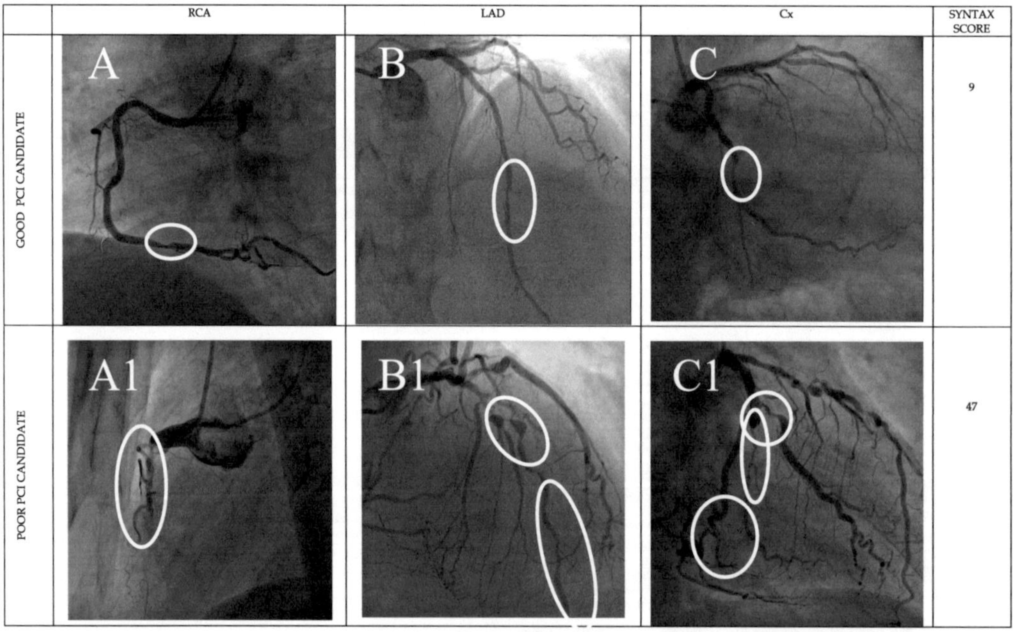

Fig. 3. Upper panel shows images of a good angiographic candidate for PCI: a stenosis on distal right coronary artery **(A)**; a stenosis on mid descending coronary artery **(B)**; a stenosis on the mid circumflex artery **(C)**. Lower panel shows images of a poor angiographic candidate to PCI: Chronic total occlusion of the right coronary artery at the first tract **(A1)**; multiple stenosis of the left descending coronary artery, also involving bifurcations and with dilated tract interposed **(B1)**; multiple stenosis of circumflex artery and its branches **(C1)**. All lesions are indicated with a circle. On the right column, the angiographic syntax score for each patient.

In the acute setting including ST-elevation myocardial infarction and non-ST-elevation myocardial infarction, PCI seems preferable as shown in AWESOME (Angina With Extremely Serious Operative Mortality Evaluation) substudy (Sedlis 2002). In patients with stable coronary artery disease, the extent of disease and non-cardiac morbidity require more careful evaluation. CABG appears more effective in terms of repeat revascularization procedures, particularly in diffuse MVD, while DES-PCI with aggressive pharmacological treatment (i.e. thienopyridines and downstream glycoprotein IIb/IIIa antagonist) is a valuable alternative in patients with less extensive disease (see figure 3).

Although PCI did not meet noninferiority against CABG in diabetic patients with 3-vessel disease, the creation of a semiquantitative method (i.e. SYNTAX score) to better characterize the three vessel disease might help to guide, in daily practice, the "clinical sense" to differentiate between patients and (non randomized) types of revascularization on a case-by-case basis. Moreover, the use of an invasive physiological assessment can add further informations to refine the most appropriate revascularization choice. The FREEDOM (Future REvascularization Evaluation in patients with Diabetes mellitus: Optimal management of Multivessel disease) trial (Farkouh 2008) will randomize more than 2000 diabetic patients with MVD to either multivessel DES-PCI or CABG, so will shed more light on the relative efficacy of CABG and DES-PCI among diabetic patients with three vessel disease. However, while awaiting the results of future trials, please, don't forget that stent will fix the lesion, CABG the vessel, but both won't fix the patient without aggressive medical therapy during the follow-up.

8. References

Baumgart D et al. for the SCORPIUS Study Investigators: One-Year Results of the SCORPIUS Study: A German Multicenter Investigation on the Effectiveness of Sirolimus-Eluting Stents in diabetic patients. J Am Coll Cardiol 2007 50: 1627-1634.

Booth J et al.; SoS Investigators: Randomized, controlled trial of coronary artery bypass surgery versus percutaneous coronary intervention in patients with multivessel coronary artery disease: six-year follow-up from the Stent or Surgery Trial (SoS). Circulation. 2008;118:381-8.

CABRI Trial Participants: First-year results of CABRI (Coronary Angioplasty versus Bypass Revascularisation Investigation). Lancet 1995;346:1179-84.

Chan C et al: A randomized comparison of sirolimus-eluting versus bare metal stents in the treatment of diabetic patients with native coronary artery lesions: the DECODE study. Catheter Cardiovasc Interv. 2008 1;72:591-600.

Cutlip DE et al.: Beyond restenosis: five-year clinical outcomes from second-generation coronary stent trials. Circulation 2004;110:1226 -1230.

Dangas G et al; TAXUS-IV Investigators : Outcomes of paclitaxel-eluting stent implantation in patients with stenosis of the left anterior descending coronary artery. J Am Coll Cardiol. 2005 Apr 19;45:1186-92.

Detre KM et al.: Coronary revascularization in diabetic patients: a comparison of the randomized and observational components of the Bypass Angioplasty Revascularization Investigation (BARI). Circulation. 1999;99:633-40.

Farkouh ME et al. Design of the Future REvascularization Evaluation in patients with Diabetes mellitus: Optimal management of Multivessel disease (FREEDOM) Trial. Am Heart J 2008;155:215-23.

Feit F et al.: Long-term clinical outcome in the Bypass Angioplasty Revascularization Investigation Registry: comparison with the randomized trial. BARI Investigators. Circulation. 2000;101:2795-802.

Freeman AM et al.: Marked improvements in outcomes of contemporary percutaneous coronary intervention in patients with diabetes mellitus. J Interv Cardiol. 2006;19:475-82.

Frye RL et al. BARI 2D Study Group: A randomized trial of therapies for type 2 diabetes and coronary artery disease. N Engl J Med. 2009;360:2503-15.

Gaede P et al.: Multi-factorial intervention and cardiovascular disease in patients with type 2 diabetes. N Engl J Med. 2003;348: 383– 393.

Hannan EL et al.: Drug-Eluting Stents vs. Coronary-Artery Bypass Grafting in Multivessel Coronary Disease. NEJM 2008;358:331-41

Hannan EL et al.: Long-term outcomes of coronary-artery bypass grafting versus stent implantation. N Engl J Med. 2005;352:2174-83.

Hillegass W: Native vessel PCI in the diabetic: DES whenever feasible. Catheterization and Cardiovascular Interventions 2008;72:608–609.

Hoffman SN et al.: A Meta-Analysis of Randomized Controlled Trials Comparing Coronary Artery Bypass Graft With Percutaneous Transluminal Coronary Angioplasty: One- to Eight-Year Outcomes. J Am Coll Cardiol 2003;41:1293–304.

Hueb W et al.: Five-year follow-up of the Medicine, Angioplasty, or Surgery Study (MASS II): a randomized controlled clinical trial of 3 therapeutic strategies for multivessel coronary artery disease. Circulation. 2007;115:1082-9.

Hueb W et al.: The medicine, angioplasty, or surgery study (MASS-II): a randomized, controlled clinical trial of three therapeutic strategies for multivessel coronary artery disease: one-year results. J Am Coll Cardiol. 2004;43:1743-51.

Kapur A et al.: Randomized comparison of percutaneous coronary intervention with coronary artery bypass grafting in diabetic patients. 1-year results of the CARDia (Coronary Artery Revascularization in Diabetes) trial. J Am Coll Cardiol. 2010;55:432-40.

Kapur A et al.: The Coronary Artery Revascularisation in Diabetes (CARDia) trial: background, aims, and design. Am Heart J. 2005;149:13-9.

Kapur A: Coronary artery revascularisation in diabetes. The CARDia trial. European Heart Journal (2008) Hotlines II. Session 1694–1695: ESC, September 1.

Kastrati A et al.: Analysis of 14 trials comparing sirolimus-eluting stents with bare-metal stents. N Engl J Med 2007;356:1030–1039.

Kim LJ et al.: Factors related to the selection of surgical versus percutaneous revascularization in diabetic patients with multivessel coronary artery disease in the BARI 2D (Bypass Angioplasty Revascularization Investigation in Type 2 Diabetes) trial. JACC Intv 2009;2:384-92.

King III SB et al. for the Emory Angioplasty Versus Surgery Trial (EAST) Investigators: Eight-year mortality in the Emory Angioplasty versus Surgery Trial (EAST). J Am Coll Cardiol 2000;35:1116-121.

King SB III et al.: A randomized trial comparing coronary angioplasty with coronary bypass surgery. N Engl J Med 1994;331:1044-1050.

Kip KE et al.: Coronary angioplasty in diabetic patients: the National Heart Lung and Blood Institute Percutaneous Transluminal Coronary Angioplasty Registry. Circulation. 1996;94:1818–1825.

Laskey WK et al.: Comparison of in-hospital and one-year outcomes in patients with and without diabetes mellitus undergoing percutaneous catheter intervention. (From the NHLBI Dynamic Registry). Am J Cardiol. 2002;90:1062–1067.

McGuire DK et al: Influence of the Bypass Angioplasty Revascularization Investigation National Heart, Lung, and Blood Institute Diabetic Clinical Alert on Practice Patterns: Results from the National Cardiovascular Network Database. Circulation 2003;107;1864-1870.

Moses JW et al; SIRIUS investigators: Sirolimus-eluting stents versus standard stents in patients with stenosis in a native coronary artery. N Engl J Med. 2003 Oct 2;349(14):1315-23.

Natali A et al.: Coronary atherosclerosis in Type II diabetes: angiographic findings and clinical outcome. Diabetologia. 2000;43:632-41.

Niles NW et al.; Northern New England Cardiovascular Disease Study Group: Department of Medicine, Dartmouth-Hitchcock Medical Center, Lebanon, New Hampshire 03756, USA. Survival of patients with diabetes and multivessel coronary artery disease after surgical or percutaneous coronary revascularization: results of a large regional prospective study. J Am Coll Cardiol. 2001;37:1008-15.

Patel A et al ADVANCE Collaborative Group.: Intensive blood glucose control and vascular outcomes in patients with type 2 diabetes. N Engl J Med. 2008;358:2560-72.

Patel MR et al: ACCF/SCAI/STS/AATS/AHA/ASNC 2009 Appropriateness Criteria for Coronary Revascularization: A Report by the American College of Cardiology Foundation Appropriateness Criteria Task Force, Society for Cardiovascular Angiography and Interventions, Society of Thoracic Surgeons, American Association for Thoracic Surgery, American Heart Association, and the American Society of Nuclear Cardiology Endorsed by the American Society of Echocardiography, the Heart Failure Society of America, and the Society of Cardiovascular Computed Tomography. J Am Coll Cardiol 2009;53:530-553.

Pereira AC et al.: Clinical Judgment and Treatment Options in Stable Multivessel Coronary Artery Disease: Results From the One-Year Follow-Up of the MASS II(Medicine, Angioplasty, or Surgery Study II). J. Am. Coll. Cardiol. 2006;48;948-953.

Rodriguez A et al.: Argentine Randomized Study: Coronary angioplasty with stenting versus coronary bypass surgery in patients with multiple-vessel disease (ERACI II): 30-day and 1-year follow-up results. ERACI II Investigators. J Am Coll Cardiol 2001; 37: 51-58.

Rodriguez A et al.: Coronary stenting versus coronary bypass surgery in patients with multiple vessel disease and significant proximal LAD stenosis: results from the ERACI II study. Heart 2003;89:184-188.

Rodriguez AE et al.: Late loss of early benefit from drug-eluting stents when compared with bare-metal stents and coronary artery bypass surgery: 3 years follow-up of the ERACI III registry. European Heart Journal 2007;28:2118–2125.

S.J Pocock et al.: Meta-analysis of randomised trials comparing coronary angioplasty with bypass surgery. The Lancet 1995;346:1184-1189.

Sabaté M et al. for the DIABETES Investigators: Randomized Comparison of Sirolimus-Eluting Stent Versus Standard Stent for Percutaneous Coronary Revascularization in diabetic patients: The Diabetes and Sirolimus-Eluting Stent (DIABETES) Trial. Circulation 2005;112:2175-2183.

Sant'Anna FM et al.: Influence of routine assessment of fractional flow reserve on decision making during coronary interventions. Am J Cardiol 2007;99:504-508

Sedlis SP et al. for the Investigators of the Department of Veterans Affairs Cooperative Study#385, the Angina With Extremely Serious Operative Mortality Evaluation (AWESOME). Percutaneous Coronary Intervention Versus Coronary Bypass Graft Surgery for Diabetic Patients With Unstable Angina and Risk Factors for Adverse Outcomes With Bypass Outcome of Diabetic Patients in the AWESOME Randomized Trial and Registry. JACC 2002;40:1555-66.

Serruys PW et al.: Arterial revascularisation therapies study part II - sirolimus-eluting stents for the treatment of patients with multivessel de novo coronary artery lesions, EuroIntervention 2005;1:147–156.

Serruys PW et al.: The ARTS study (Arterial Revascularization Therapies Study). Semin Interv Cardiol. 1999;4:209-19.

Serruys PW et al.; Lescol Intervention Prevention Study (LIPS) Investigators: Fluvastatin for prevention of cardiac events following successful first percutaneous coronary intervention: a randomized controlled trial. JAMA. 2002;287:3215-22.

Serruys PW et al.; SYNTAX Investigators. Percutaneous coronary intervention versus coronary-artery bypass grafting for severe coronary artery disease. N Engl J Med. 2009;360:961-72.

SoS Investigators: Coronary artery bypass surgery versus percutaneous coronary intervention with stent implantation in patients with multivessel coronary artery disease (the Stent or Surgery trial); a randomized controlled trial. Lancet 2002; 360: 965-970.

Spaulding C et al.: A pooled analysis of data comparing sirolimus-eluting stents with bare-metal stents. N Engl J Med 2007;356:989–997.

Srinivas VS et al.: Contemporary percutaneous coronary intervention versus balloon angioplasty for multivessel coronary artery disease: a comparison of the National Heart, Lung and Blood Institute Dynamic Registry and the Bypass Angioplasty Revascularization Investigation (BARI) study. Circulation. 2002;106:1627-33.

Stettler C et al.: Drug eluting and bare metal stents in people with and without diabetes: collaborative network meta-analysis BMJ 2008;337:a1331

Stettler C et al.: Outcomes associated with drug-eluting and bare-metal stents: a collaborative network meta-analysis. Lancet 2007;370:937–948.

Tarantini G et al.: PCI versus CABG for multivessel coronary disease in diabetics. Catheterization and Cardiovascular Interventions 2009;73:50-58.

The BARI investigators: Influence of diabetes on 5-year mortality and morbidity in a randomized trial comparing PTCA and CABG in patients with multivessel disease: the Bypass Angioplasty Revascularization Investigation (BARI). Circulation 1997; 96: 1761-1769.

The Bypass Angioplasty Revascularization Investigation (BARI) Investigators: Comparison of Coronary Bypass Surgery with Angioplasty in Patients with Multivessel Disease. N Engl J Med 1996;335:217-25.

The Scandinavian Simvastatin Survival Study Group: Randomized trial of cholesterol lowering in 4444 patients with coronary heart disease: the Scandinavian Simvastatin Survival Study (4S). Lancet 1994;344:1383-1389

Tonino PA et al.: Fractional flow reserve versus angiography for guiding percutaneous coronary intervention. N Engl J Med 2009;360:213-224.

UK Prospective Diabetes Study Group: Intensive blood-glucose control with sulphonylureas or insulin compared with conventional treatment and risk of complications in patients with type 2 diabetes (UKPDS 33). Lancet 1998;352:837– 853.

Van Belle E et al.: Patency of percutaneous transluminal coronary angioplasty sites at 6-month angiographic follow-up: A key determinant of survival in diabetics after coronary balloon angioplasty. Circulation. 2001;103:1218-24.

Writing Group for the Bypass Angioplasty Revascularization Investigation (BARI) Investigators: Five-year clinical and functional outcome comparing bypass surgery and angioplasty in patients with multivessel coronary disease. A multicenter randomized trial. JAMA. 1997;277:715-21.

Yusuf S et al.: Effects of angiotensin-converting-enzyme inhibitor, ramipril, on cardiovascular events in high-risk patients. The Heart Outcomes Prevention Evaluation Study investigators. N Engl J Med 2000;342:145–153.

12

Diastolic Heart Failure After Cardiac Surgery

Ahmed A. Alsaddique[1], Colin F. Royse[2],
Mohammed A. Fouda[3] and Alistair G. Royse[4]
[1]*Professor of Cardiac Surgery King Fahad Cardiac Center,*
College of Medicine, King Saud University, Riyadh,
[2]*Professor of Anaesthesia and Pain Management Unit*
Department of Pharmacology, University of Melbourne
[3]*Professor of Cardiac Surgery King Fahad Cardiac Center,*
College of Medicine, King Saud University, Riyadh,
[4]*Associate Prof Department of Cardiac Surgery,*
The Royal Melbourne Hospital, Parkville,
[1,3]*Saudi Arabia*
[2,4]*Australia*

1. Introduction

It appears that for some time diastole was taken for granted and largely ignored. Systole was thought of as the only function that truly predicted cardiac risk. The fact that diastolic heart failure (DHF) was referred to at one point as "heart failure with normal ejection fraction (EF)" lends credence to this assumption. It has been proven since that cardiac relaxation is an active energy-dependent process that begins in late systole and extends into early or mid-diastole (Shah & Pai, 1992). The fact that diastolic dysfunction contributes to up to half of the cases of heart failure dispelled the myth that systolic function is the only factor to consider in cardiac risk assessments (Bhatia etal., 2006, Owan etal., 2006, Vasan etal., 1995). Cardiologists are ahead of surgeons in recognizing the importance of diastolic function in clinical practice. They have noticed that changes in diastolic filling pattern are of a prognostic value following myocardial infarction. Left ventricular remodeling following acute myocardial infarction (AMI) is a well known phenomenon occurring in the earliest post infarction phase and continuing for weeks or months. A restrictive transmitral filling pattern which is a marker of diastolic dysfunction provides significant information in these patients. A short initial deceleration time (DT) < 150 ms obtained as early as 1 day after AMI can identify patients who are likely to undergo LV remodeling in the following year (Otasević ,2001). Remodeling is a precursor of heart failure and a strong predictor of mortality. Therefore, an early restrictive filling pattern as evidenced by a short DT identifies patients who are likely to develop progressive LV dilation and dysfunction. Persistence of a restrictive filling pattern is the most powerful independent predictor of severe dilation and late mortality (Temporelli etal, ,2004, Whalley etal, 2006). The importance of diastolic dysfunction to the surgeon became apparent when it was established that it is a predictor of difficult weaning off cardiopulmonary bypass and mortality (Bernard etal, 2001, Salem etal,

2006). Finally, the impact of diastolic dysfunction affects the anesthesiologist as these patients may tolerate acute preload reduction with induction of anesthesia poorly leading to low cardiac output and hypotension. This patient population presents difficult anesthetic challenges and places these patients at high risk of perioperative morbidity and mortality (Couture etal, 2009 Sanders etal, 2009). In short, diastolic dysfunction has touched every facet of clinical practice. This chapter will predominantly focus on DHF (with normal EF) as distinct to the combined systolic and diastolic failure.

2. Clinical spectrum

Diastolic dysfunction can be defined as the inability of the left ventricle to adequately fill at low or normal atrial pressures unrelated to intrinsic valve disease or pericardial pathology. This dysfunction can result either from an impairment in LV compliance (passive mechanism) or from an alteration in LV relaxation (active process).

Since not all patients who undergo heart surgery have a normal EF, the classical definition of DHF of heart failure with normal EF does not always apply. It is therefore necessary not to overlook the status of the preoperative EF when assessing the DHF in the postoperative heart. With this understanding DHF in the postoperative state is better defined as a clinical syndrome of heart failure with a preserved left ventricular EF in the absence of major valve disease or pericardial pathology (Vasan & Levy, 2000 Vasan, 2003). It is associated with abnormalities of diastolic distensibility, filling, or relaxation of the left ventricle (Gaasch & Zile, 2004) clinically; DHF is usually accompanied by severe reduction of exercise capacity, neuroendocrine activation, and poor quality of life. Typically the ventricle has thick walls and a small cavity (increased left ventricular mass/volume ratio) (Kitzman etal, 2000). In contrast to systolic heart failure, DHF affects women more frequently. DHF can occur alone or in combination with systolic heart failure. In isolated DHF (characterized as a small stiff heart), the only abnormality in the pressure-volume relationship occurs during diastole, when there are increased diastolic pressures with a low end diastolic volume. In systolic heart failure, the abnormalities in the pressure-volume relationship during systole include decreased EF, stroke volume and stroke work. If there are in addition, changes in the diastolic portion of the pressure-volume relationship that leads to increased diastolic pressures, the implication then is that there is both systolic and diastolic cardiac failure (Zile &, Brutsaert , 2002; Deswal, 2005; Burkhoff etal. 2003).These concepts are depicted in Figure 1, using simplified pressure-volume loops, and showing the left ventricular end-diastolic pressure-volume curves. The normal left ventricle is shown with (LVEDP) < 16 mmHg. For DHF, the loop is smaller indicating reduced stroke volume, and shifted up and to the left, with LVEDP > 16 mmHg. It is important to note, that the end-diastolic volume in DHF is at the lower range of normal. In contrast, the end-diastolic volume in patients with systolic failure is increased.

3. Mechanics of diastole

Ventricular relaxation is an active energy-dependent process that begins in late systole and extends into early or mid-diastole (van Kraaij et al.2003). Relaxation can be defined as the time period during which the myocardium loses its ability to generate force and further shortening, and returns to an unstressed length and force (Zile &, Brutsaert, 2002) Diastole begins at the closure of the aortic valve and lasts until closure of the mitral valve

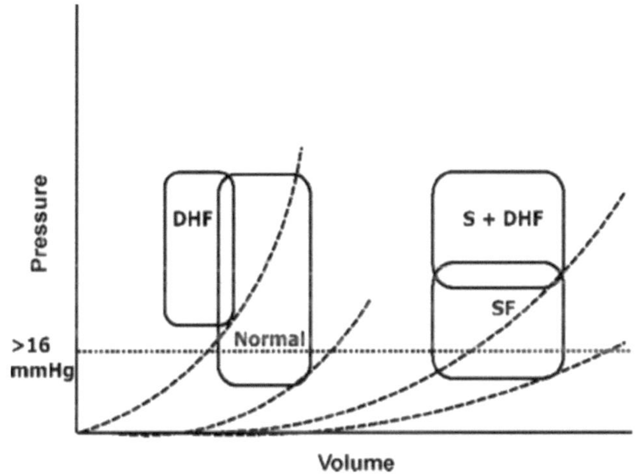

Fig. 1. Pressure–volume loop diagram indicating the position of the end-diastolic pressure–volume on curve for DHF; normal diastolic function (Normal); systolic failure (SF), and systolic and diastolic failure (S+DHF). A horizontal dashed line at >16 mmHg indicates division between normal and raised end-diastolic pressure. Adapted with permission from Elsevier Publishing (Alsaddique etal 2009]

(Kawaguchi et al, 2003). Broadly speaking, diastole can be looked at as two phases; isovolumetric relaxation corresponds to LV pressure decline at constant volume, that lasts from the closure of the aortic valve to opening of the mitral valve. The second phase is auxotonic relaxation corresponding to LV filling lasting until closure of the mitral valve. LV filling depends mainly on the pressure gradient between the LA and LV which is influenced by ventricular compliance, active relaxation, and augmented by atrial contraction towards end-diastole. Traditionally however, diastole is divided into four distinct phases: isovolumetric relaxation, early rapid ventricular filling, diastasis and atrial systole. The isovolumic relaxation time is a continuum of systole and is dependent on it. The early rapid ventricular filling phase is dependent on LV relaxation and compliance. Diastasis is dependent on both the heart rate and chamber compliance. The atrial contraction depends on the chamber compliance, left atrial (LA) function and the conduction system of the heart. At the cellular level, diastole begins when adenosine triphosphate hydrolyzes and actin-myosin cross bridges unlink, leading to sarcomeric relaxation. This is related to decreases in cytoplasmic Ca^{2+} and the subsequent dissociation of Ca^{2+} from troponin C. The majority of cytosolic Ca^{2+} is actively resequestered into the sarcoplasmic reticulum via the sarcoplasmic reticulum Ca^{2+}ATPase (SERCA2). The remaining cytosolic calcium is removed by the sarcolemmal sodium calcium exchanger and other mechanisms (Groban, 2005). Diastolic function depends on the passive elastic recoil properties of the LV as well as active relaxation. Impaired active myocardial relaxation causes a slow decline in the left ventricular intracavity pressure. The mitral valve opens later, as left atrial filling needs to increase in order to provide a positive gradient across the mitral valve. In severe cases, an increased left atrial pressure state is developed so as to exceed the (increased) left ventricular intracavity pressure (Aurigemma & Gaasch , 2004). An increase in passive chamber compliance can also produce the same pattern and result in elevated LVEDP, thereby necessitating an increased left atrial pressure to provide a driving gradient (Zile et al, 2004). The mechanisms that cause diastolic dysfunction are multifactorial (Kiss etal, 2004). However, they can be broadly categorized as intrinsic (that is affecting the ventricular muscle) or extrinsic (any process that can cause external compression of the left ventricle). A summary of these causes is shown in Table 1. Whilst many of these causes are not reversible in the short term, it is important for clinicians to understand potentially reversible causes so that they can be readily identified and treated. An example of extrinsic pathology is a distended abdomen caused by dilated stomach and bowels actively pushing on the diaphragm, compressing the heart and interfering with cardiac filling, thereby leading to or exacerbating the development of DHF. The major factors that affect diastolic function are ventricular relaxation and compliance. Other factors that influence diastolic function to a lesser degree include systolic function, left atrial pressure, the pericardium, and intrathoracic pressure (Wu &Yu , 2005). In diastolic dysfunction relaxation abnormalities appear early and the inability of the left ventricle to fill in early diastole significantly affect the rapid filling phase resulting in a compensatory increase in filling with atrial contraction. The other factor that determines LV filling is chamber compliance (distensibility of the ventricles), defined as the change in volume over the change in pressure (dV/dP). It can be derived using the relationship between changes in end diastolic pressure (EDP) and end diastolic volume (EDV) by using the formula:

$$\text{Compliance} = \Delta\,\text{EDV} \,/\, \Delta\,\text{EDP}$$ (Gilbert &,Glantz, 1989; Lewis &, Gotsman, 1976)

When ventricular compliance begins to decrease the EDP rises, but the EDV remains unchanged. The increase in EDP reduces the pressure gradient across the mitral valve leading to reduced ventricular filling culminating in decreased cardiac output. Diastolic relaxation is more sensitive to ischemia than systolic contraction, and may lead to subtle relaxation abnormalities without systolic impairment (Garcia-Fernandez etal, 1999). In coronary artery disease, ventricular relaxation as reflected in the early diastolic filling rate may be impaired at rest.

4. Contributing factors

Primary diastolic failure is typically seen in patients with hypertensive or valvular heart disease as well as in hypertrophic or restrictive cardiomyopathy but can also occur in a variety of other clinical situations. The main risk factors for this form of heart failure are advancing age, hypertension, and diabetes mellitus (- Zile & Gaasch 2001). There is a high incidence of diastolic dysfunction among normotensive patients with diabetes mellitus (Boyer etal, 2004). Increased matrix collagen, interstitial fibrosis, myocardial microangiopathy, and myocytes hypertrophy are common findings in the diabetic heart that can lead to diastolic dysfunction. Tight glycemic control decreases the risk of heart failure in patients with diabetes (Iribarren etal, 2001; Liu etal, 2001).The defect in DHF is a combination of impaired ventricular relaxation and a decrease in passive ventricular distensibility (Aurigemma & Gaasch, 2004; Zile etal, 2004). The low cardiac output associated with DHF is due to inadequate ventricular filling, not impaired systolic contraction, and is an important point to remember when managing these patients. LV filling depends mainly on the pressure gradient between the LA and LV which is influenced by compliance, active relaxation, and at end diastole by atrial contraction (Appleton etal, 2000). There are number of predisposing factors that can contribute to DHF in the postoperative cardiac surgical patient. The mechanisms by which these factors exert their

Intrinsic causes	
Cause	**Comment**
Delay in active relaxation	Any cause that interferes with myofilament cross-bridge detachment. Includes poor calcium sequestration, abnormal calcium sensitivity, myocardial ischemia, abnormal sodium/calcium exchanger or alteration in the myocyte calcium-handling proteins
Abnormal "cardiac spring"	During contraction, molecular springs such as Titan molecules are compressed, and during diastole contribute to chamber expansion via mechanical elastic recoil. Abnormalities of these molecules may cause diastolic heart failure. It also underlines the importance of systolic function in early diastolic recoil.
Myocardial fibrosis	Abnormalities of collagen, or other infiltrative processes (such as amyloid), may increase ventricular wall stiffness by a variety of mechanisms
Left ventricular hypertrophy	This is associated but not necessarily causative of diastolic dysfunction. Chronic increased load such as hypertension or aortic stenosis may also cause changes in collagen composition.
Acute myocardial ischemia	Active relaxation is highly energy dependent, and acute myocardial ischemia will lead to (reversible) diastolic dysfunction
Extrinsic causes	
Right ventricle pressure or volume overload	The right ventricle physically compresses the left ventricle. In severe cases, the left ventricle becomes D-shaped rather than O-shaped. Any course of pressure or volume overload, including pulmonary hypertension will exacerbate left-sided diastolic dysfunction.
Pericardium	Pericardial fluid or restrictive pericardial disease will limit ventricular filling or physically compress the left ventricle.
Pleural fluid	A large pleural effusion may compress the heart
Hyper inflated lungs	Pressure from the lungs is transmitted via the pericardium to the heart. Severe lung hyperinflation mimics pericardial tamponade. High levels of PEEP are similar.
Distended abdomen	Fluid, fat, or gaseous distension can cause myocardial compression, particularly in the supine patient

Table 1. Causes of diastolic dysfunction

effect are briefly explained. Atrial fibrillation is a common occurrence in the postoperative period. It causes loss of atrial contraction that results in impaired diastolic filling. Myocardial hypertrophy is another predisposing factor found in some of the valvular lesions and in hypertensive patients. Its presence interferes with the passive late phase of diastolic filling of the LV contributing to diastolic dysfunction. Myocardial ischemia in the postoperative cardiac surgical patient significantly slows active myocardial relaxation during early diastole. It may also lead to rhythm disturbances that will further aggravate LV diastolic dysfunction. Tachyarrhythmias impair LV filling by shortening the diastolic phase of the cardiac cycle resulting in impaired LV filling (- Zile & Brutsaert, **2002).** The effect of positive pressure ventilation (to which virtually all of open heart surgery patients are subjected to postoperatively) on cardiac performance is complex involving changes in preload and afterload for both right and left ventricles. Positive pressure ventilation can lower ventricular filling, and may also reduce afterload, enhancing ventricular emptying during systole. The effect on cardiac output depends on whether the effect on preload or afterload predominates. If the patient is normovolemic and intrathoracic pressure are within normal the effect on afterload reduction predominates resulting in an increase in the cardiac output. The increase in stroke volume leads to increase in systolic blood pressure during lung inflation results in a phenomenon known as reverse pulsus paradoxus. The beneficial effects of positive pressure ventilation on cardiac output are reversed by hypovolemia leading to decreased cardiac output and hypotension (Pinsky , 2005 2007)]. Pericardial constriction or tamponade causes increased resistance to diastolic filling and physiologically is "acute severe extrinsic diastolic failure" whereby the heart becomes physically compressed by the pericardial effusion. Renal insufficiency results in volume overload that leads to a slowing of myocardial relaxation potentially contributing to DHF (Tsuyuk etal, 2001). Chronic anemia is usually accompanied by an increase in cardiac mass due to volume overload. In the animal model, chronic anemia resulted in increased left ventricular end-diastolic pressure and decreased functional reserve which in turn can lead to diastolic dysfunction. It can also lead to tachycardia that it turn shortens diastole resulting in diastolic dysfunction. The anemia that is seen in the postoperative period due to excessive postoperative blood loss is transient, acute and is often rapidly corrected in these patients leading to very little if any effect on the diastolic function (Rakusan, etal **2001)**. Chronically uncontrolled hypertension is by far the most common predisposing factor in for DHF. It can lead to DHF through a number of ways; one of them is by causing LV hypertrophy that can results in a delayed LV relaxation with all its attendant effects on diastolic filling. The other mechanism is related to a reduced arterial compliance that can also contribute to diastolic dysfunction (Mottram etal, 2005). Hypertension that is seen at times in the postoperative period is usually transient is quickly managed and therefore does not pose the same risk of the more common form of hypertension. At times one may need to pace the heart in the post operative period; as most pacing wires placed at surgery are ventricular, pacing under these circumstances would affect diastolic filling bringing about diastolic dysfunction or could even trigger DHF in some instances. This is largely due to the loss of the atrial contribution to LV filling (Alsaddique, 2008). It is therefore better to keep this possibility in mind and make the extra effort of placing both atrial and ventricular wires for sequential pacing. There seems to be some evidence that Nitric Oxide (NO) metabolism plays a role in acute diastolic dysfunction following episodes of ischemia and reperfusion. It is thought that NO could have a beneficial role as pretreatment with cyclic guanosine monophosphate (cGMP) donors, or with NO donors protects myocytes from relaxation failure in animal models (Schlüter etal, 1994; Draper & Shah, 1997; du Toit etal, 1998).

5. Assessment of diastolic function

5.1 Echocardiography evaluation

Transthoracic echocardiography (TTE) or transesophageal echocardiography (TEE) play a major role in the assessment of diastolic function. A combination of 2-dimensional echocardiography, pulsed wave Doppler, Color M-mode (CMM) and Tissue Doppler imaging (TDI) are used in combination to categorize the grade of diastolic dysfunciton.

2-D echocardiography is used to assess ventricular dimensions, LV mass, EF and LA size. Pulsed wave Poppler (PWD) measures the velocity of blood at the cursor position. The mitral inflow Doppler spectral display is composed of an E (early) wave for passive diastolic filling followed by an A (atrial) wave for atrial systole. Mitral blood flow is affected by LV relaxation, LV compliance, and the LA-LV pressure gradient. PWD is used to assess transmitral flow velocity recording and pulmonary vein flow velocity variables in the evaluation of diastolic dysfunction (Hunt etal, 2001; Vasan & Levy, 2000). The four useful variables from mitral flow are: peak early diastolic transmitral flow velocity (E), peak late diastolic transmitral flow velocity (A), early filling deceleration time (DT) and A wave duration [Adur] (Myśliński etal, 2002; Appleton etal, 1988). A normal E/A ratio is considered to be between 0.75 and 1.5. Early filling DT reflects LV compliance in early diastole. The normal DT is usually less than 200 milliseconds in young patients and may exceed 200 ms in patients over 60 years of age (Garcia etal, 1998). Pulmonary venous (PV) flow is composed of systolic and diastolic waves, and an atrial contraction reversal wave. The normal patterns is systolic predominance, but this is reversed when the LAP is elevated. In high LAP, the atrial reversal wave increased in duration such that it exceeds the mitral A wave duration. The major problem with the use of PV flow variables is the difficulty in obtaining adequate measurement when using TTE. The Doppler flow parameters are influenced by a variety of factors including altered loading conditions and heart rate, and not all patients "fit the pattern" (Appleton etal, 2001; Pirracchio etal, 2007). In the operative and critical care settings, the loading conditions and heart rates change frequently, and the patterns may alter without significant change in chamber compliance. Therefore, the results from these measurements may be inconsistent and accordingly inconclusive in the postoperative cardiac surgical patient. Color M-mode (CMM) Doppler flow propagation velocity (Vp) is an easily obtained diastolic index. It displays velocity information a long a line that extends from the mitral valve to the LV apex, providing superior temporal resolution (5 milliseconds), spatial resolution (1mm) and velocity resolution (5 cm/s). The commonly used variable for CMM Doppler is the Vp into the LV which is the velocity at which the blood travels from the mitral valve to the LV apex. In sinus rhythm CMM is characterized by 2 distinct waves, one corresponds to the E wave and the second one to the A wave.

Vp relates well to LV relaxation and is claimed to be relatively load independent. A Vp value of less than 45 cm / s is consistent with diastolic dysfunction in patients older than 30 years of age < 55 cm/s in patients less than 30 years of age (Onose etal, 1999; Dumesnil etal, 1991). However, a major limitation of Vp is that it is heart rate dependent and in the perioperative setting, heart rate changes frequently.

Tissue Doppler imaging (TDI) is an ultrasound imaging modality that directly measures myocardial velocity during the cardiac cycle and allows wall movement to be directly analyzed (Vitarelli &, Gheorghiade, 1998; Dokainish, 2004). The myocardial portion commonly studied is above the mitral annulus at either the septal or lateral walls. Three wave forms are described, Peak systolic wave, early diastolic wave (Ea) and the end diastolic wave (a') related to the atrial contraction. The Ea wave is relatively independent of loading state and is used to assess LV relaxation, a cut off of 8 cm /s for septal Ea or < 10 cm/s for lateral wall Ea measurement is now widely accepted as a sign of diastolic dysfunction (Sohn etal, 1997). It is easy to perform and available in the majority of patients even if the 2-D imaging is poor, and holds promise as a method to quantify change in diastolic function. When measuring TDI, Khouri and associates measure only early diastolic myocardial velocity (e') at the lateral corner of the mitral annulus, because it has been noted that the lateral annular velocity is more reproducible than the septal annular velocity (Khouri etal, 2004). Figure 2 reveals Echocardiographic findings typical of DHF pattern. Transthoracic echocardiography (TTE) is not always possible in the postoperative situation, due to hemodynamic instability, mediastinal air, the close proximity to a fresh surgical wound, presence of drains and dressings, or due to the inability to position the patient in an optimum way. In addition, mechanical ventilation with high positive end-expiratory pressure, pacing wires, ECG leads further add to the obstacles for the desired examination window resulting in a poor image quality.

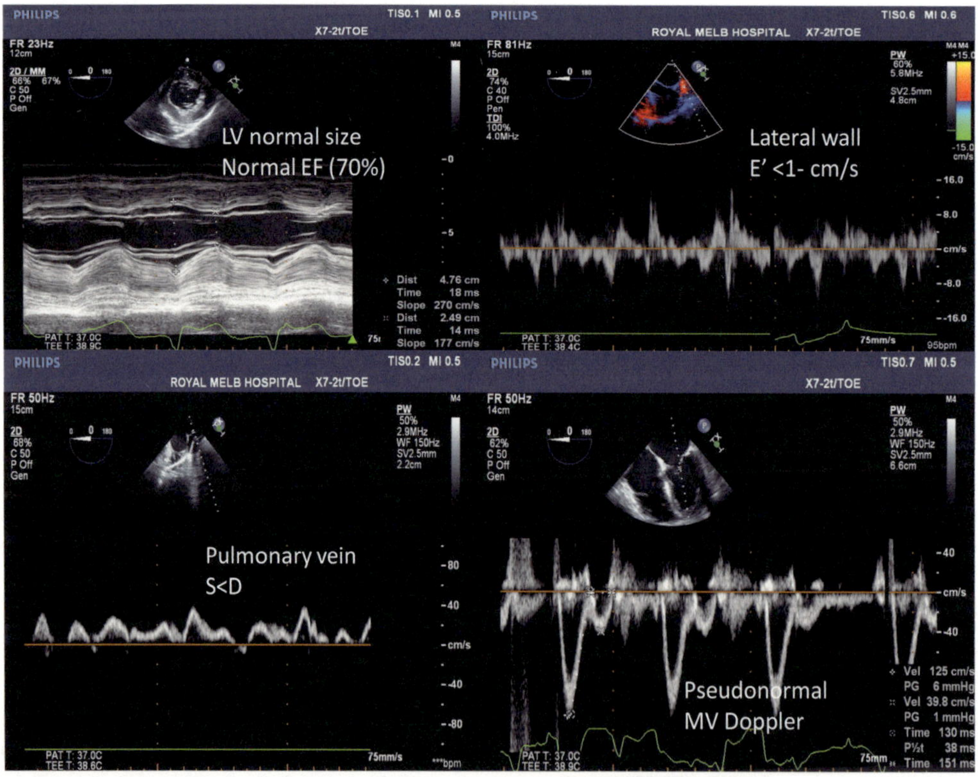

Fig. 2 Typical diastolic failure (small stiff heart) typically Grade 2 American Society of Echocardiography (ASE).
This is a common pattern in the periopertive setting. Typically Cardiac Index (CI) 1.8-2.2 l/min/m^2 Pulmonary Artery Wedge Pressur(PCWP) > 15 mmHg

5.2 Use of Transesophageal Echocardiography (TEE)

TEE has a well established role in cardiac surgery as it has proved to be a valuable tool for intraoperative decisions particularly in valve surgery (Eltzschig etal, 2008). In addition, it has also proved to be useful in the field of intensive care for the assessment of hemodynamics and to track its variations after therapeutic interventions. Repeated measurements of left ventricular end-diastolic dimension are recommended in order to accurately track the hemodynamic changes, as a single determination is not felt to be reliable. TEE can adequately assess right ventricular function and left ventricular filling pressure using combined Doppler modalities (Vignon, 2005). The same parameters that are described for assessing diastolic function utilizing TTE can be achieved using TEE (Groban& Dolinski , 2005; Klein etal, 1999) though caution should be exercised as many of the Doppler parameters have not been extensively validated in sedated and ventilated patients.

5.3 Identifying a high left atrial pressure

A simple way to conceptualize diastolic failure is to recognize that if high left atrial pressure is present, then clinically important diastolic failure is present, as the body has had to adapt to a stiff ventricle by raising the LAP sufficient to provide an adequate transmitral driving gradient to fill the LV. Figure 3 High LAP can be diagnosed by invasive monitoring (such as a pulmonary artery catheter), or non-invasively with TTE or TEE. A simple pattern that can be easily recognized is that of a tense left atrium, evident by a fixed curve of the interatrial septum pointing from the left to the right atria. When the LAP is normal, the interatrial septum changes direction to point to the left atrium during mid-systole. Once a high LAP is detected, then echocardiography is focused on the chamber dimensions and EF to determine if it is DHF (small LV with normal EF), or systolic and diastolic failure (large heart with reduced EF).

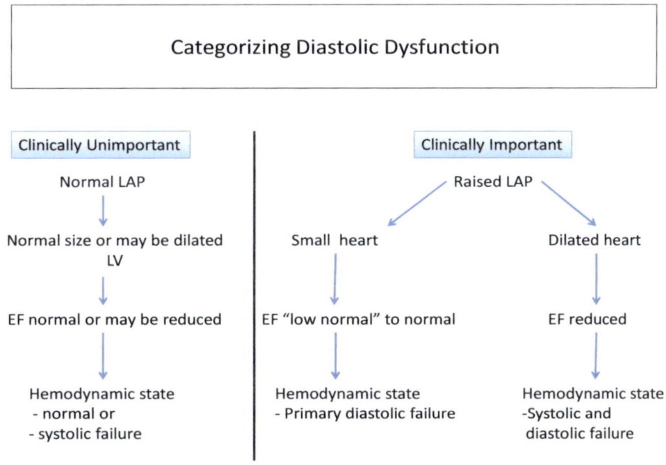

Fig. 3. Flow chart to categorize diastolic dysfunction. Clinically important diastolic failure is associated with raised left atrial pressure. Diastolic dysfunction with normal left atrial pressure does not usually affect hemodynamic stability.The key is to identify high LAP and then identify if the LV volume is small to normal or dilated, in order to differentiate primary diastolic failure form systolic and diastolic failure.

5.4 Natriuretic peptides

B-type Natriuretic peptide (BNP) is a marker of systolic left ventricular dysfunction and heart failure. It however increases in subjects with diastolic dysfunction (mean 20.3+/-4.7 pg/ml vs. control 9.6+/-0.5 pg/ml, $p<0.001$). A normal BNP level virtually excluded the presence of diastolic dysfunction and concomitant left ventricular hypertrophy (LVH). Increased BNP concentrations in subjects with diastolic dysfunction are strongly related to LVH (Lukowicz etal, 2005).] In patients with normal systolic function, elevated BNP levels and diastolic filling abnormalities might help to reinforce the diagnosis diastolic dysfunction (Lubien etal, 2002; Krishnaswamy etal, 2001) A-type atrial, natriuretic peptide (ANP) is secreted from the atria in response to dilatation. Brain-type (B-type) natriuretic peptide (BNP) is a neurohormone that is released by the cardiac myocytes when left ventricular wall stress increases. After secretion the pro-hormone is cleaved to the biologically active hormone (BNP) and an inactive N-terminal fragment (N-BNP) Plasma levels of BNP increase in direct relation to increase in ventricular end-diastolic volume and end-diastolic pressure of both right and left side(Stewart, 2005). A rise in BNP produces vasodilatation and increase in renal sodium excretion (Maisel etal, 2002). Atrial natriuretic peptide and brain natriuretic peptide are known to be indices for heart failure. Postoperative ANP plateaus on the third postoperative day and decreases gradually down to the preoperative level by one month Postoperative BNP plateaus, showing very slow decrease and it never returning to the preoperative level (Song etal, 2004; Bail etal, 2004)]. This pattern of changes in the BNP and ANP levels after cardiac surgery makes it rather impractical to use them as markers for heart failure in the immediate postoperative setting of these patients.

5.5 Cardiac catheterization

The characteristic finding of DHF is an elevated left ventricular end diastolic pressure (LVEDP) over 16 mm Hg in the presence of a normal LV chamber size (van Heerebeek etal 2006; Kitzman etal, 2002) Vasan and Levy recommended cardiac catheterization as a prerequisite for making the diagnosis of a definite DHF (Vasan & Levy 2000). In the post-operative setting of a fresh open heart surgery cardiac, catheterization is probably not warranted and the diagnosis can be made by less invasive means.

5.6 Multidetector CT (MDCT) of the heart

Cardiac MDCT is most commonly performed for the purpose of noninvasive cardiac angiography. Image data are acquired continuously during a single breath-hold scan, typically 10 to 15 seconds in duration. Contrast is required for angiography and for endocardial border definition, with typical doses in the range of 60 to 80 mL per scan, quite comparable to a diagnostic cardiac catheterization. Patients with cardiomyopathies of all etiologies represent a large and growing population that stands to benefit from advanced imaging techniques (Sibley & Lima, 2008). Electron-beam computed tomography (EBCT) has been shown to be a reliable tool for the assessment of ventricular diastolic function and to detect constrictive filling pattern (Kloeters etal, 2008; Rumberger, 2000). These tools cannot be utilized in the assessment of the post operative heart for logistical reasons

5.7 Cardiac magnetic resonance

Cardiac magnetic resonance (CMR) is the latest addition to the diagnostic tools. The specific advantage of cardiac magnetic resonance (CMR) over echocardiography is the possibility to acquire images in any selected plane or along any selected axis. A routine CMR examination in the setting of heart failure will acquire short access images covering the entire heart from base to apex in addition, to the long access slices. It can also provide a range of LV filling parameters almost similar to those obtained by echocardiography (Rademakers & Bogaert , 2006; Hauser etal, 2004) . CMR is considered as a valid alternative for echocardiography when an adequate echocardiographic assessment cannot be obtained. It is the diagnostic modality of choice for assessing small changes in LA or LV volumes and in LV mass (Rademakers, 2003). Clinical use of CMR is expanding and starting to address diastolic LV dysfunction. It is not of course practical to obtain CMR in the fresh postoperative cardiac surgical patient suspected to have DHF.

6. Diagnosis of DHF in postoperative heart

In an ICU environment, the diagnostic criteria are usually based on invasive hemodynamic measurements. As ventricular compliance begins to decrease, the end-diastolic pressure (EDP) rises but the end-diastolic volume (EDV) remains unchanged. The increase in EDP reduces the pressure gradient necessary for ventricular filling and this eventually leads to a lower EDV resulting in a decrease in cardiac output via the Frank-Starling mechanism. The usual method of assessing cardiac failure by the relationship between ventricular filling pressure and stroke volume does not distinguish between systolic and DHF. The end-diastolic pressure (EDP) is elevated in both types of heart failure. The end-diastolic volume (EDV) is increased in systolic heart failure and is decreased in DHF thus it is the parameter that will distinguish systolic from DHF (Aurigemma & Gaasch, 2004). The measurement that is most often utilized to distinguish between diastolic and systolic heart failure is the EF. The EF is normal or near normal in patients with DHF and is reduced in systolic heart failure.

Pulmonary artery catheter with a fast response thermistor can measure the EF of the right ventricle. These catheters are able to register the temperature (T) changes during each cardiac cycle. The change in temperature is due to dilution of the indicator fluid by venous blood that fills the ventricle during diastole. The amount of blood that fills the ventricle during diastole is equal to the stroke volume, the temperature differences between each plateau on the curve (T_1 - T_2) is the thermal equivalent of the stroke volume (SV) (Figure 4). Temperature T_1 is the thermal marker for end-diastolic volume (EDV). The EF becomes equivalent to the ratio $T_1 - T_2 / T_1$ or [SV/EDV] (Spinale etal, 1990,1991). Once the EF is measured the stroke volume can be calculated by dividing the cardiac output by heart rate. The EDV can be determined by rearranging the EF formula EDV = SV/ EF. The normal RV Right ventricular (RV) EF using thermodilution method is 0.45 to 0.50 which is about 10% lower than the EF measured by radionuclide imaging (Kay etal, 1983). The accepted normal for RVEDV is [80 to 140ml/m^2] (Siniscalchi etal, 2005).

The chief points to help in the diagnosis of DHF in the postoperative heart are: (1) Hemodynamic evidence of heart failure (2) Mean pulmonary capillary wedge pressure >12 mmHg (Paulus etal, 2007) (3) Echocardiographic evidence of raised left atrial pressure (LAP) as evidenced by a distended LA with the interatrial septum displaying a fixed curvature towards the right atrium (Kusumoto etal 1993; Royse etal, 2004). (4) Echocardiographic evidence of a small LV in the absence of hypovolemia and valvular heart disease (5) Low EDV as determined by the pulmonary artery catheter (6) EF better or similar to the preoperative one. Table 2.

- Increased PACWP
- EF ≥ Preop [a]
- Evidence of raised LAP [a]
- Small LV [a]
- Low EDV [b]
- Absence of significant pericardial effusion [a]

[a] Revealed by echocardiography. [b] As determined by pulmonary artery catheter.

Table 2. Features that would suggest DHF in a postoperative heart.PACWP: pulmonary artery capillary wedge pressure; CI: cardiac index; LAP: left atrial pressure; EF:; EDV: end diastolic volume. Adapted with permission from Elsevier Publishing (Alsaddique, 2008)

Indeed according to the European criteria, a normal cardiac index in the face of pulmonary edema suggests DHF (Paulus et al, 2007). Echocardiography is a useful tool to diagnose DHF. In the postoperative heart suspected to have DHF it is not always possible to get an adequate assessment. In addition, air trapped within the postoperative mediastinum creates poor acoustic windows through which ultrasounds waves cannot pass. An echocardiography study that would simply establish that the left ventricular function has not deteriorated compared to the preoperative one and rules out the presence of cardiac tamponade or significant pericardial effusion can usually be done and would probably suffice under the circumstances. If the hemodynamics allow, one can probably use TEE to diagnose of DHF, it remains however an invasive procedure that should only be carried out by an experienced operator. Published guidelines for performance of TEE should be followed (Nihoyannopoulos et al, 2007; Cheiltin et al, 2003; Benjamin et al, 1998). The information gained by TEE should be integrated with the rest of the hemodynamic parameters (pulmonary artery occlusion pressures or pulmonary artery end-diastolic pressures), LA dimensions, and conventional Doppler imaging of mitral inflow in conjunction with TDI of the lateral mitral annular wall.

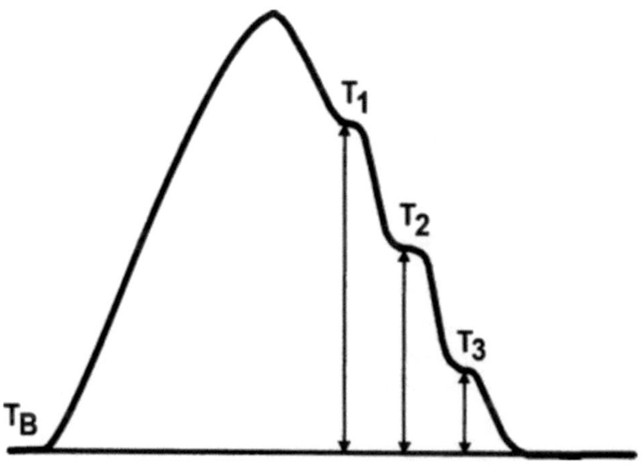

Fig. 4. Thermodilution EF for the right ventricle. T_B baseline blood temperature. T_1, T_2 and T_3 are successive temperature plateaux. (Adapted with permission from Elsevier)

As it has been determined that objective measurement of LV diastolic function serves to confirm rather than establish the diagnosis of DHF. The diagnosis of DHF can be assumed without the measurement of the various parameters that reflect LV diastolic function in the presence of acute pulmonary edema associated with indirect signs of elevated left atrial pressure (Zile eta, 2001).

7. Perioperative management of DHF

Management begins by anticipating the problem before it actually happens. In the preoperative period, it is important to identify patients who may have or are at risk of DHF. Any prior history of DHF is important to identify and attention should be paid to patients who are likely to develop it in order to prevent any further deterioration of diastolic function in the post operative period. Chronically uncontrolled hypertension is a common cause of DHF it should be sought and aggressively treated prior to surgery to reduce the risk of perioperative heart failure (Kostis etal, 1997). Hypertension leads to DHF because of LV hypertrophy and decreased arterial compliance (Mottram etal, 2005). Diabetes mellitus, especially with poor glycemic control, is independently associated with abnormal LV relaxation, is similar in severity to that associated with systemic hypertension. The combination of diabetes and hypertension is associated with greater abnormality than patients with either condition alone. Aggressive control of diabetes, as well as of hypertension, should be considered an important component of the management in the pre operative period. Tight glycemic control decreases the risk of heart failure in patients with diabetes (Iribarren etal, 2001; Liu etal, 2001) . It is helpful to avoid hypovolemia, tachycardia and tachyarrhythmias as they impair LV filling by shortening the diastolic phase of the cardiac cycle resulting in suboptimal LV filling (Zile & Brutsaert, 2002) . Any reversible predisposing factors is to be corrected prior to surgery. Echocardiography is helpful in the preoperative assessment of patients especially those with compromised cardiac performance in order to identify the nature of heart failure. Risk factors for DHF include elderly patients, the female gender, hypertension, increased left ventricular mass, diabetes, obesity, and ischemic heart disease (Klapholz etal, 2004)

8. Intraoperative and postoperative management

The key to managing DHF is to maintain preoperative parameters as closely as possible. Managing DHF is analogous to walking on a tightrope. Any minor deviation from the "normal parameters tightrope" could lead to hypotension and low cardiac output, or pulmonary venous congestion. The second key principle is to maintain operating volume. As shown in Figure 1, the left ventricle with DHF operates at "just adequate" volume. If the volume is reduced, then a marked reduction in stroke volume will occur leading to low cardiac output and hypotension. It is also important to realize that it is difficult to achieve normal volume in DHF because of the relaxation abnormality. Although the left ventricular volume appears low, it is in the setting of an elevated left atrial pressure. Management of DHF is therefore a process of maintaining a delicate balance and avoiding the contributing and triggering factors that can lead to poor hemodynamic outcome. A summary of these contributing factors is shown in Figure 5. Reduced LV volume (such as blood loss or vasodilation) rapidly leads to hypotension. Tachycardia shortens the diastolic filling time, thereby reducing left ventricular volume and stroke volume (Zile & Brutsaert, 2002). High-dose inotropes initially may increase blood pressure, but as tachycardia ensues, it would cause progressive reduction in left ventricular volume producing a hyperdynamic empty ventricle. High levels of positive end expiratory pressure (PEEP), obesity, pericardial or pleural effusions cause extrinsic compression of the heart and worsen diastolic function. Conversely, excessive administration of fluid in an attempt to improve cardiac output may not produce an increase in stroke volume but will produce an increase in end-diastolic pressure. This may exacerbate pulmonary venous congestion. Excessive hypertension or vasoconstriction will reduce EF and increase left ventricular end-diastolic volume. This has the effect of shifting up the end-diastolic pressure-volume curve where a small increase in volume will produce a large increase in end-diastolic pressure, increasing the risk of pulmonary edema. Bradycardia increases diastolic filling time, and will lead to an increase in the peak LVEDP. DHF can lead to pulmonary hypertension due to elevated pressure transmitted back through the pulmonary veins (Owan etal, 2006). Hypercapnea and hypoxia are potent causes of pulmonary hypertension in the perioperative setting.

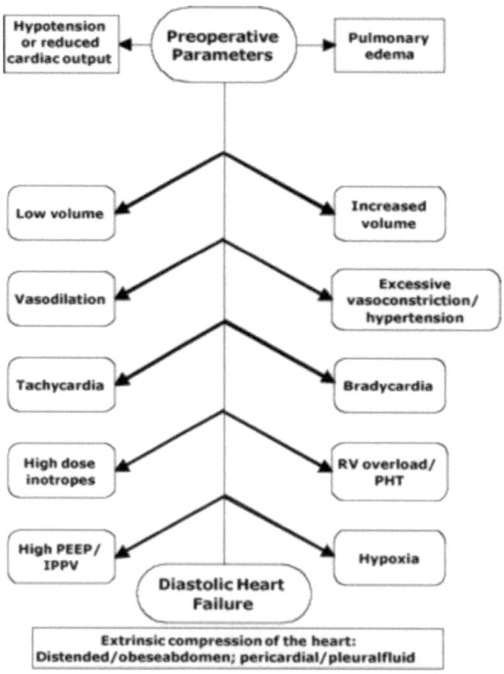

Fig. 5. Contributing factors to hemodynamic instability in patients with DHF. Deviation from normal parameters can lead to either hypotension/reduced cardiac output, or to pulmonary edema. (Adapted with permission from Elsevier)

9. Management strategies

A summary of clinical strategies is shown in Figure 6. The mainstay of treatment is to be realistic about hemodynamic goals, and to return the patient to normal preoperative parameters. Potential reversible causes (particularly extrinsic causes) should be identified and managed like pericardial tamponade and significant pericardial effusion as they cause resistance to LV filling leading to acute DHF. These conditions should therefore be suspected in the event of unexplained DHF in the postoperative patient. Echocardiography is the most effective clinical tool to diagnose and monitor DHF. It can even gives indications about the hemodynamic profile of the patient, a raised left atrial pressure can be identified by enlarged atria, and a fixed curvature of the interatrial septum bowing from left to right (Royse et al 2001). One has to assess the different hemodynamic parameters of the patient to find out the cause for the imbalance that led to failure. For example, in the setting of reduced volume, administration of fluids, avoidance of tachycardia and reducing high dose inotropes will improve left ventricular end-diastolic volume. Vasoconstrictors may be required to counteract the effect of vasodilation which is seen during and immediately after cardiac surgery, thereby returning systemic vascular resistance to normal. Mechanical ventilation may affect hemodynamic performance in DHF. The mechanism is complex involving changes in preload and afterload for both right and left ventricles. Positive pressure ventilation may reduce venous return thereby reducing preload; and it also may reduce afterload enhancing ventricular ejection. This may have a variable effect on cardiac output. If the patient is normovolemic and intrathoracic pressure is normal, then the effect on afterload reduction may increase cardiac output. The beneficial effects of positive pressure ventilation on cardiac output are reversed by hypovolemia leading to decreased cardiac output and hypotension. Mechanical ventilation is beneficial in order to avoid hypercapnea, and PEEP can help reduce pulmonary venous congestion (Pinsky 2005, 2007). The use of continuous positive airway pressure (CPAP) by a face mask in the spontaneously breathing patient is reported to be effective in the treatment of diastolic dysfunction and may therefore be a useful ventilatory support under these circumstances (Benjelid etal, 2005; Moritz etal, 2003; Bersten etal, 1991)

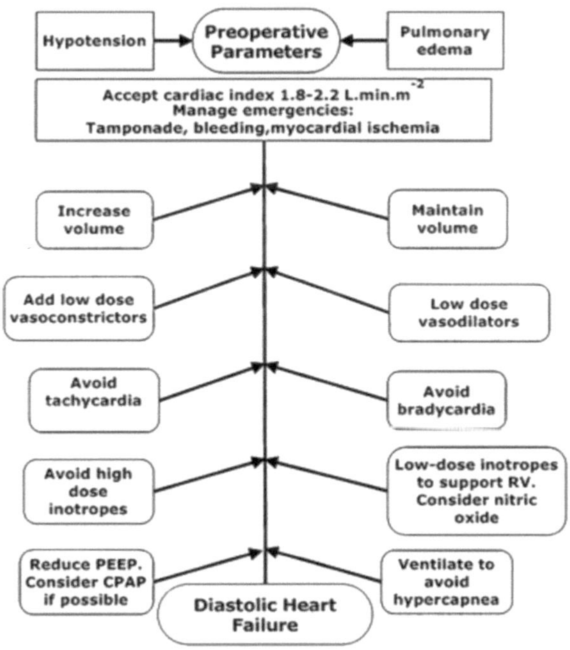

Fig. 6. Strategies to treat DHF in the perioperative setting. Treatment strategies are aimed to return to preoperative parameters. RV is right ventricle, PEEP is positive end-expiratory pressure; CPAP is continuous positive airway pressure. (Adapted with permission from Elsevier)

10. The contributing factors

Acute renal failure leads to volume overload and can trigger DHF (Tsuyuki etal 2001) Excessive fluid administration has the same effect and can be a contributing factor for post operative DHF. Atrial fibrillation (AF) leads to loss of effective atrial contraction, changes LV filling pattern and results in a slowing of myocardial relaxation thereby triggering DHF. Pharmacological or electrical cardioversion may be necessary to restore sinus rhythm or at least rate control. In the postoperative coronary artery bypass patient unexplained DHF should lead to the suspicion of acute graft malfunction, which could happen in the absence of any signs of ischemia. Postoperative myocardial ischemia is an important reversible cause of diastolic dysfunction in the postoperative period as ischemia significantly slows active myocardial relaxation during early diastole affecting thereby LV filling. Ischemia could also lead to rhythm disturbances that will further aggravate LV diastolic dysfunction. It is well known that tachycardia and dysrhythmias shorten diastole leading to impaired left ventricular filling. Restoration of sinus rhythm should always be a priority in management (Zile & Brutstaert, (Piaarcchio 2002). If pacing is required, then atrio-ventricular sequential pacing will enhance ventricular filling. Ventricular pacing alone leads to loss of the atrial contribution (Alsaddique, 2008) and right ventricular pacing may induce dyssynchronous contraction. Pain may induce tachycardia and hypertension with the potential of triggering DHF through these mechanisms.Sepsis can exacerbate DHF, as it affects both systolic and diastolic function of the heart. In case of DHF developing late in the postoperative period sepsis should be considered as one of the possibilities. The role of sepsis in causing diastolic failure was identified by using pressure-volume loops in anesthetized endotoxemic rabbits. Left ventricular diastolic properties were shown to be altered; with prolonged relaxation, decreased compliance leading to increased end-diastolic pressure. Diastolic dysfunction can contribute to the development of cardiogenic septic shock (Pirracchio etal, 2007). Other factors that can contribute to DHF include a large pleural effusion or any other process that causes extrinsic compression of the heart or that could potentially impair or delay ventricular filling could contribute to or trigger DHF. This includes pericardial tamponade which is in effect "acute extrinsic DHF".

11. Additional management considerations

The incidence of pure DHF in the postoperative heart in not known. Many cases of failure that are thought of as systolic failure are in reality diastolic in nature. There is no consensus on management of diastolic failure in the postoperative heart or intensive care environment in general. Echocardiography can be used not only to diagnose but also to monitor therapy and the hemodynamic changes. These points deserve emphasis:

1. The management of DHF is based on the strategy of avoiding pulmonary congestion whilst maintaining adequate cardiac output, and correction of any predisposing factors. As the systolic function is maintained in diastolic failure positive inotropes have little role in the management. The exception is where there is "low normal" EF or evidence of RV dysfunction or RV strain in the setting of pulmonary hypertension. In these situations, **low dose** inotrope therapy may improve cardiac output and hemodynamic stability. High dose inotrope therapy will induce tachycardia, and shorten diastolic filling time, leading to progressive reduction in LV preload and deterioration in hemodynamics.
2. In diastolic failure ventricular filling is impaired, diuretic therapy leads to volume depletion that will further impair ventricular filling resulting in a more reduction of the cardiac output.

3. Vasodilation is the enemy of DHF. Though vasodilation facilitates ejection, the heart empties but is unable to adequately re-fill, leading to progressive reduction in preload and deterioration in hemodynamic conditions. Normalizing systemic vascular resistance with a vasoconstrictor helps to maintain hemodynamic stability and normotension.
4. Many patients with DHF also have pulmonary hypertension. Hypotension in this setting leads to compromise of RV blood flow and relative RV ischemia, thereby causing RV failure. The RV fails by dilating, which leads to further compression of the LV and worsening DHF. This can lead to a spiral of progressive hypotension. In these circumstances a vasoconstrictor to preserve blood pressure and maintain LV preload, and in addition low dose inotrope (such as dobutamine) to support RV function, can improve hemodynamic stability. If the situation remains refractory it is worth considering nitric oxide (NO) to selectively treat right ventricular pressure overload. There is to our knowledge no published work on the use NO in DHF but it remains as an option if all else fails (Granton & Moric, 2008; Natori etal, 2003).

12. Use of diuretics

Diuretics should be used with caution, as high filling pressure is required to maintain cardiac output. Diuresis may result in hypotension in patients with DHF because of the steep shape of the left ventricular end-diastolic pressure-volume relationship, where small changes in end-diastolic volume will lead to reduced stroke volume. The use of diuretics must be countered by increased vigilance of hemodynamic variables, as indiscriminate use can be counter-productive (Zile & Burstaert, 2002; Aurigemma & Gaasch 2004).

13. Antiarrhythmics

Intravenous digoxin is a commonly used therapy for the management atrial fibrillation and paroxysmal atrial tachycardia. Other therapeutic agents include calcium antagonists such as verapamil, beta-blockers such as esmololol sotolol for acute rhythm control, or amiodarone. The current evidence supports the use of amiodarone for AF occurring after cardiac surgery. Amiodarone also reduces perioperative ventricular tachyarrhythmias and strokes, and helps reduce duration of hospitalization (Bagshaw etal,2006; Saltman, 2003). Nevertheless digoxin continues to be valuable in long-term therapy of atrial flutter and fibrillation. More recently digoxin has been the subject of different studies to determine its effects on all forms of heart failure (HF). It has been shown that digoxin at serum concentration of 0.5-0.9 ng/mL reduces mortality and hospitalizations in all HF patients, including those with DHF. At higher serum levels, digoxin reduces HF hospitalization but has no effect on mortality or all-cause hospitalizations (Ahmed etal, 2006). The recommendation went further to suggest that the results of the DIG trial may provide support for the use of digoxin in patients who have heart failure with preserved EF, because a trend toward reduction in hospitalizations for heart failure was observed with digoxin in the ancillary trial (Ahmed, 2006)]. However the guidelines of the American College of Cardiology–American Heart Association Task Force for the management of heart failure and the Task Force for the Diagnosis and Treatment of Chronic Heart Failure of the European Society of Cardiology do not recommend the use of digoxin in patients who have heart failure with preserved EF (Hunt etal 2005; Swedberg etal, 2005).

13.1 Use of inotropes

Agressive use of positive inotropic agents have little role in the management of DHF, though low dose inotropes may improve stability in the setting of low-normal EF or where there is pulmonary hypertension as described earlier [such as a combination of 3-5mcg/kg/min dobutamine and norepinepherine 3-5 mcg/min] (Little & Brucks, 2005; Wu & Yu, 2005). This is a very common pattern in DHF in the perioperative setting and may be exaccerbated by poor cardioprotection (especially to the right heart), myocardial edema or reperfusion injury. Pharmacologically, the use of high dose inotropes leads to an increase in heart rate, which causes shortening of diastolic filling time leading to reduced ventricular volume and a gradual worsening of cardiac output. Therefore, in DHF it is probably wise to accept less than ideal hemodynamics provided adequate perfusion is maintained. It is therefore suggested that a cardiac **index between 1.8 and 2.2 L.min.m-2** is acceptable. Aiming for higher levels of cardiac index may not be readily achieved, and the strategy used would necessitate higher doses of inotropes and volume, with potential for greater pulmonary venous congestion. The danger of increasing inotrope use is that if the patient deteriorates, the typical response is to increase the inotropic dose leading to further tachycardia and shortened diastolic filling, thereby further reducing stroke volume and worsening cardiac performance, effectively creating a vicious circle of deterioration. The art of managing these patients is to achieve the delicate balance between hypotension and pulmonary venous congestion by judicious use of vasopressors, low-dose inotropes and fluids, such that their baseline hemodynamic state is maintained until the recovery processes following surgery abate.

13.2 Role of Vasodilators

It is important to appreciate that vasodilators facilitate ventricular ejection, and in the setting of a stiff left ventricle, makes it difficult to re-fill. This is especially important if there is associated tachycardia , as this will further exacerbate the inability to adequately refill the ventricle. If vasodilators are used they could make the ventricle operates at a lower end-diastolic volume further contributing to the low cardiac output. Under these circumstances a vasoconstrictor may actually be helpful by reducing EF and increasing the end diastolic volume. Vasodilators (especially inodilators) are appropriate for secondary DHF (systolic and diastolic failure). It is important to remember, however, the goal of maintaining preoperative hemodynamics, which means that the level of vasodilation should not depart considerably from baseline. In practice, most patients will have a vasodilation state after surgery, and are already excessively dilated. Vasodilator use in this setting can be counterproductive. If using inodilators, then add norepinepherine to control excessive vasodilation, and return it towards normal.

13.3 Role of vasoconstrictors:

Vasoconstrictors should be considered as part of the management of DHF, if vasodilation is manifest in the postoperative course. Vasodilation is common both during and immediately after cardiac surgery, and is part of the sterile inflammatory response syndrome seen following cardiac surgery. Diastolic abnormality prevents adequate filling of the left ventricle so that the end-diastolic volume progressively declines. Low-dose vasoconstrictors are protective in this setting with the aim of normalizing but not increasing vascular resistance.

13.4 Other pharmacological agents.

The value of beta-blockers in the perioperative period has recently been questioned because of the POISE trial that has examined their effect on non-cardiac surgery patients (POISE study group, 2008). Nevertheless one could extrapolate that the same would probably happen in a cohort of cardiac surgery patients. Beta blockers offer cardiac protection in the shape of a reduction of myocardial infarction (Andersen etal, 2008; Everly etal, 2004). Conversely, the incidence of stroke and its resulting patient disability was increased in the treatment group leading to increased mortality (Sear etal, 2008). Caution should be exercised with aggressive use of perioperative beta blockade. Beta blockers in the postoperative heart are used for control of tachycardia in the presence of adequate volume. An ultra short acting agent given intravenously (e.g. esmolol or landiolol that have a very short half life can be helpful (Mitchell etal, 2002; Kirshenbaum etal 1985; Yoshida etal, 2008). They can also help in case of fast atrial fibrillation to achieve an initial rate control in the process of stabilizing the hemodynamics (Kobayashi etal, 2004). Verapamil, a calcium channel blocker, can also be used intravenously to control heart rate and to treat fast atrial fibrillation (Abernethy & Schwartz, 1999). Calcium channel blockers in general are effective in DHF caused by idiopathic hypertrophic cardiomyopathies (Setaro etal 1990), but they do not offer the same benefits to diastolic failure caused by other factors (Nishimura etal, 1993). There are no drugs specifically marketed for the treatment of diastolic dysfunction. Inodilators may improve diastolic function in systolic and DHF, or bi-ventricular failure, as they will maintain stroke volume at a lower left ventricular end-diastolic volume. This has the effect of the heart working at a lower end-diastolic pressure. Unloading of the right ventricle will reduce the effect of left ventricular compression via the interventricular septum.

Long-term (outpatient) treatment that addresses myocardial remodeling includes ACE-inhibitors and angiotensin receptor blockers, calcium channel blockers, careful use of diuretics such as spironolactone, carvidelol, control of hypertension and treatment of myocardial ischemia (Yip etal, 2008; Yamamoto etal, 2005;Bergstrom etal, 2004; Yoshhida etal, 2004) Future strategies are likely to address disorders of calcium handling, as well as modulating myocardial proteins and collagen subtypes (Kass etal, 2004)

13.5 Cardiac resynchronization therapy

Cardiac-resynchronization therapy (CRT) has been shown to improve the rate of survival, quality of life, exercise capacity, and functional status in patients with a prolonged QRS interval and moderate-to-severe heart failure that is resistant to optimal medical therapy. CRT is thought to improve the left ventricular EF and functional status by minimizing regional left ventricular delay caused by prolonged ventricular conduction, reducing mitral regurgitation and left ventricular reverse remodeling, and normalizing neurohormonal factors. Current guidelines support the use of CRT in patients with an EF of 35% or less, moderate or severe heart failure (New York Heart Association [NYHA] class III or IV), and a prolonged QRS interval [≥120 msec] (Abraham etal, 2002; (Leclercq etal, 2002). CRT did not improve peak oxygen consumption in patients with moderate-to-severe heart failure with narrow QRS intervals providing evidence these patients may not benefit from this form of therapy (Beshai etal, 2007). The effects on diastolic function have been the subject of recent studies by load-dependent pulsed-wave Doppler transmitral indices. A number of studies have shown that in heart failure patients receiving CRT, improvement in LV diastolic function is coupled to the improvement in LV systolic function (Waggoner etal, 2005). The specific value of CRT for the treatment of the DHF as distinct from systolic and diastolic failure has not however, been extensively investigated.

14. Summary

5. DHF is " a small stiff heart" with high left atrial pressure, whereas systolic and diastolic failure is a dilated heart with reduced EF and a high left atrial pressure, and echocardiography is the best way to differentiate these two conditions.
6. The key operating principle in DHF is to maintain their preoperative haemodynamic state and maintain operating volume
7. The key operating principle of systolic and diastolic failure is to improve stroke volume at a lower operating volume
8. The cardiac index in DHF is not great - but is enough. Do not "shoot for the stars".
9. Low dose inotropes and enough vasoconstrictors to normalise vascular resistance can improve hemodynamic stability
10. High dose inotropes are often counterproductive
11. Excessive vasodilation is the enemy of DHF.

15. References

Abernethy DR, Schwartz JB 1999 Calcium-antagonist drugs. *N Engl J Med.* 4;341(19):1447-57

Abraham WT, Fisher WG, Smith AL, Delurgio DB, Leon AR, Loh E, Kocovic DZ, Packer M, Clavell AL, Hayes DL, Ellestad M, Trupp RJ, Underwood J, Pickering F, Truex C, McAtee P, Messenger J; MIRACLE Study Group. Multicenter In Sync Randomized Clinical Evaluation Cardiac resynchronization in chronic heart failure. N Engl Med. 2002 ;346(24):1845-53.

Ahmed A, Rich MW, Fleg JL, Zile MR, Young JB, Kitzman DW, Love TE, Aronow WS, Adams KF Jr, Gheorghiade M Effects of digoxin on morbidity and mortality in diastolic heart failure: the ancillary digitalis investigation group trial. Circulation. 2006;114(5):397-403

Ahmed A, Rich MW, Love TE, Lloyd-Jones DM, Aban IB, Colucci WS, Adams KF, Gheorghiade M Digoxin and reduction in mortality and hospitalization in heart failure: a comprehensive post hoc analysis of the DIG trial. Eur Heart J. 2006 (2):178-86.

Alsaddique AA Recognition of diastolic heart failure in the postoperative heart. Eur J Cardiothorac Surg. 2008 Dec;34(6):1141-8. Epub 2008 Jun 24

Alsaddique AA, Recognition of diastolic heart failure in the postoperative heart, Eur J Cardiothorac Surg (2008), doi:10.1016/j.ejcts.2008.05.030

Alsaddique AA, Royse AG, Royse CF, Fouda MA.Management of diastolic heart failure following cardiac surgery. Eur J Cardiothorac Surg. 2009 Feb;35(2):241-9. Epub 2008 Dec 11

Andersen SS, Hansen ML, Gislason GH, Folke F, Schramm TK, Fosbøl E, Sørensen R, Rasmussen S, Abildstrøm SZ, Madsen M, Køber L, Torp-Pedersen C.Mortality and

Reinfarction among Patients Using Different Beta-Blockers for Secondary Prevention after a Myocardial Infarction. Cardiology. 2008 9;112(2):144-150. [Epub ahead of print]

Appleton CP, Firstenberg MS, Garcia MJ, Thomas JD The echo-Doppler evaluation of left ventricular diastolic function. A current perspective. Cardiol Clin. 2000;18:513-46, ix

Appleton CP, Hatle LK, Popp RL Relation of transmitral flow velocity patterns to left ventricular diastolic function: new insights from a combined hemodynamic and Doppler echocardiographic study. J Am Coll Cardiol. 1988;12:426-40

Aurigemma GP, Gaasch WH Clinical practice. Diastolic heart failure. N Engl J Med. 2004 9;351(11):1097-105.

Aurigemma GP, Gaasch WH. Clinical practice, Diastolic heart failure N Eng J Med 2004;351:1097-105

Aurigemma GP, Gaasch WH. Clinical practice. Diastolic heart failure. N Engl J Med 2004;351:1097-1105.

Aurigemma GP, Gaasch WH. Diastolic heart failure. N Engl J Med 2004; 351: 1097–105

Bagshaw SM, Galbraith PD, Mitchell LB, Sauve R, Exner DV, Ghali WA Prophylactic amiodarone for prevention of atrial fibrillation after cardiac surgery: a meta-analysis. Ann Thorac Surg. 2006 ;82(5):1927-37

Bail DH, Kofler M, Ziemer G. Brain natriuretic peptide (BNP) in patients undergoing coronary artery bypass grafting. Thorac Cardiovasc Surg. 2004;52:135-40

Bendjelid K, Schütz N, Suter PM, Fournier G, Jacques D, Fareh S, Romand JA. Does continuous positive airway pressure by face mask improve patients with acute cardiogenic pulmonary edema due to left ventricular diastolic dysfunction? Chest. 2005 ;127(3):1053-8

Benjamin E, Griffin K, Leibowitz AB, Manasia A, Oropello JM, Geffroy V, DelGiudice R, Hufanda J, Rosen S, Goldman M. Goal-directed transesophageal echocardiography performed by intensivists to assess left ventricular function: comparison with pulmonary artery catheterization. J Cardiothorac Vasc Anesth. 1998 Feb;12(1):10-5

Bergstrom A, Andersson B, Edner M, Nylander E, Persson H, Dahlstrom U. Effect of carvedilol on diastolic function in patients with diastolic heart failure and preserved systolic function. Results of the Swedish Doppler-echocardiographic study (SWEDIC). Eur J Heart Fail 2004;6:453-461.

Bernard F, Denault A, Babin D, Goyer C, Couture P, Couturier A, Buithieu J. Diastolic dysfunction is predictive of difficult weaning from cardiopulmonary bypass. Anesth Analg. 2001;92:291-8

Bersten AD, Holt AW, Vedig AE, Skowronski GA, Baggoley CJ. Treatment of severe cardiogenic pulmonary edema with continuous positive airway pressure delivered by face mask. N Engl J Med. 1991 26;325(26):1825-30

Beshai JF, Grimm RA, Nagueh SF, Baker JH 2nd, Beau SL, Greenberg SM, Pires LA, Tchou PJ; RethinQ Study Investigators. Cardiac-resynchronization therapy in heart failure with narrow QRS complexes. N Engl J Med. 2007;357(24):2461-71.

Bhatia RS, Tu JV, Lee DS, Austin PC, Fang J, Haouzi A, Gong Y, Liu PP. Outcome of heart failure with preserved ejection fraction in a population-based study. N Engl J Med. 2006 355:260-9

Boyer JK, Thanigaraj S, Schechtman KB, Perez JE. Prevalence of ventricular diastolic dysfunction in asymptomatic, normotensive patients with diabetes mellitus. Am J Cardiol 2004;93:870-875

Burkhoff D, Maurer MS, Packer M. Heart failure with a normal EF: is it really a disorder of diastolic function? Circulation. 2003; 11;107(5):656-8

Cheitlin MD, Armstrong WF, Aurigemma GP, Beller GA, Bierman FZ, Davis JL, Douglas PS, Faxon DP, Gillam LD, Kimball TR, Kussmaul WG, Pearlman AS, Philbrick JT, Rakowski H, Thys DM. ACC/AHA/ASE 2003 guideline update for the clinical application of echocardiography--summary article: a report of the American College of Cardiology/American Heart Association Task Force on Practice Guidelines (ACC/AHA/ASE Committee to Update the 1997 Guidelines for the Clinical Application of Echocardiography). J Am Coll Cardiol. 2003 Sep 3;42(5):954-70.

Couture P, Denault AY, Shi Y, Deschamps A, Cossette M, Pellerin M, Tardif JC Effects of anesthetic induction in patients with diastolic dysfunction. Can J Anaesth. 2009 May;56(5):357-65. Epub 2009 Apr 2

Deswal A. Diastolic dysfunction and diastolic heart failure: mechanisms and epidemiology. Curr Cardiol Rep. 2005 ;7(3):178-83

Dokainish H. Doppler tissue imaging in the evaluation of left ventricular diastolic function. Curr Opin Cardiol. 2004;19:437-41.

Draper NJ, Shah AM Beneficial effects of a nitric oxide donor on recovery of contractile function following brief hypoxia in isolated rat heart. J Mol Cell Cardiol. 1997;29:1195-205

du Toit EF, McCarthy J, Miyashiro J, Opie LH, Brunner F Effect of nitrovasodilators and inhibitors of nitric oxide synthase on ischemic and reperfusion function of rat isolated hearts. Br J Pharmacol. 1998 ;123:1159-67

Dumesnil JG, Gaudreault G, Honos GN, Kingma JG Jr Use of Valsalva maneuver to unmask left ventricular diastolic function abnormalities by Doppler echocardiography in patients with coronary artery disease or systemic hypertension. Am J Cardiol. 1991;68:515-9

Eltzschig HK, Rosenberger P, Löffler M, Fox JA, Aranki SF, Shernan SK. Impact of intraoperative transesophageal echocardiography on surgical decisions in 12,566 patients undergoing cardiac surgery. Ann Thorac Surg. 2008 Mar;85(3):845-52

Everly MJ, Heaton PC, Cluxton RJ Jr Beta-blocker underuse in secondary prevention of myocardial infarction. Ann Pharmacother. 2004 ;38(2):286-93.

Gaasch WH, Zile MR. Left ventricular diastolic dysfunction and diastolic heart failure. Annu Rev Med 2004;55:373-394.

Garcia MJ, Thomas JD, Klein AL New Doppler echocardiographic applications for the study of diastolic function. J Am Coll Cardiol. 1998;32:865-75

Garcia-Fernandez MA, Azevedo J, Moreno M, Bermejo J, Perez-Castellano N, Puerta P, Desco M, Antoranz C, Serrano JA, Garcia E, Delcan JL. Regional diastolic function in ischaemic heart disease using pulse wave Doppler tissue imaging. Eur Heart J. 1999 Apr;20(7):496-505

Gilbert JC, Glantz SA Determinants of left ventricular filling and of the diastolic pressure-volume relation. Circ Res. 1989; 64:827-52

Granton J, Moric J. Pulmonary Vasodilators-Treating the Right Ventricle. Anesthesiol Clin. 2008 ;26(2):337-353

Groban L, Dolinski SY. Transesophageal echocardiographic evaluation of diastolic function. Chest. 2005 Nov;128(5):3652-63.

Groban L. Diastolic dysfunction in the older heart. J Cardiothorac Vasc Anesth 2005;19:228-236.

Hauser TH, McClennen S, Katsimaglis G, Josephson ME, Manning WJ, Yeon SB. Assessment of left atrial volume by contrast enhanced magnetic resonance angiography. J Cardiovasc Magn Reson. 2004;6:491-7.

How to diagnose diastolic heart failure: a consensus statement on the diagnosis of heart failure with normal left ventricular EF by the Heart Failure and Echocardiography Associations of the European Society of Cardiology. Eur Heart J. 2007;28:2539-50.

Hunt SA, Abraham WT, Chin MH, Feldman AM, Francis GS, Ganiats TG, Jessup M, Konstam MA, Mancini DM, Michl K, Oates JA, Rahko PS, Silver MA, Stevenson LW, Yancy CW, Antman EM, Smith SC Jr, Adams CD, Anderson JL, Faxon DP, Fuster V, Halperin JL, Hiratzka LF, Jacobs AK, Nishimura R, Ornato JP, Page RL, Riegel B; American College of Cardiology; American Heart Association Task Force on Practice Guidelines; American College of Chest Physicians; International Society for Heart and Lung Transplantation; Heart Rhythm Society. ACC/AHA 2005 Guideline Update for the Diagnosis and Management of Chronic Heart Failure in the Adult: a report of the American College of Cardiology/American Heart Association Task Force on Practice Guidelines (Writing Committee to Update the 2001 Guidelines for the Evaluation and Management of Heart Failure): developed in collaboration with the American College of Chest Physicians and the International Society for Heart and Lung Transplantation: endorsed by the Heart Rhythm Society Circulation. 2005;112(12):e154-235.

Hunt SA, Baker DW, Chin MH, Cinquegrani MP, Feldman AM, Francis GS, Ganiats TG, Goldstein S, Gregoratos G, Jessup ML, Noble RJ, Packer M, Silver MA, Stevenson LW, Gibbons RJ, Antman EM, Alpert JS, Faxon DP, Fuster V, Jacobs AK, Hiratzka LF, Russell RO, Smith SC Jr; American College of Cardiology/American Heart Association. ACC/AHA guidelines for the evaluation and management of chronic heart failure in the adult: executive summary. A report of the American College of Cardiology/American Heart Association Task Force on Practice Guidelines (Committee to revise the 1995 Guidelines for the Evaluation and Management of Heart Failure). J Am Coll Cardiol. 2001 Dec;38(7):2101-13

Iribarren C, Karter AJ, Go AS, Ferrara A, Liu JY, Sidney S, Selby JV. Glycemic control and heart failure among adult patients with diabetes Circulation. 2001;103:2668-73

Iribarren C, Karter AJ, Go AS, Ferrara A, Liu JY, Sidney S, Selby JV. Glycemic control and heart failure among adult patients with diabetes. Circulation 2001;103:2668-2673.

Kass DA, Bronzwaer JG, Paulus WJ. What mechanisms underlie diastolic dysfunction in heart failure? Circ Res 2004;94:1533-1542.

Kawaguchi M, Hay I, Fetics B, Kass DA Combined ventricular systolic and arterial stiffening in patients with heart failure and preserved EF: implications for systolic and diastolic reserve limitations. Circulation. 2003;107:714-20

Kay HR, Afshari M, Barash P, Webler W, Iskandrian A, Bemis C, Hakki AH, Mundth ED Measurement of ejection fraction by thermal dilution techniques. J Surg Res. 1983;34:337-46

Khouri SJ, Maly GT, Suh DD, Walsh TE. A practical approach to the echocardiographic evaluation of diastolic function. J Am Soc Echocardiogr. 2004;17:290-7

Kirshenbaum JM, Kloner RA, Antman EM, Braunwald E Use of an ultra short-acting beta-blocker in patients with acute myocardial ischemia. Circulation. 1985 ;72(4):873-80

Kitzman DW, Little WC, Brubaker PH, Anderson RT, Hundley WG, Marburger CT, Brosnihan B, Morgan TM, Stewart KP. Pathophysiological characterization of isolated diastolic heart failure in comparison to systolic heart failure. Jama 2002;288:2144-2150.

Kitzman DW, Little WC, Brubaker PH, Anderson RT, Hundley WG, Marburger CT, Brosnihan B, Morgan TM, Stewart KP..Pathophysiological characterization of isolated diastolic heart failure in comparison to systolic heart failure. JAMA. 2002;288:2144-50

Klapholz M, Maurer M, Lowe AM, Messineo F, Meisner JS, Mitchell J, Kalman J, Phillips RA, Steingart R, Brown EJ, Jr., Berkowitz R, Moskowitz R, Soni A, Mancini D, Bijou R, Sehhat K, Varshneya N, Kukin M, Katz SD, Sleeper LA, Le Jemtel TH. Hospitalization for heart failure in the presence of a normal left ventricular ejection fraction: results of the New York Heart Failure Registry. J Am Coll Cardiol 2004;43:1432-1438.

Klein AL, Canale MP, Rajagopalan N, White RD, Murray RD, Wahi S, Arheart KL, Thomas JD Role of transesophageal echocardiography in assessing diastolic dysfunction in a large clinical practice: a 9-year experience. Am Heart J. 1999 Nov;138(5 Pt 1):880-9

Kloeters C, Dushe S, Dohmen PM, Meyer H, Krug LD, Hermann KG, Hamm B, Konertz WF, Lembcke A Evaluation of left and right ventricular diastolic function by electron-beam computed tomography in patients with passive epicardial constraint. J Comput Assist Tomogr. 2008 Jan-Feb;32(1):78-85

Kobayashi M, Machida N, Mitsuishi M, Yamane Y. Beta-blocker improves survival, left ventricular function, and myocardial remodeling in hypertensive rats with diastolic heart failure. Am J Hypertens 2004;17:1112-1119.

Kostis JB, Davis BR, Cutler J, Grimm RH, Jr., Berge KG, Cohen JD, Lacy CR, Perry HM, Jr., Blaufox MD, Wassertheil-Smoller S, Black HR, Schron E, Berkson DM, Curb JD, Smith WM, McDonald R, Applegate WB. Prevention of heart failure by antihypertensive drug treatment in older persons with isolated systolic hypertension. SHEP Cooperative Research Group. Jama 1997;278:212-216.

Krishnaswamy P, Lubien E, Clopton P, Koon J, Kazanegra R, Wanner E, Gardetto N, Garcia A, DeMaria A, AS Utility of B-natriuretic peptide levels in identifying patients with left ventricular systolic or diastolic dysfunction. Am J Med. 2001 Sep;111 (4):274-9

Kusumoto FM, Muhiudeen IA, Kuecherer HF, Cahalan MK, Schiller NB Response of the interatrial septum to transatrial pressure gradients and its potential for predicting pulmonary capillary wedge pressure: an intraoperative study using transesophageal echocardiography in patients during mechanical ventilation J Am Coll Cardiol. 1993;21:721-8.

Leclercq C, Kass DA. Retiming the failing heart: principles and current clinical status of cardiac resynchronization. J Am Coll Cardiol 2002;39:194-201

Lewis BS, Gotsman MS. Left ventricular diastolic pressure-volume relations in man S Afr Med J. 1976;50:97-1

Little WC, Brucks S Therapy for diastolic heart failure. Prog Cardiovasc Dis. 2005; 47(6):380-8.

Liu JE, Palmieri V, Roman MJ, Bella JN, Fabsitz R, Howard BV, Welty TK, Lee ET, Devereux RB. The impact of diabetes on left ventricular filling pattern in normotensive and hypertensive adults: the Strong Heart Study. J Am Coll Cardiol. 2001;37:1943-9

Liu JE, Palmieri V, Roman MJ, Bella JN, Fabsitz R, Howard BV, Welty TK, Lee ET, Devereux RB. The impact of diabetes on left ventricular filling pattern in normotensive and hypertensive adults: the Strong Heart Study. J Am Coll Cardiol 2001;37:1943-1949.

Lubien E, DeMaria A, Krishnaswamy P, Clopton P, Koon J, Kazanegra R, Gardetto N, Wanner E, Maisel AS. Utility of B-natriuretic peptide in detecting diastolic dysfunction: comparison with Doppler velocity recordings. Circulation. 2002 Feb 5; 105(5):595-601.

Lukowicz TV, Fischer M, Hense HW, Döring A, Stritzke J, Riegger G, Schunkert H, Luchner A; MONICA Investigators. BNP as a marker of diastolic dysfunction in the general population: Importance of left ventricular hypertrophy. Eur J Heart Fail. 2005 Jun; 7(4):525-31.

Maisel AS Krishnaswamy P, Nowak RM, McCord J, Hollander JE, Duc P, Omland T, Storrow AB, Abraham WT, Wu AH, Clopton P, Steg PG, Westheim A, Knudsen CW, Perez A, Kazanegra R, Herrmann HC, McCullough PA; Breathing Not Properly Multinational Study Investigators Rapid measurement of B-type natriuretic peptide in the emergency diagnosis of heart failure. N Engl J Med. 2002 Jul 18;347(3):161-7

Mitchell RG, Stoddard MF, Ben-Yehuda O, Aggarwal KB, Allenby KS, Trillo RA, Loyd R, Chang CT, Labovitz AJ Esmolol in acute ischemic syndromes. Am Heart J. 2002;144(5):E9

Moritz F, Benichou J, Vanheste M, Richard JC, Line S, Hellot MF, Bonmarchand G, Muller JM Boussignac continuous positive airway pressure device in the emergency care of acute Eur J Emerg Med. 2003 ;10(3):204-8

Mottram PM, Haluska BA, Leano R, Carlier S, Case C, Marwick TH. Relation of arterial stiffness to diastolic dysfunction in hypertensive heart disease. Heart. 2005;91:1551-6

Myśliński W, Mosiewicz J, Biłan A, Makaruk B, Jaszyna M, Hanzlik J. Prognostic value of the atrial pulsed Doppler recordings of transmitral flow in the assessment of left ventricular diastolic dysfunction. Ann Univ Mariae Curie Sklodowska [Med]. 2002;57:23-32

Natori S, Hasebe N, Jin YT, Matsusaka T, Ido A, Matsuhashi H, Ihara T, Kikuchi K. Inhaled nitric oxide modifies left ventricular diastolic stress in the presence of vasoactive agents in heart failure. Am J Respir Crit Care Med. 2003 15;167(6):895-901

Nihoyannopoulos P, Fox K, Fraser A, Pinto F; Laboratory Accreditation Committee of the EAE EAE laboratory standards and accreditation. Eur J Echocardiogr. 2007 Jan;8(1):80-7

Nishimura RA, Schwartz RS, Holmes DR Jr, Tajik AJ Failure of calcium channel blockers to improve ventricular relaxation in humans. J Am Coll Cardiol. 1993;21(1):182-8

Onose Y, Oki T, Tabata T, Yamada H, Ito S Assessment of the temporal relationship between left ventricular relaxation and filling during early diastole using pulsed Doppler echocardiography and Doppler tissue imaging. Jpn Circ J. 1999;63:209-15

Otašević P, Nesković AN, Popović Z, Vlahović A, Bojić D, Bojić M, Popović AD. Short early filling deceleration time on day 1 after acute myocardial infarction is associated with short and long term left ventricular remodeling. Heart. 2001 May;85(5):527-32

Owan TE, Hodge DO, Herges RM, Jacobsen SJ, Roger VL, Redfield MM. Trends in prevalence and outcome of heart failure with preserved ejection fraction. N Engl J Med. 2006;355:251-9

Owan TE, Hodge DO, Herges RM, Jacobsen SJ, Roger VL, Redfield MM. Trends in prevalence and outcome of heart failure with preserved ejection fraction. N Engl J Med. 2006; 355(3):251-9

Paulus WJ, Tschöpe C, Sanderson JE, Rusconi C, Flachskampf FA, Rademakers FE, Marino P, Smiseth OA, De Keulenaer G, Leite-Moreira AF, Borbély A, Edes I, Handoko ML, Heymans S, Pezzali N, Pieske B, Dickstein K, Fraser AG, Brutsaert DL
Paulus WJ, Tschöpe C, Sanderson JE, Rusconi C, Flachskampf FA, Rademakers FE, Marino P, Smiseth OA, De Keulenaer G, Leite-Moreira AF, Borbély A, Edes I, Handoko ML, Heymans S, Pezzali N, Pieske B, Dickstein K, Fraser AG, Brutsaert DL
Pinsky MR Cardiovascular issues in respiratory care. Chest. 2005;128(5 Suppl 2):592S-597S
Pinsky MR Heart-lung interactions Curr Opin Crit Care. 2007;13(5):528-31.
Pirracchio R, Cholley B, De Hert S, Solal AC, Mebazaa A Diastolic heart failure in anaesthesia and critical care. Br J Anaesth. 2007;98:707-21.
Pirracchio R, Cholley B, De Hert S, Solal AC, Mebazaa A Diastolic heart failure in anaesthesia and critical care. Br J Anaesth. 2007; 98(6):707-21
POISE Study Group, Devereaux PJ, Yang H, Yusuf S, Guyatt G, Leslie K, Villar JC, Xavier D, Chrolavicius S, Greenspan L, Pogue J, Pais P, Liu L, Xu S, Málaga G, Avezum A, Chan M, Montori VM, Jacka M, Choi P. Effects of extended-release metoprolol succinate in patients undergoing non-cardiac surgery (POISE trial): a randomized controlled trial. Lancet. 2008 31;371(9627):1839-47.
Rademakers FE, Bogaert J Cardiac dysfunction in heart failure with normal ejection fraction: MRI measurements. Prog Cardiovasc Dis. 2006;49:215-27
Rademakers FE. Magnetic resonance imaging in cardiology. Lancet 2003; 361:359–360.
Rakusan K, Cicutti N, Kolar F Effect of anemia on cardiac function, microvascular structure, and capillary hematocrit in rat hearts. Am J Physiol Heart Circ Physiol. 2001;280:H1407-14
Royse CF, Royse AG, Bharatula A, Lai J, Veltman M, Cope L, Kumar A Substernal epicardial echocardiography: a recommended examination sequence and clinical evaluation in patients undergoing cardiac surgery. Ann Thorac Surg. 200478:613-9; discussion 619.
Royse CF, Royse AG, Soeding PF, Blake DW. Shape and movement of the interatrial septum predicts change in pulmonary capillary wedge pressure. Ann Thorac Cardiovasc Surg 2001;7:79-83.
Rumberger JA. Use of electron beam tomography to quantify cardiac diastolic function. Cardiol Clin. 2000 Aug;18(3):547-56
Salem R, Denault AY, Couture P, Bélisle S, Fortier A, Guertin MC, Carrier M, Martineau R. Left ventricular end-diastolic pressure is a predictor of mortality in cardiac surgery independently of left ventricular ejection fraction. Br J Anaesth. 2006;97:292-7.
Saltman AE. Is it time to choose amiodarone for postoperative atrial fibrillation? J Thorac Cardiovasc Surg. 2003;125(6):1202-3
Sanders D, Dudley M, Groban L.Diastolic dysfunction, cardiovascular aging, and the anesthesiologist. Anesthesiol Clin. 2009 Sep;27(3):497-517Anesthesiol Clin. 2009 Sep;27(3):497-517
Schlüter KD, Weber M, Schraven E, Piper HM. NO donor SIN-1 protects against reoxygenation-induced cardiomyocyte injury by a dual action Am J Physiol. 1994;267:H1461-6.
Sear JW, Giles JW, Howard-Alpe G, Foëx P. Perioperative beta-blockade, 2008: what does POISE tell us, and was our earlier caution justified? Br J Anaesth. 2008 ;101(2):135-8.

Setaro JF, Zaret BL, Schulman DS, Black HR, Soufer R Usefulness of verapamil for congestive heart failure associated with abnormal left ventricular diastolic filling and normal left ventricular systolic performance. Am J Cardiol. 1990 ;66(12):981-6.

Shah PM, Pai RG. Diastolic heart failure. Curr Probl Cardiol. 1992 Dec;17(12):781-868.

Sibley CT, Lima JA. Assessment of ventricular structure and function with multidetector CT and MRI. Curr Cardiol Rep. 2008 Feb; 10(1):67-71

Siniscalchi A, Pavesi M, Piraccini E, De Pietri L, Braglia V, Di Benedetto F, Lauro A, Spedicato S, Dante A, Pinna AD, Faenza S Right ventricular end-diastolic volume index as a predictor of preload status in patients with low right ventricular ejection fraction during orthotopic liver transplantation. Transplant Proc. 2005;37:2541-3

Sohn DW, Chai IH, Lee DJ, Kim HC, Kim HS, Oh BH, Lee MM, Park YB, Choi YS, Seo JD, Lee YW Assessment of mitral annulus velocity by Doppler tissue imaging in the evaluation of left ventricular diastolic function. J Am Coll Cardiol. 1997;30:474-80

Song MH, Kobayashi Y, Michi H. Clinical implication of atrial and brain natriuretic Peptide in coronary artery bypass grafting. Asian Cardiovasc Thorac Ann. 2004; 12:41-6.

Spinale FG, Zellner JL, Mukherjee R, Crawford FA Placement considerations for measuring thermodilution right ventricular ejection fractions. Crit Care Med. 1991;19:417-21.

Spinale FG, Zellner JL, Mukherjee R, Ferris SE, Crawford FA Thermodilution right ventricular ejection fraction. Catheter positioning effects. Chest. 1990;98:1259-65

Stewart RA. Broader indications for B-type natriuretic peptide testing in coronary artery disease. Eur Heart J. 2005;26:207-9

Swedberg K, Cleland J, Dargie H, Drexler H, Follath F, Komajda M, Tavazzi L, Smiseth OA, Gavazzi A, Haverich A, Hoes A, Jaarsma T, Korewicki J, Lévy S, Linde C, Lopez-Sendon JL, Nieminen MS, Piérard L, Remme WJ; Task Force for the Diagnosis and Treatment of Chronic Heart Failure of the European Society of Cardiology. Guidelines for the diagnosis and treatment of chronic heart failure: executive summary (update 2005): The Task Force for the Diagnosis and Treatment of Chronic Heart Failure of the European Society of Cardiology. Eur Heart J. 2005 (11):1115-40.

Temporelli PL, Giannuzzi P, Nicolosi GL, Latini R, Franzosi MG, Gentile F, Tavazzi L, Maggioni AP; GISSI-3 Echo Substudy Investigators. Doppler-derived mitral deceleration time as a strong prognostic marker of left ventricular remodeling and survival after acute myocardial infarction: results of the GISSI-3 echo sub study. J Am Coll Cardiol. 2004 May 5;43(9):1646-53

Tsuyuki RT, McKelvie RS, Arnold JM, Avezum A Jr, Barretto AC, Carvalho AC, Isaac DL, Kitching AD, Piegas LS, Teo KK, Yusuf S Acute precipitants of congestive heart failure exacerbations. Arch Intern Med. 2001;161:2337-42

Tsuyuki RT, McKelvie RS, Arnold JM, Avezum A Jr, Barretto AC, Carvalho AC, Isaac DL, Kitching AD, Piegas LS, Teo KK, Yusuf S Acute precipitants of congestive heart failure exacerbations. Arch Intern Med. 2001;161:2337-42

van Heerebeek L, Borbély A, Niessen HW, Bronzwaer JG, van der Velden J, Stienen GJ, Linke WA, Laarman GJ, Paulus WJ Myocardial structure and function differ in systolic and diastolic heart failure. Circulation. 2006 25;113:1966-73.

van Kraaij DJ, van Pol PE, Ruiters AW, de Swart JB, Lips DJ, Lencer N, Doevendans PA. Diagnosing diastolic heart failure. Eur J Heart Fail. 2002 Aug;4(4):419-30.

Vasan RS, Benjamin EJ, Levy D. Prevalence, clinical features and prognosis of diastolic heart failure: an epidemiologic perspective. J Am Coll Cardiol 1995;26:1565-1574

Vasan RS, Levy D. Defining diastolic heart failure: a call for standardized diagnostic criteria. *Circulation* 2000;101: 2118-21

Vasan RS.Diastolic heart failure. BMJ. 2003 Nov 22;327(7425):1181-2

Vignon P Hemodynamic assessment of critically ill patients using echocardiography Doppler. Curr Opin Crit Care. 2005 Jun;11(3):227-34

Vitarelli A, Gheorghiade M Diastolic heart failure: standard Doppler approach and beyond. Am J Cardiol. 1998 Jun 18;81(12A):115G-121G.

Waggoner AD, Faddis MN, Gleva MJ, de las Fuentes L, Dávila-Román VG. Improvements in left ventricular diastolic function after cardiac resynchronization therapy are coupled to response in systolic performance. J Am Coll Cardiol. 2005 ;46(12):2244-9

Waggoner AD, Faddis MN, Gleva MJ, De Las Fuentes L, Osborn J, Heuerman S, Davila-Roman VG. Cardiac resynchronization therapy acutely improves diastolic function. J Am Soc Echocardiogr. 2005;18(3):216-20

Whalley GA, Gamble GD, Doughty RN. Restrictive diastolic filling predicts death after acute myocardial infarction: systematic review and meta-analysis of prospective studies. Heart. 2006 Nov;92(11):1588-94.

Wu EB, Yu CM Management of diastolic heart failure--a practical review of pathophysiology and treatment trial data. Int J Clin Pract. 2005 ;59(10):1239-46

Yamamoto K, Mano T, Yoshida J, Sakata Y, Nishikawa N, Nishio M, Ohtani T, Hori M, Miwa T, Masuyama T. ACE inhibitor and angiotensin II type 1 receptor blocker differently regulate ventricular fibrosis in hypertensive diastolic heart failure. J Hypertens 2005;23:393-400.

Yip GW, Wang M, Wang T, Chan S, Fung JW, Yeung L, Yip T, Lau ST, Lau CP, Tang MO, Yu CM, Sanderson JE. The Hong Kong diastolic heart failure study: a randomized controlled trial of diuretics, irbesartan and ramipril on quality of life, exercise capacity, left ventricular global and regional function in heart failure with a normal EF. Heart 2008;94:573-580.

Yoshida J, Yamamoto K, Mano T, Sakata Y, Nishikawa N, Nishio M, Ohtani T, Miwa T, Hori M, Masuyama T. AT1 receptor blocker added to ACE inhibitor provides benefits at advanced stage of hypertensive diastolic heart failure. Hypertension 2004;43:686-691.

Yoshida Y, Terajima K, Sato C, Akada S, Miyagi Y, Hongo T, Takeda S, Tanaka K, Sakamoto A.Clinical role and efficacy of landiolol in the intensive care unit J Anesth. 2008;22(1):64-9.

Zile MR, Baicu CF, Gaasch WH. Diastolic heart failure -- abnormalities in active relaxation and passive stiffness of the left ventricle. N Engl J Med 2004;350:1953-1959.

Zile MR, Brutsaert DL. New concepts in diastolic dysfunction and diastolic heart failure: Part II: causal mechanisms and treatment. Circulation 2002;105:1503-1508.

Zile MR, Brutsaert DL. New concepts in diastolic dysfunction and diastolic heart failure: Part I: diagnosis, prognosis, and measurements of diastolic function. Circulation 2002;105:1387-93

Zile MR, Gaasch WH, Carroll JD, Feldman MD, Aurigemma GP, Schaer GL, Ghali JK, Liebson PR. Heart failure with a normal ejection fraction: is measurement of diastolic function necessary to make the diagnosis of diastolic heart failure? Circulation. 2001;104:779-82

13

Spinal Cord Stimulation for Managing Angina from Coronary Artery Disease

Billy Huh
Department of Anesthesiology, Duke University Medical Center, USA

1. Introduction

Despite the recent advances in managing angina pectoris, many patients with coronary artery disease suffer from intractable pain. For those patients who have already failed optimal medical and surgical therapy, very few, if any, therapeutic options are available. However, spinal cord stimulation (SCS) may play a unique role in managing such refractory anginal pain.

The analgesic effect of SCS has been known since 1967 when Norman Shealy was able to show electrical stimulation of the dorsal column of spinal cord suppressed the response to noxious stimulation in animal study and abolished pain in a patient with terminal cancer (Shealy et.al. 1967). The rationale for this technique was based on the "gate theory" of pain proposed by Melzack and Wall (Melzack &Wall 1965). The SCS has been used mostly in patients suffering chronic low back pain but has also been used successfully in a variety of other conditions including radiculopathy, complex regional pain syndrome, post-herpetic neuralgia, multiple sclerosis, and other types of neuropathic pain. Moreover, several studies were able to demonstrate the pain relieving effect of SCS in peripheral vascular disease, associated with an increase in local blood flow as well as angina pectoris (Augustinsson et.al., 1985; Cook et.al., 1976; Jacobs et.al., 1990; Murphy et.al., 1987).

The use of electrical stimulation to manage angina was initially reported by Mannheimer et.al. (1982). The study showed that patients with severe angina pectoris treated with transcutaneous electrical nerve stimulation (TENS) reported decreased frequency and severity of anginal attacks, improved exercise tolerance, and a reduction in ST segment depression in electrocardiogram. But TENS unit is not suitable for long term therapy due to skin irritation and the stimulation equipment often restricted physical activity.

Murphy et.al. (1987) placed SCS in the dorsal column in 10 patients with intractable angina pectoris. All patients were suffering with severe intractable angina pectoris, unresponsive to maximal medical therapy and not suitable for coronary artery bypass surgery, and all had angina at rest or on minimal exertion. Three patients had suffered myocardial infarction previously, and five patients had previously undergone coronary artery bypass surgery. The patients were typically on β-blocker, calcium channel blocker, diuretics, and topical or sublingual nitroglycerin as needed.

All patients reported excellent results following the implantation with a significant decrease in both severity and frequency of angina attacks. All patients were able to reduce sublingual nitroglycerin requirement. One patient has returned to work. Three patients who experienced recurrence of angina, one had previously documented myocardial infarction (MI) and coronary artery bypass graft (CABG). He had two episodes of angina pectoris after almost 3 years after the implant.

In another patient angina recurred for the first time 2 years after SCS. A third patient complained of a return of angina in a new location, not covered by the area of dorsal column stimulation. Insertion of an additional electrode succeeded in relieving the new angina. Three patients have died of complications related to their ischemic heart disease, 5 to 32 months after the SCS implant. Another patient died of cardiogenic shock from MI nearly 7 months after the implantation.

Mannheimer et.al. (1988 & 1998) showed that SCS increased patients' tolerance to elevated heart rate under the controlled pacing. At the heart rate comparable to that producing angina, myocardial lactate production diminished, ST segment depression decreased, time to ST depression increased, and time to recovery from ST depression decreased respectively. SCS also reduced coronary sinus blood flow and myocardial oxygen consumption. Myocardial lactate level increased and the magnitude and duration of ST segment depression increased to the same values as during control pacing, indicating that myocardial ischemia during treatment with SCS can give rise to anginal pain. Thus spinal cord stimulation has an anti-anginal and anti-ischemic effect in severe coronary artery disease. These effects seem to be secondary to a decrease in myocardial oxygen consumption, and SCS does not mask the patient of a warning signal.

Similarly, Sanderson et. al. (1992) studied effectiveness of SCS in 14 patients with severe intractable angina unresponsive to standard therapies including bypass grafting. After implantation of SCS units, the patients were assessed by a symptom questionnaire, treadmill exercise, and atrial pacing. There was a significant improvement of angina, and nitroglycerine usage decreased markedly. SCS increased exercise duration from a mean of 414 to 478 seconds, and total ST segment depression was decreased both at maximum exercise (7.1 vs. 5.6 mm) and at 90% of the maximum control heart rate (3.5 vs. 2.6 mm). During the right atrial pacing, the maximum heart rate was reached before onset of angina (143 vs. 150 per min), and total ST segment depression was less at all heart rates. Benefit has persisted in some patients for over 2 years

A retrospective analysis of patients from the Italian Multicenter Registry (Romano et.al. 2000) showed that SCS is an effective therapy in patients with refractory angina pectoris, especially for those who cannot undergo revascularization procedure. One hundred and thirty patients (83 males, 47 females, mean age 74.8) were given SCS implantation for refractory angina and followed for 31.4 +/- 25.9 months. The follow-up data of 116 patients (89.2%) showed that SCS resulted in significant decrease in New York Heart Association (NYHA) functional class from 2.5 to 1.5 ($p < 0.01$). During the follow-up 41 patients (35.3%) died, and 14.2% developed a new acute MI. The annual total mortality rate was 6.5%, whereas the cardiac mortality rate was 5%. Compared to the survivors, patients who died showed a higher incidence of left ventricular dysfunction, previous MI and bypass surgery at implantation.

2. Outcome studies

A first long term outcome study performed by Sanderson et.al. (1994) confirmed that SCS is an effective and safe form of alternative therapy for the patient whose angina is unresponsive to conventional therapies. The results were from follow-up study over a period of 62 months on 23 patients who had SCS implanted for intractable angina unresponsive to standard therapy. Symptomatic improvement was good and persisted with a mean change of NYHA grade from 3.1 pre-operatively to 2.0 (P < 0.01) immediately after operations. Nitrite consumption fell markedly. Mean treadmill exercise time increased from 407 to 499 sec (P < 0.01). Forty-eight hour ST segment monitoring in those with SCS showed a reduction of frequency and duration of ischemic events. There were three deaths, none of which were sudden or unexplained. Two patients had a myocardial infarction, which was associated with typical pain and not masked by the treatment.

In a prospective, controlled study, Hautvast et.al. (1998) randomized patients with chronic intractable angina pectoris to 13 treatment and 12 control groups. Inclusion criteria included chronic intractable angina pectoris class III or IV based on the NYHA criteria, unresponsive to beta-blocking agents, calcium antagonists, and nitrates. Myocardial ischemia was documented by ≥0.1 mV ST depression during a treadmill exercise test, and coronary artery disease was documented by angiogram. Moreover, patients were not suitable for percutaneous coronary angioplasty or coronary artery bypass grafting. Exclusion criteria were the inability to perform an exercise test, cardiac stress test, and the anatomically unsuitable for stimulator implantation. The efficacy of SCS was evaluated for 6-week follow-up of daily intermittent stimulation compared with baseline and with a control group. Compared with control, SCS group exercise duration and time to angina increased; anginal attacks and sublingual nitrate consumption and ischemic episodes on 48-hour electrocardiogram (ECG) decreased. ST-segment depression on the exercise ECG decreased at comparable workload. Anginal attacks and consumption of sublingual nitrates decreased, perceived quality of life increased, and pain decreased.

In a larger prospective study, Mannheimer et.al. (1998) randomized 104 patients into SCS and CABG groups (SCS, 53; CABG, 51). The patients were assessed with respect to symptoms, exercise capacity, ECG changes during exercise, heart rate-blood pressure product, mortality, and cardiovascular morbidity before and 6 months after the operation. Both groups had satisfactory symptom relief (P<.0001), and there was no difference between SCS and CABG group. The CABG group had an increase in exercise capacity (*P*=.02), less ST-segment depression on maximum (*P*=.005) and comparable (*P*=.0009) workloads, and an increase in the heart rate-blood pressure product both at maximum (*P*=.0003) and similar (*P*=.03) workloads compared with the SCS group. Eight deaths occurred during the follow-up period, 7 in the CABG group and 1 in the SCS group. On an intention-to-treat basis, the mortality rate was lower in the SCS group (*P*=.02). Cerebrovascular morbidity was also lower in the SCS group (*P*=.03). They concluded that efficacy of CABG and SCS to be equivalent in terms of symptom relief in this group of patients and concluded that SCS may be a good alternative for patients with an increased risk of surgical complications.

3. Mechanism

The mechanism of SCS induced anti-nociceptive response is not well understood. Several theories have been proposed and elucidated based on the previous investigations on both animal model and patients treated with SCS.

3.1 Sympathetic blockade

The perception of pain during myocardial infarction is thought to be mediated by sympathetic afferent nerve fibers (Bonica et.al., 1990). Therefore, high thoracic epidural analgesia with local anesthetic can block cardiac afferent sympathetic fibers resulting in improved analgesia during myocardial infarction (Blomberg et. al., 1989). Mannheimer et. al. (1982; 1985) suggested that improved pain relief results in decreased sympathetic activity leading to improved blood flow.

In animal study, stimulation of spinal cord at weak to moderate intensity (50 Hz; 0.2 msec; amplitude 2/3 of evoking muscle contraction) improved ischemic conditions by suppressing sympathetic activity to the effector organ (Linderoth et.al., 1991a). In peripheral ischemic model, sympathectomy prior to SCS implant abolished benefits (Linderoth et.al. 1991b), and blockade of sympathetic preganglionic with hexamethnium or guanethidine totally abolished vasodilator effects of SCS (Linderoth et.al. 1991b, 1994a). Moreover, selective pharmacological blockade of autonomic transmission with an α-1 antagonist prazosine also prevented increase in blood flow with SCS.

However at higher intensity stimulation (90% of motor threshold) Croom (1996a, 1996b) showed that SCS produced increased microvascular flow independent of hexamethomium or phentolamine, a α-1 adrenergic receptor antagonist (Croom et.al., 1997). Under the similar stimulation intensity, Foreman et.al. (1998) showed that SCS attenuated intrinsic cardiac neuronal activity, and the markedly decreased activity of neurons during local occlusion of coronary blood flow to the left ventricle. In another animal study, Olgin et.al. (2002) demonstrated that thoracic SCS slowed the sinus rate and prolonged atrioventricular (AV) nodal conduction time. This effect was not eliminated by bilateral sympathectomy, while bilateral vagal transection completely eliminated effect. In addition, thoracic SCS did not change nitric oxide (NO) level at the coronary sinus. Hence, they attributed decreased sinus rate and prolonged AV conduction to activation of parasympathetic system by SCS mediated via the vagus nerve.

Similarly, anti-anginal effect can be also achieved by SCS at higher intensity in human. Murphy et.al. (1987) first demonstrated a successful treatment of otherwise intractable angina pectoris at the range of amplitude: 3-7 volts, frequency: 80-100 Hz, and pulse width: 250-500/sec. However, Sanderson et.al. (1995) used TENS in healthy volunteers and found weak association between TENS and an anti-sympathetic effect. Norsell et.al. (1997) have evaluated effect of SCS on myocardial and sympathetic tone in angina patients with SCS using norepinephrine (noradrenaline) spillover techniques. Their result showed very little effect of SCS in reducing cardiac sympathetic activity. Although overall sympathetic activity was decreased, they postulated this to reduced oxygen demand. In addition, Robertson et.al. (1983) studied plasma catecholamine levels in 10 patients with frequent spontaneous episodes of coronary artery spasm to evaluate the role of the sympathetic nervous system. Patients were evaluated for peripheral venous norepinephrine in supine and upright postures, urinary excretion of catecholamines, and functional testing of the sympathetic nervous system. Results showed that there were no changes in arterial and coronary sinus levels of norepinephrine and epinephrine drawn early in ischemia compared to the control. Plasma epinephrine levels, higher in arterial than coronary sinus samples, rose significantly only late in ischemia, hence generalized sympathetic nervous system activation is unlikely to be the sole cause of angina. Hence association between SCS induced relief of angina and anti-sympathetic effect is not robust.

3.2 Blood flow

Although SCS proved to have beneficial effects such as decreased anginal time, decreased duration and magnitude of ST segment depression during exercise compared with control values, but there were no significant changes in regional myocardial perfusion, as measured by positron emission tomography (PET) during exercise (De Landsherre, 1992). The previous studies have shown that TENS treatment failed to increase coronary sinus blood flow for patients with angina pectoris although anti-ischemic effect has been shown with improved myocardial lactate metabolism.(Cohen et.al., 1966; Emanuelssonm 1987; Mannheimer, 1989). Thus, literature studies do not support the hypothesis that the anti-ischemic effect of SCS is due to increase in coronary artery blood flow.

3.3 Oxygen demand and supply balance

The coronary venous oxygen tension is relatively constant during changes in myocardial oxygen consumption, and number of literature studies hinted that the coronary blood flow depends largely on autoregulatory mechanisms (Mosher, 1964; Miller, 1979). The animal study by Knabb (1983) showed a linear correlation between myocardial oxygen consumption and coronary blood flow. Coronary physiology study by Feigl (1983) showed that β-blockade gives rise to a reduction in both oxygen consumption and blood flow but did not affect the relation between these variables. It is possible that myocardial hypoxia leads to an increased concentration of adenosine, which produces arteriolar vasodilatation and an increase in blood flow, thus compensating for the decrease in myocardial oxygen tension. If SCS results in decrease in myocardial oxygen consumption, there will also be reduction in coronary blood flow.

3.4 Direct pain inhibition

Based on the original "gate theory" proposed by Melzack &Wall (1965), there is also reason to believe that spinal cord stimulation has a direct pain inhibiting effect on angina. The animal study by Chandler et. al. (1993) found that spinal cord stimulation attenuated anginal pain by reducing the activity of the spinal thalamic tract neurons which transmit nociceptive somatic and cardiac impulses. Two other studies (Kroger, 1989; Blomberg, 1989) suggested that treatment which has a direct pain inhibiting effect also decreases the activity in the cardiac sympathetic nerves, hence decreases the myocardial oxygen requirement. Nevertheless, direct pain inhibiting effect theory seems valid but not the singular interpretation of the analgesic effect of SCS.

3.5 Endogenous opioids

In animal study, Oliveras et.al (1977) showed that the analgesic effects obtained in the cat by central inferior raphe nucleus stimulation are greatly reduced by the administration of a specific opiate antagonist, naloxone. Moreover, Tonelli et.al. (1988) showed 50% increase in cerebrospinal β-endorphin and β-lipotropin levels for patients receiving good pain relief from SCS. These studies suggested link between SCS and endogenous opioid release, and implicated the β-endorphin response to SCS could have clinical value in predicting the success of treatment. On the contrary, Myerson et.al. (1977) showed that the pain relief produced by SCS is not reversed by naloxone.

The release of endogenous opioid via SCS may depend on stimulation frequency. Han et.al, (1991) studied two groups of patients receiving low-frequency (2 Hz) and high-frequency (100 Hz) transcutaneous nerve stimulation (TENS). The cerebrospinal fluid (CSF) sample obtained before and after stimulation showed that low frequency stimulation resulted in a significant increase (367%, $P < 0.05$) of met-enkephalin but not dynorphin A, whereas high-frequency (100 Hz) produced a 49% increase in dynorphin A ($P < 0.01$) but not met-enkephalin. This is consistent with findings observed by Fei et.al. (1987) in animal experiments where low-frequency stimulation releases Met-enkephalin and high-frequency stimulation dynorphin A. The analgesia induced by low-frequency stimulation was readily reversed by naloxone and, therefore, probably mediated via mu-receptors; whereas analgesia induced by high-frequency stimulation required much higher doses of naloxone for reversal but was easily reversed by a kappa-receptor antagonist, indicating that the effects were mediated via kappa-receptors (Han et.al., 1986). Since dynorphins are preferred ligands for kappa-receptors, these studies strongly suggested that the opioid mechanism stimulated by high-frequency stimulation may be dynorphinergic.

3.6 Amino acids and peptides

The previous studies have shown that SCS can induce release of inhibitory amino acids such as substance P (SP), serotonin (5HT), γ-amino butyric acid (GABA), and glycine in the cerebral spinal fluid (CSF) (Linderoth et.al.1992, 1994b; Myerson et.al., 1985; Duggan & Foong 1985; Simpson et.al., 1993). The antinociceptive properties of these substances are well documented depending on the location of administration in the central nerve system (CNS). Stiller et.al.(1996) showed that dysfunction of the spinal GABA system caused by the nerve damage in rats displayed tactile allodynia with significantly lower GABA in the dorsal horn compared to the control; while those responded to SCS showed dramatic increase in GABA and normalized withdrawal threshold. Moreover, the beneficial effect of SCS on allodynia could be reversed by the intrathecal injection of GABA-B antagonist; while the animals which failed to normalize tactile threshold due to the nerve lesion, intrathecal injection of GABA agonist (e.g., baclofen) increased threshold (Cui et.al., 1996).

The benefit of SCS may not be limited to the increased release of inhibitory neurotransmitters. Kangra et.al. (1991) and Hao (1993) showed that SCS can also decrease release of excitatory amino acids such as glutamate and aspartate in the dorsal horn; hence further modulating pain transmission. Cui et.al. (1997 & 1998) showed that SCS can also activate release of adenosine, and simultaneous activation of GABA-B and adenosine A-1 receptors may exert synergistic action. The beneficial effect of SCS is completely abolished when both of these receptors are blocked at the same time. They have also observed that injection of GABA-B and adenosine simultaneously can potentiate the effect of SCS on animals, however human trial data is equivocal.

3.7 Redistribution of blood flow

Hautvast et. al. (1996) has shown that spinal cord stimulation at T1 induces the redistribution of myocardial blood flow, resulting in a decrease in angina pectoris attacks.

The study demonstrated that spinal cord stimulation modulates regional cerebral blood flow (rCBF) in brain areas known to be involved in cardiovascular control and in areas associated with nociception. They postulated that the anti-anginal effect of SCS may therefore be the result of centrally mediated analgesic effects.

Mobilia et.al. (1998) studied 15 patients who already had SCS implanted for refractory angina pectoris. Eight patients had a previous MI and four patients had undergone a revascularization procedure. All patient underwent two positron emission tomographies (PET) with nitrogen-13-ammonia as the perfusion tracer. The first one was performed with the stimulator switched off for at least 20 hours, and the second one with the stimulator switched on for at least 4 hours. The quantitative evaluation of regional mean blood flow (MBF) showed an increase in regional myocardial perfusion with the stimulator was observed in 47 (62%) out of 75 regions studied. Hence they concluded that the beneficial effects of SCS in refractory angina may be associated with an increase in mean MBF and to a redistribution of MBF between the regions with low or normal basal flow and the regions with high basal flow.

Murray et.al, (2000) has elegantly explained redistribution model of SCS on myocardial blood flow citing findings by Crea et.al. (1989) and Gaspardone et.al. (1993). The similarities between SCS and theophylline in angina treatment are such that both seem to improve exercise capacity, and anti-ischemic action does not appear to be mediated by systemic hemodynamic effects or by stenosis dilation. Therefore, the improvement of myocardial ischemia from SCS is probably due to redistribution of coronary blood flow toward the underperfused areas of myocardium.

At present the exact mechanism of action of neurostimulation is not known. All of the above mechanisms have been sought, and it is possible that more than one of them is responsible for the results of neurostimulation.

4. Surgical technique and stimulation equipment

The SCS lead is typically implanted in the operating room using sterile technique. Under the fluoroscopy guided technique, upper thoracic (T4 toT6 interspace) interspace is entered using Touhy needle to access epidural space. Usually single SCS lead is advanced up to C7 to T2 level. The procedure is performed under local anesthesia to allow the patient to communicate with the physician during the intraoperative testing. The electrode position is adjusted during the intraoperative testing such that the patient feels a paresthesia in the region of anginal pain. The ideal position is when the stimulation produces a paresthesia in the precordial area and spreading into the left arms as the current intensity is increased.

In order to enter epidural space at T4 to T5 interspace, skin entry point of Touhy needles is marked approximately 1 to 2 vertebral levels inferiorly. A 5 to 7 cm vertical skin incision is made from the needle entry point approximately one finger breadth lateral to the midline. The subcutaneous tissues are then cut down deep using bovie until dorsal column fascia is visualized. Then at the top of the incision, a Touhy needle is advanced toward epidural space 1 to 1 ½ levels above the entry site using paramedian approach at no greater than 45 degree approach using loss of resistance technique. The electrode tip is typically placed a few millimeters to the left of midline at the level of C7 to T2 (Figure 1) under the fluoroscopy guidance. Following the successful intraoperative testing, the electrode is sutured to the fascia using anchoring device. The pulse generator is typically placed in a subcutaneous pocket below the left costal arch or gluteal region. The lead is then tunnelled subcutaneously from the anchor site to the generator site. The pulse generator is then interrogated to ensure good lead connection. Antibiotic prophylaxis is required for implantable devices. Prophylactic antibiotics must be administered to the patient within 1 hour prior to surgical incision. Studies show that a single preoperative dose of antibiotic is as effective as a 5-day course of postoperative therapy assuming an uncomplicated procedure. Duration of prophylaxis beyond 24 hours or use of post operative antibiotics are generally not recommended (*The Medical Letter* 2004; Fabian et.al., 1992; Bozorgzadeh et.al., 1999; Luchette et.al., 2006).

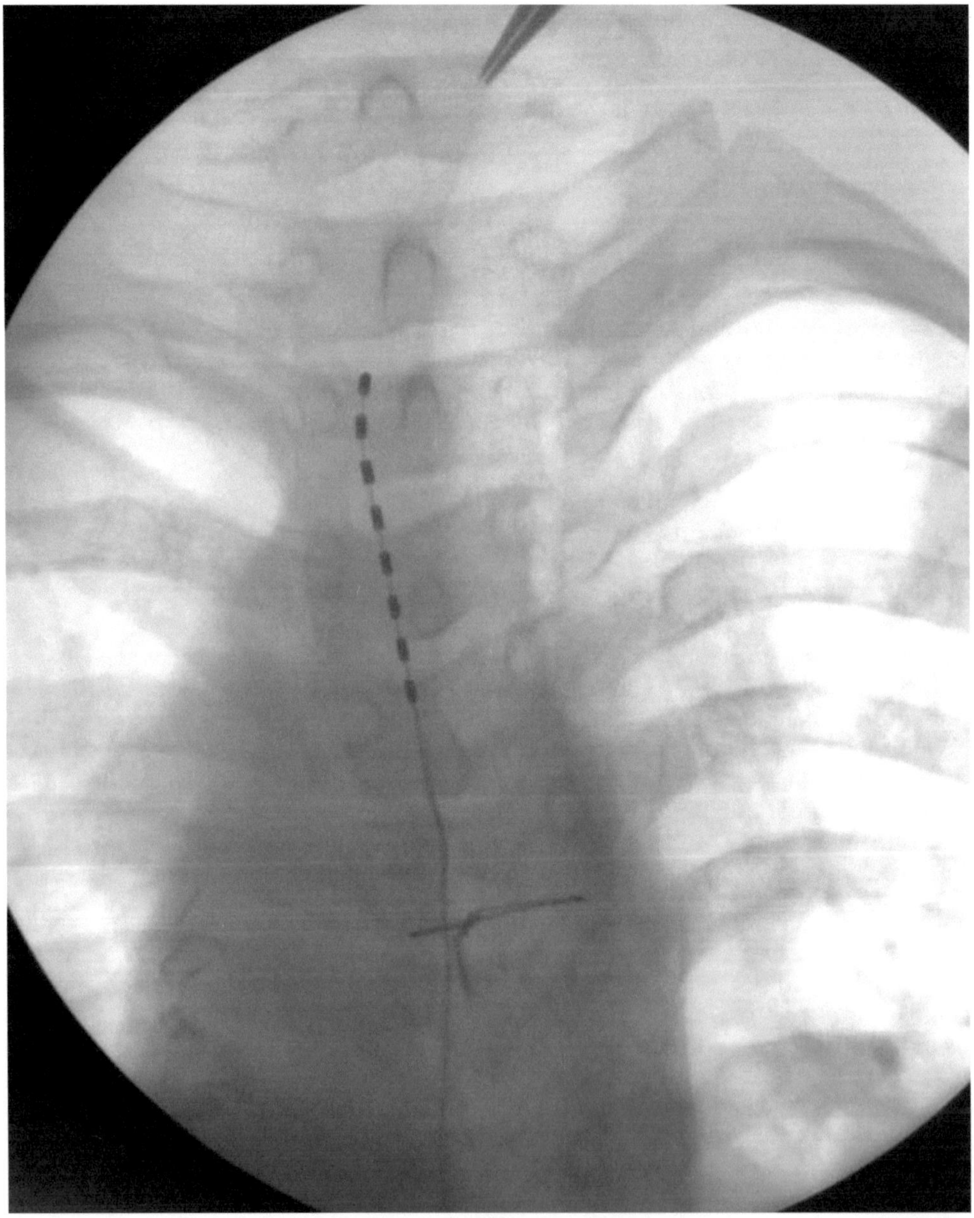

Fig. 1. SCS lead placement at upper thoracic spine.

5. Indications and patient selection

The patients with refractory angina pectoris referred to our pain clinic by cardiologist usually has exhausted optimal therapeutic modalities including pharmacotherapy (β-blocker, calcium channel antagonist, vasodilator), surgical (e.g., coronary artery bypass graft (CABG), percutaneous transluminal coronary angioplasty (PTCA), stent placement, etc), and often maintained on anticoagulant and potent opioid analgesics which referring physicians are uncomfortable sustaining. Therefore, these patients are considered inoperable and untreatable. The inclusion and exclusion criteria are well described in Table 1 (De Vries et al 2007). The algorithmic approach to angina pectoris depicted in Figure 2 (Kleef et.al. 2011) shows that SCS has its niche as the last resort treatment for managing refractory angina.

In the United States, use of SCS for angina is still considered "off label." Hence there are considerable obstacles to obtaining health insurance preauthorization. The prior treatment history is rigorously scrutinized, and often requires peer to peer review between the treating physician and physicians representing insurance company. Such process leads to further delay in providing treatment in a timely manner, and patients tend to become sub-optimal for the procedure. Therefore, the use of SCS for angina is not as common in the United States compared to Europe.

Inclusion criteria

1. Severe chest pain (NYHA classes III–IV or VAS score >7)
2. Optimal tolerated pharmacological therapy
3. Significant coronary artery disease (i.e. >1 stenosis of 75%)
4. Not eligible for Percutaneous Transluminal Intervention or Coronary Artery Bypass Surgery
5. No prognostic benefit from surgical revascularization (according to guidelines)
6. Patient considered intellectually capable to manage the SCS device
7. No acute coronary syndrome during last 3 months

Exclusion criteria

1. Myocardial infarction within the last 3 months
2. Uncontrolled disease such as hypertension or diabetes mellitus
3. Personality disorders or psychological instability
4. Pregnancy
5. Implantable cardioverter defibrillator (ICD) and pacemaker dependency
6. (Local) infections
7. Insurmountable spinal anatomy
8. Contraindication to withheld anti-platelet agents or coumadins
9. Addictive behavior

*De Vries et.al. (2007). With permission

Table 1. Inclusion and exclusion criteria SCS for ischemic heart disease (IHD)*

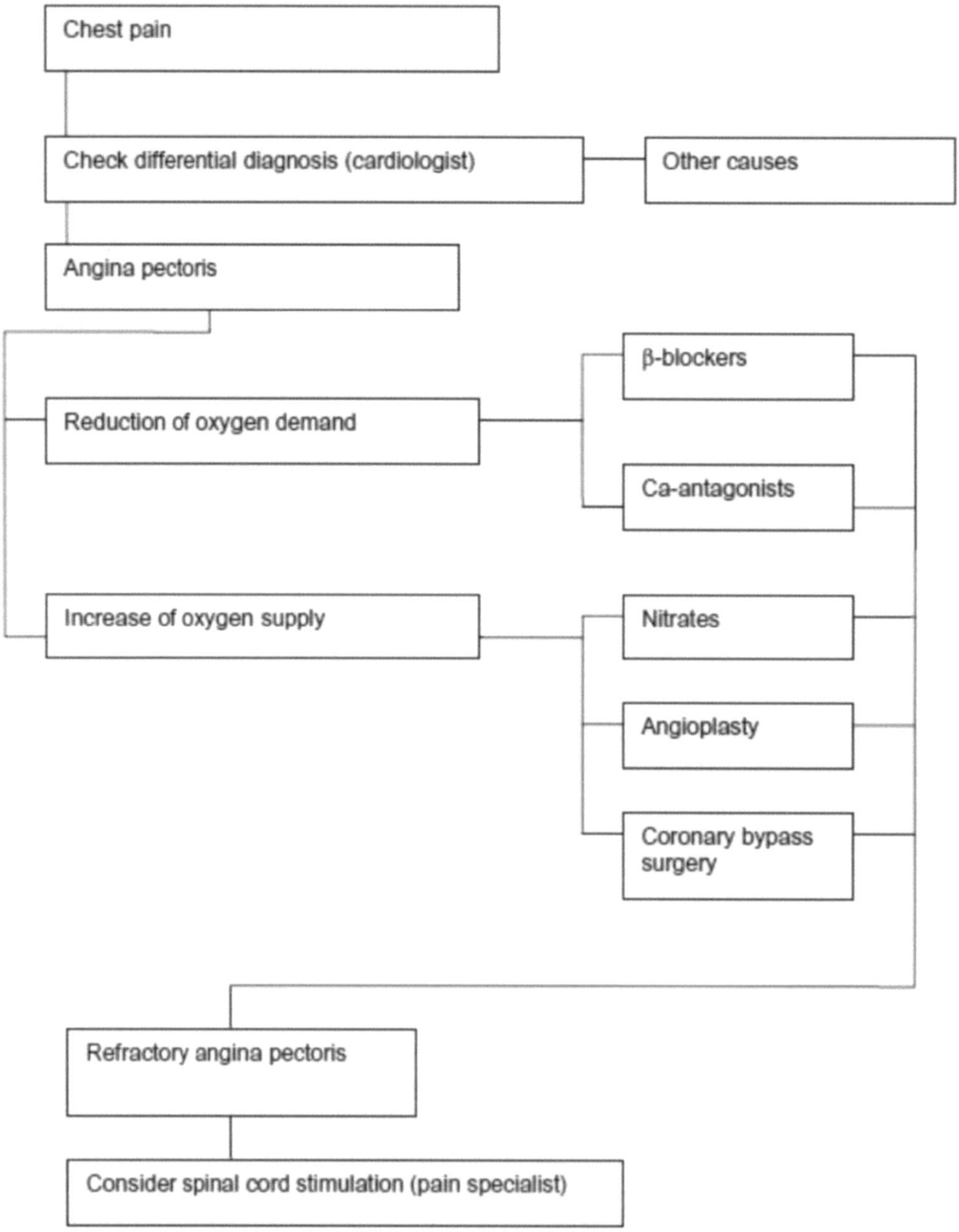

Fig. 2. Algorithm for the treatment of refractory angina pectoris (Kleef et.al. 2011). With permission.

6. Cost effectiveness

The cost-effectiveness of spinal cord stimulation in patients with intractable angina has been assessed by Merry et.al. (2001). The cost of healthcare utilization by patients suffering from intractable angina, unsuitable for coronary revascularization, before and after treatment with spinal cord stimulation on eight patients. Information on consumption of specified medical resources for the twelve months preceding implantation, the implantation period, and the twelve months following implantation was collected. Where available, data were also collected for the eighteen months preceding and following treatment.

The six patients with successful stimulation spent fewer days in hospital (p=0.028) and consumed fewer resources (p=0.046) following implantation than in the period before implantation. The two patients for whom spinal cord stimulation was unsuccessful spent more days in hospital and consumed more resources in the twelve months following, than in the twelve months preceding attempted implantation. Extrapolation of data for all eight patients suggests that, on average, the cost of implanting a spinal cord stimulator will be recovered in approximately fifteen months.

The retrospective study by Rasmussen et.al. (2004) assessed economic significances of SCS treatment on 18 consecutive patients. Before implantation of the SCS system, the patients were in a TENS treatment for 2–11 months. At the time of implant all patients were in NYHA functional group III/IV. The study is based on cost data from the year prior to start of TENS treatment compared with the year after implantation of the SCS system. They found that SCS is effective in reducing hospital and non-hospital related expenses.

Several additional studies have also showed cost effectiveness following the SCS implantation. The 2-year follow-up of the 104 patients participating in the Electrical Stimulation versus Coronary Artery Bypass Surgery in Severe Angina Pectoris (ESBY) study by Andréll et.al. (2003) found that SCS is less expensive than coronary artery bypass grafting in treating angina pectoris. The SCS group had fewer hospitalization days related to the primary procedure and to cardiac events. A systematic review by Taylor et. al. (2004) demonstrated that the initial costs of the SCS are offset by a reduction in post-implant healthcare demand and costs.

Murray et al. (1999) showed that the average time the patients were in the hospital after revascularization was 8.3 days per year versus 2.5 days per year after SCS. The authors confirmed that SCS was effective in preventing hospital admissions in patients with refractory angina.

7. Stimulation parameter

Stimulation parameters are usually different for each patient as stimulation is individualized to produce optimal relief in each patient. Our own experience and published parameter range for angina vary widely. For the purpose of reference, the range of stimulation parameters published is: pulse amplitude 1-10 volt, frequency 80-100 Hz, pulse width 150 to 500 µsec (Murphy et.al. 1987; Hautvast et. al. 1997; Gersbach et.al. 2001).

8. Complications

The major complications of SCS implant are rare, and most complications are minor and limited to superficial infection, lead migrations, battery failure and electrode fractures (De jongste et.al. 1994 &2000). The overall complication rate in the literature is up to 12% (Borjesson et.al. 2008), but the complication rate is highly dependent on implanter's experience, technique, and patient factor. It seems logical to expect higher complication rate from the inexperienced implanter. The earlier studies showed higher incidence of lead migration (De Jongste and

Staal, 1993; Jessurun et.al., 1997). But our own experience over last 10 years show dramatic decrease in lead migration in part attributed to improved lead anchor technologies.

Discomfort at implantable electrical pulse generator (IPG) sites is not uncommon and often results in persistent pain in patients with spinal cord stimulator. The IPG is most frequently implanted in the gluteal region to take advantage of the natural cushion provided by the abundance of adipose tissue in the buttock area. However, IPG sites are subject to unrelenting pressure and trauma of daily activities such as sitting, lying down, and bending leading to cutaneous hyperalgesia. Often, patients require additional analgesics or revision of the IPG pocket to control pain. A retrospective review of 20 patients at our institution (Huh and Kuo, 2011) who underwent revision due to painful IPG site (9 relocation versus 11 deep implantation at the same site) showed that decrease in pain score was significant within each group ($p < 0.001$), but no significant difference in pain was found between the two techniques ($p = 0.5779$). However, we recommend deep re-implantation of the IPG at the original site over the relocation due to the simplicity of the procedure. Re-implantation does not require creating a new pocket, and it is not limited by the length of the electrode.

9. Conclusion

Spinal cord stimulation (SCS) is an alternative therapy for patients with intractable angina who has not responded to standard therapies. Studies shows that SCS provide relief from the angina pain, decrease use of analgesia and nitrates, decrease incidence of ischemic attacks, improve heart function and quality of life

Although there is abundant evidence from Europe to show the benefits of SCS for refractory angina pectoris, the use of SCS in the United States is still considered experimental. Hence at large academic institutions, CABG is still the most commonly performed procedure for severe CAD. Health insurance coverage for SCS is challenging for angina pectoris. The scope of the disease process is enormous, and future direction begs to invest in a large multicenter prospective study to obtain Food and Drug Administration approval to benefit patients

10. References

Andréll P, Ekre O, Eliasson T, Blomstrand C, Börjesson M, Nilsson M, Mannheimer C. Cost-Effectiveness of Spinal Cord Stimulation versus Coronary Artery Bypass Grafting in Patients with Severe Angina Pectoris – Long-Term Results from the ESBY Study. *Cardiology* 2003;99:20-24.

Augustinsson LE, Carlsson CA, Holm J, Jivegird L. Epidural electrical stimulation in severe limb ischemia. *Ann Surg* 1985;202:104-10.

Blomberg S, Curelaru I, Emanuelsson H, Herlitz J, Ponten J, Rickten SE. Thoracic epidural anesthesia in patients with unstable angina pectoris. *Eur Heart J* 1989;10: 437-44.

Bonica JJ. *The management of pain. Vol II.* 2nd ed .Philadelphia: Lea and Febiger, 1990;1001-30.

Borjesson M, Andrell P, Lundberg D, Mannheimer C. Spinal cord stimulation in severe angina pectoris – A systemic review based on the Swedish Council on Technology assessment in health care report on long-standing pain. *Pain* 2008;140:501-508.

Bozorgzadeh A, Pizzi WF, Barie PS, et.al. The duration of antibiotic administration in penetrating abdominal trauma. *Am J Surg* 1999;177:125-31.

Chandler MJ, Brennan TJ, Garrison DW, Kim KS, Schwartz PJ, Forman RD. A mechanism of cardiac pain suppression by spinal cord stimulation: implications for patients with angina pectoris. *Eur Heart J* 1993;14:96-105.

Cohen LS, Elliott WC, Klein MD, Gorlin R. Coronary heart disease. Clinical cinearteriographic and metabolic correlations. *Am J Cardiol* 1966;17: 153-68.
Cook AW, Oygar A, Baggenstos P, Pacheco S, Kleriga E. Vascular disease of extremities. Electrical stimulation of spinal cord and posterior roots. *NY StateJMed* 1976;76:366-8.
Crea F, Pupita G, Galassi A, *et al.* Effect of theophylline on myocardial ischaemia. *Lancet* 1989;i:683–6.
Croom JE. Mechansims for cutaneous vasodiltation due to electrical stimulation of the dorsal surface of the spinal cord. *Thesis.* University of Oklahom, Oklahoma City 1996a:173.
Croom JE, Barron KW, Chandler MJ, Foreman RD. Cutaneous blood flow increases in the rat hind paw during dorsal column stimulation. *Brain Res* 1996b:728:281-286.
Croom JE, Foreman RD, Chandler MJ, Barron KW. Cutaneous vasodilation during dorsal column stimulation is mediated by dorsal roots and CGRP. *Am J Physiol* 1997:272:H950-H957.
Cui J-G, Linderoth B, Meyerson BA. Effects of spinal cord stimulation on touch-evoked allodynia involve GABAergic mechanism. An experimental study in the mononeuropathic rat. *Pain* 1996;66:287-295.
Cui J-G, Sollevi A, Linderoth B, Meyerson BA. Adenosine receptor activation suppresses tactile hypersensitivity and potentiates effect of spinal cord in mononeuopathic rats. *Neurosci Lett* 1997;223:173-176.
Cui J-G, Meyerson BA, Sollevi A, Linderoth B. Effects of spinal cord stimulation on tactile hypersensitivity in mononeuropathic rats is potentiated by $GABA_B$ and adenosine receptor activation. *Neurosci Lett* 1998;247:183-186.
De Jongste MJ, Staal MJ. Preliminary results of a randomized study on the clinical efficacy of spinal cord stimulation for refractory angina pectoris. Acta Neurochir Suppl 1993;58:161–4.
DeJongste MJL, Nagelkerke D., Hooyschuur CM, Journke HL, Meyler WJ, Staal M J, de Jonge PJ, Lie KI. Stimulation characteristics, complications, and efficacy of spinal cord stimulation systems in patients with refractory angina. A prospective feasibility study. *PACE* 1994; 17:1751-1760.
DeJongste MJ. Spinal cord stimulation for ischemic heart disease. *Neurol Res* 2000;22:293–298.
De Landsherre C, Mannheimer C, Habets A, Guillame M, Bourgeois I, Augustinsson L-E, et al. Effect of spinal cord stimulation on regional myocardial perfusion assessed by positron emission tomography. *Am J Cardio*l, 1992 ;69:1143-9.
De Veries J, De Jongste MJL, Spincemaille G, Staal M. Spinal cord stimulation for ischemic heart disease and peripheral vascular disease. *Advances and Technical Standards in Neurosurgery* 2007; 32;64-84.
Duggan AW, Foong FW. Bicuculline and spinal inhibition produced by dorsal column stimulation in the cat. *Pain* 1985;22:249-250.
Emanuelsson H, Mannheimer C, Waagitein F, Wilhelmsson C. Catecholamine metabolism during pacing-induced angina pectoris and the effect of transcutaneouse elctrical nerve stimulation. *Am Heart J* 1987;114:1360-6.
Fabian TC, Croce MA, Payne LW, et.al. Duration of antibiotic therapy for penetrating abdominal trauma: a prospective trial. *Surgery* 1992;112:788-95.
Fei H, Xie GX, Han JS. Low and high frequency electroacupuncture stimulation release met 5-enkaphalin and dynorphin A and B in rat spinal cord. *Chin Sci Bull* 1987;32:1496-1501.

Feigl EO. Coronary physiology. *PhysiolRev* 1983;63:1-205.

Foreman RD, Ardell JL, Armour JA et.al. High thoracic spinal cord stimulation attenuates intrinsic cardiac neuronal actvity in the dog: Implication for treating refractory angina pectoris. *Soc Neuroscit Abstr* 1998;24(part I):394 (No. 154:19).

Gaspardone A, Crea F, Iamele M, *et al.* Bamiphylline improves exercise-induced myocardial ischaemia through a novel mechanism of action. *Circulation* 1993;88:502–8.

Gersbach PA, Hasdemi MG, Eeckhout, von Segesser LK. Spinal Cord Stimulation Treatment for Angina Pectoris: More Than a Placebo? *Ann Thorac Surg* 2001;72:S1100–4.

Han JS, Dingh XZ, Fan SG. The frequency as the cardinal determinant for electroacupuncture analgesia to be reversed by opioid antagonist. *Acta physiol Sin* 1986;38:475-482.

Han JS, Chen XH, Sun SL et.al. Effect of low and high-frequency TENS on Met-enkephalin-Arg-Phe and dynorphin. A immunoreactivity in human lumbar CSF. *Pain* 1991;47:295-298.

Hao J. Photochemically induced spinal ischemia: behavioral, electrophysiological and morphological studies with special emphasis on sensory function. Thesis, Karolinska Institute, Stockholm 1993.

Hautvast, R. W. M., Blanksma, P. K., DeJongste, M. J. L., Pruim, J., van der Wall, E. E., Vaalburg, W. and Lie, K. I. Effect of spinal cord stimulation on myocardial blood flow assessed by positron emission tomography in patients with refractory angina pectoris. *Am. J. Cardiol.,* 1996; 77:462-467.

Hautvast RWM, Horst GJT, DeJong BM, DeJongste MJL, Blanksma PK, Paans AMJ, and Korf J. Relative Changes in Regional Cerebral Blood Flow During Spinal Cord Stimulation in Patients with Refractory Angina Pectoris, *European Journal of Neuroscience,* 1997; 9:1178-1183.

Hautvast RWM, DeJongste MJL, et.al. Spinal cord stimulation in chronic intractable angina pectoris: A randomized, controlled efficacy study. *Am Heart J.,* 1998; 136:1114-20.

Huh BK, Kuo CP. Comparing the Efficacy of Two Revision Techniques for Reducing Pain at Spinal Cord Stimulator Implantable Pulse Generator Sites. American Society of Anesthesiologist Annual Meeting *Abstract* #950. October 16, 2011.

Jacobs MJHM, Jorning PJG, Beckers RCY, Ubbink DT, van Kleef M, Slaaf DW, et al. Foot salvage and improvements of microvascular blood flow as a result of epidural spinal cord electrical stimulation. *J Vasc Surg* 1990; 12: 354-60.

Jessurun GA, TenVaarwerk IA, DeJongste MJ, Tio RA, Staal MJ. Sequelae of spinal cord stimulation for refractory angina pectoris. Reliability and safety profile of long-term clinical application. *Coronary Artery Dis* 1997;8:33–8.

Kangra I, Jing M, Randic M. Actions of baclofen on rat dorsal horn neurons. *Brain Res* 1991;562:265-275.

Kleef MV, Staats P, Mekhail N, Huygen F, Chronic Refractory Angina Pectoris. *Pain Practice.* early on line publication, March 2011.

Knabb RM, Ely SW, Bacchus AN, Rubio R, Berne RM. Consistent parallel relationships among myocardial oxygen consumption, coronary blood flow, and pericardial infuate adenosine concentration with various interventions and β-blockade in the dog. *Circ Res* 1983; 53:33-41.

Kroger K, Schipke J, Thimer V, Heusch G. Poststenotic ischaemic myocardial dysfunction induced by peripheral nociceptive stimulation. *Eur Heart J* 1989;10:179-82.

Linderoth B, Fedorcsak I, Meyerson BA. Peripheral vasodilation after spinal cord stimulation: animal studies of putative effector mechanisms. *Neurosurgery* 1991a;28:187-195.

Linderoth B, Gunasekera L, Meyerson B. Effects of sympathectomy on skin and muscle microcirculation during dorsal column stimulation: animal studies. *Neurosurgery* 1991b:29:874-879.

Linderoth B, Gazelius B, Franck J, Brodin E. Dorsal column stimulation induces release of serotonin and substance P in the cat dorsal horn. *Neurosurgery* 1992;31:289-297.

Linderoth B, Herregodts P, Meyerson B. Sympathetic mediation of peripheral vasodilatation induced by spinal cord stimulation: animal studies of the role of cholinergic and adrenergic receptor subtypes. *Neurosurgery* 1994a;35:711-719.

Linderoth B., Stiller CO, Gunasekera L, O'Connor WT, Ungerstedt U, Brodin E. Gamma-aminobutyric acid is released in the dorsal horn by electrical spinal cord stimulation: an in vivo microdialysis study in the rat. *Neurosurg* 1994b;34:484-489.

Luchette FA, Borzotta AP, Croce MA, et.al. Practice management guidelines for prophylactic antibiotic use in penetrating abdominal trauma. Available online at: http://www.east.org. [Accessed 09 October 2006].

Mannheimer C, Carlsson CA, Ericson K, Vedin A, Wilhelmsson C. Transcutaneous electrical nerve stimulation in severe angina pectoris. *Eur Heart J*, 1982;3:297-302.

Mannheimer, C., Carlsson, C.A., Emanuelsson, H., Vedin. A., Waagstein, F. et al.. The effects of transcutaneous electrical nerve stimulation in patients with severe angina pectoris. *Circulation*, 71 (1985) 308-316.

Mannheimer C, Augustinsson L-E, Carlsson C-A, Manhem K, Wilhelmsson C. Epidural spinal electrical stimulation in severe angina pectoris. *Br Heart J*, 1988; 59:56-61.

Mannheimer C, Emanuelsson H, Waagstein F, Wilhelmsson C. Influence of naloxone on the effects of transcutaneous electrical nerve stimulation (TENS) in pacing-induced angina pectoris. *Br Heart J*. 1989;62:36-42.

Mannheimer C, Eliasson T, Augustinsson LE, et al. Electrical stimulation versus coronary artery bypass surgery in severe angina pectoris: the ESBY study. *Circulation* 1998;97:1157–1163.

Melzack R, Wall P, Pain mechanisms: A new theory. *Science* 1965; 150:971-9.

Merry AF, Smith WM, Anderson DJ, Emmens DJ, Choong CK, Cost-effectiveness of spinal cord stimulation in patients with intractable angina. *N Z Med J* 2001 Apr 27;114(1130):179-81.

Miller WL, Belardinelli L, Bacchus A, Foley DH, Rubio R, Berne RM. Canine myocardial adenosine and lactate production, oxygen consumption, and coronary blood flow during stellate ganglia stimulation. *Circ Res*, 1979; 45:708-18.

Mobilia G., Zuin G. Zanco P., DiPede F., Pinato G., Neri G., Caranel S., Raviele A., Ferlin G., Buchberger R., Effects of spinal cord stimulation on regional myocardial blood flow in patients with refractory angina. A positron emission tomography study. *G Ital Cardiol*. 1998 (10):1113-9.

Mosher P, Ross J, McFate PA, Show RF. Control of coronary blood flow by an auto regulatory mechanism. *Circ Res* 1964;14:250-9.

Murphy DF, Giles KE. Dorsal column stimulation for pain relief from intractable angina pectoris. *Pain* 1987;28:365-368.

Murray S, Carson KG, Ewings PD, Collins PD, James MA. Spinal cord stimulation significantly decreases the need for acute hospital admission for chest pain in patients with refractory angina pectoris. *Heart* 1999;82:89-92.

Murray S, Collins PD, James MA. Neurostimulation treatment for angina pectoris. *Heart* 2000;83:217–220.

Myerson BA, Bothius J, Terenius L, Wahlstrom A. Endorphine mechanisms in pain relief with intracerebral and dorsal column stimulation, in 3rd Meeting of the European Society of Stereotactic and Functional Neurosurgery. Freiburg, Germany 1977 (Abstract).

Myerson BA, Brodin E. Linderoth B. Possible neurohumoral mechanisms in CNS stimulation for pain suppression. *Appl Neurophysiol* 1985;48:175-180.

Norsell H, Eliasson T, Mannheimer C, *et al*. Effects of pacing induced myocardial stress and spinal cord stimulation on whole body and cardiac norepinephrine spillover. *Eur Heart J* 1997;18:1890–6.

Olgin JE, Takahashi T, Wilson E et.al. Effects of thoracic spinal cord stimulation on cardiac autonomic regulation of the sinus and atrioventricular nodes. *J Cariovasc Electrophysiol* May 2002;13:4475-481.

Oliveras, J.L., Hosobuchi, Y., Redjemi, F. and Guilbaud, G., Opiate antagonist, naloxone, strongly reduces analgesia by stimulation of raphe nucleus (centralis inferior), *Brain Res* 1977;120:211-229.

Rasmussen MB, Hole P, Andersen C, Electric Spinal Cord Stimulation in the Treatment of Angina Pectoris: A Cost-Utility Analysis. *Neuromodulation* 2004; 7: 89-97.

Robertson RM, Bernard Y, Robertson D. Arterial and coronary sinus catecholamines in the course of spontaneous coronary artery spasm. *Am Heart J* 1983;105:901-6.

Romano M, Auriti A, Cazzin R. et. al. Epidural spinal stimulation in the treatment of refractory angina pectoris. Its clinical efficacy, complications and long-term mortality. An Italian multicenter retrospective study. *Ital Heart J Supp* 2000 Jan;1(1):97-102.

Sanderson JE, Brooksby P, Waterhouse D, Palmer RBG, Neubauer K. Epidural spinal electrical stimulation for severe angina: a study of its effects on symptoms, exercise tolerance and degree of ischaemia. *Eur Heart J* 1992;13:628-33

Sanderson JE, Ibrahim B, Waterhouse D, Palmer RB. Spinal electrical stimulation for intractable angina--long-term clinical outcome and safety. *Eur Heart J* 1994 Jun:15(6):810-4.

Sanderson JE, Tomlinson B, Lau MJW, *et al*. The effects of transcutaneous nerve stimulation (TENS) on the autonomic nervous system. *Clin Auton Res* 1995;5:81–84.

Shealy CN, Mortimer JT, Reswick JB. Electrical inhibition of pain by stimulation of the dorsal columns. *Anesth Anaig* 1967;46:489-91.

Simpson RD, Robertson CS, Goodman JC. Glycine: a potential mediator of electrically induced pain modification. *Biomed lett* 1993;48:193-207.

Stiller CO, Cui J-G, O'Connor WT, Brodin E, Meyerson BA, Linderroth B. Release of GABA in the dorsal horn and suppression of tactile allodynia by spinal cord stimulation in mononeuropathic rats. *Neurosurgery* 1996;39:367-375.

Taylor R, Taylor RJ, Van Buyten JP, Buchser E. North R, Bayliss S. The cost effectiveness of spinal cord stimulation in the treatment of pain: a systematic review of the literature. *J Pain Symptom Manage* 2004;27:370-337.

The Medical Letter. Antibiotic prophylaxis for surgery. Treatment guidelines. 2004;2(20):27-32.

Tonelli L, Setti T, Falasca A et.al, investigation on cerebrospinal fluid opioid and neurotransmitters related to spinal cord stimulation. *Appl Neurophysiol* 1988;51:324-332.